COLLINS GEM

CALORIE COUNTER

for
Branded
Foods

COLLINS GEM

CALORIE COUNTER

for Branded Foods

COLLINS
London and Glasgow

First published 1984
Second Edition 1987
Reprint 10 9 8 7 6 5 4 3 2

ISBN 0 00 458830 4
Printed in Great Britain

CONTENTS

INTRODUCTION

Diets come and diets go, but still the most reliable way of losing weight – or of maintaining a sensible weight – is by counting Calories.

The energy the body needs to survive is generated from the nutrients – carbohydrates, fats, proteins and vitamins – in the food we eat. When we consume in this form more energy than our bodies use up in our daily life, then we put on weight. About half the energy used up by the body in a day is needed to enable it just to survive – this is the basic metabolism rate – while the other half is taken up by activity, by work or play. Generally speaking, people who do more need more and can consume more. A miner expends more energy than an office worker, a docker more than a driver, a squash player more than a golfer. In the following pages there are tables which give the average energy used in a day doing certain jobs, and the energy used in an hour taking part in certain activities. But, for reasons still not perfectly understood by scientists, not everyone uses up the same amount of energy doing the same job or playing the same game; we each have to determine our own energy needs and decide for ourselves how much food energy we need to consume.

Also included among the tables are those for desirable weights according to height and frame. It has been calculated that one pound of body fat is equal to 3500 Calories, so for every pound required to be lost, 3500 Calories must come out of the diet – but not all at once! Anyone considering trying to lose a lot of weight should consult their doctor, and those just keen not to overdo it should remember that the best way to lose weight – or not to put it on – is to eat a sensible diet and to eat in moderation.

The most convenient form of measurement of the energy value of food for non-scientific use is the kilocalorie, or Calorie, which is what is given here. The foods are listed in **bold roman type** in alphabetical order in the left-hand column of each page; the name of the manufacturer is in the second column; and the energy values are given per 100 grams (3.5 ounces) in the third column. Where at all possible and available, in the last column Calorie values per portion or pack are given. If such information is not available, then the Calorie value per ounce has been given. Unbranded foods and Calorie values listed in ***bold italic type*** have been obtained with permission from *The Composition of Foods*, published by Her Majesty's Stationery Office.

The publishers are grateful to all the manufacturers who gave information on their products. The list of foods included is as up to date as it was possible to make it, but it should be remembered that new food products are frequently put on the market and existing ones withdrawn, so it has not been possible to include everything. If you cannot find a particular food here, you can still, however, obtain a guideline figure by finding an equivalent product from a different manufacturer.

Weights and measures

Imperial to Metric

1 ounce (oz) = 28.35 grams (g)
1 pound (lb) = 453.60 grams (g)
1 fluid ounce (fl. oz) = 29.57 millilitres (ml)
1 pint = 0.568 litre

Metric to Imperial

100 grams (g) = 3.53 ounces (oz)
1 kilogram (kg) = 2.2 pounds (lb)
100 millilitres (ml) = 3.38 fluid ounces (fl. oz)
1 litre = 1.76 pints

Average daily Calorie expenditure, by occupation

Men		**Women**	
Sedentary			
Retired	2300	Elderly	
Office workers	2500	housewives	1980
Lab technicians	2850	Middle-aged	
Drivers, pilots,		housewives	2075
teachers, journalists,			
professional people,			
shop workers	2700		
Building workers	3000		
Moderately active			
University students	2950	Lab technicians	2125
Light industry,		Shop workers	2250
railway workers,		Univ. students	2300
postmen, joiners,		Factory workers	2320
farm workers	3000	Office workers	2200
Very active			
Steel workers	3250	Bakery workers, some	
Some farm workers	3450	factory workers	2500
Army cadets and			
recruits	3500		
Miners, forestry			
workers, dockers, some			
building workers	3600		

Average hourly Calorie requirement, by activity:

	Women	Men
Bowling	207	270
Cycling: moderate	192	256
hard	507	660
Dancing: ballroom	264	352
Domestic work	153	200
Driving	108	144
Eating	84	112
Gardening: active	276	368
Golf	144	192
Ironing	120	160
Office work: active	120	160
Rowing	600	800
Running: moderate	444	592
hard	692	900
Sewing and knitting	84	112
Sitting at rest	84	112
Skiing	461	600
Squash	461	600
Swimming: moderate	230	300
hard	480	640
Table tennis	300	400
Tennis	336	448
Typing	108	144
Walking: moderate	168	224

Desirable weights of adults

Small frame: men and women
Height without shoes

		Men					Women		
ft in	m	st lb	st lb	kgs		st lb	st lb	kgs
4 8	1.42					6 8–	7 0	41.7–44.5
4 9	1.45					6 10–	7 3	42.6–45.8
4 10	1.47					6 12–	7 6	43.6–47.2
4 11	1.50					7 1–	7 9	44.9–48.5
5 0	1.52					7 4–	7 12	46.3–49.9
5 1	1.55	8 0–	8 8	50.8–54.4		7 7–	8 1	47.6–51.3
5 2	1.58	8 3–	8 12	52.2–56.3		7 10–	8 4	49 –52.6
5 3	1.60	8 6–	9 0	53.5–57.2		7 13–	8 7	50.4–54
5 4	1.63	8 9–	9 3	54.9–58.5		8 2–	8 11	51.7–55.8
5 5	1.65	8 12–	9 7	56.3–60.3		8 6–	9 1	53.5–57.6
5 6	1.68	9 2–	9 11	58.1–62.1		8 10–	9 5	55.3–59.4
5 7	1.70	9 6–	10 1	59.9–64		9 0–	9 9	57.2–61.2
5 8	1.73	9 10–	10 5	61.7–65.8		9 4–	10 0	59 –63.5
5 9	1.75	10 0–	10 10	63.5–68		9 8–	10 4	60.8–65.3
5 10	1.78	10 4–	11 0	65.3–69.9		9 12–	10 8	62.6–67.1
5 11	1.80	10 8–	11 4	67.1–71.7				
6 0	1.83	10 12–	11 8	69 –73.5				
6 1	1.85	11 2–	11 13	70.8–75.8				
6 2	1.88	11 6–	12 3	72.6–77.6				
6 3	1.91	11 10–	12 7	74.4–79.4				

Desirable weights of adults

Medium frame: men and women
Height without shoes

			Men			Women		
ft	in	m	st lb	st lb	kgs	st lb	st lb	kgs
4	8	1.42				6 12–	7 9	43.6–48.5
4	9	1.45				7 0–	7 12	44.5–49.9
4	10	1.47				7 3–	8 1	45.8–51.3
4	11	1.50				7 6–	8 4	47.2–52.6
5	0	1.52				7 9–	8 7	48.5–54
5	1	1.55	8 6–	9 3	53.5–58.5	7 12–	8 10	49.9–55.3
5	2	1.58	8 9–	9 7	54.9–60.3	8 1–	9 0	51.3–57.2
5	3	1.60	8 12–	9 10	56.3–61.7	8 4–	9 4	52.6–59
5	4	1.63	9 1–	9 13	57.6–63.1	8 8–	9 9	54.4–61.2
5	5	1.65	9 4–10	3	59 –64.9	8 12–	9 13	56.3–63.1
5	6	1.68	9 8–10	7	60.8–66.8	9 2–10	3	58.1–64.9
5	7	1.70	9 12–10	12	62.6–69	9 6–10	7	59.9–66.7
5	8	1.73	10 2–11	2	64.4–70.8	9 10–10	11	61.7–68.5
5	9	1.75	10 6–11	6	66.2–72.6	10 0–11	1	63.5–70.3
5	10	1.78	10 10–11	11	68 –74.8	10 4–11	5	65.3–72.1
5	11	1.80	11 0–12	2	69.9–77.1			
6	0	1.83	11 4–12	7	71.7–79.4			
6	1	1.85	11 8–12	12	73.5–81.7			
6	2	1.88	11 13–13	3	75.8–83.9			
6	3	1.91	12 4–13	8	78 –86.2			

Desirable weights of adults

Large frame: men and women
Height without shoes

		Men			Women		
ft in	m	st lb	st lb	kgs	st lb	st lb	kgs
4 8	1.42				7 6–	8 7	47.2–54
4 9	1.45				7 8–	8 10	48.1–55.3
4 10	1.47				7 11–	8 13	49.4–56.7
4 11	1.50				8 0–	9 2	50.8–58.1
5 0	1.52				8 3–	9 5	52.2–59.4
5 1	1.55	9 0–10	1	57.2–64	8 6–	9 8	53.5–60.8
5 2	1.58	9 3–10	4	58.5–65.3	8 9–	9 12	54.9–62.6
5 3	1.60	9 6–10	8	59.9–67.1	8 13–10	2	56.7–64.4
5 4	1.63	9 9–10	12	61.2–69	9 3–10	6	58.5–66.2
5 5	1.65	9 12–11	2	62.6–70.8	9 7–10	10	60.3–68
5 6	1.68	10 2–11	7	64.4–73	9 11–11	0	62.1–69.9
5 7	1.70	10 7–11	12	66.7–75.3	10 1–11	4	64 –71.7
5 8	1.73	10 11–12	2	68.5–77.1	10 5–11	9	65.8–73.9
5 9	1.75	11 1–12	6	70.3–78.9	10 9–12	0	67.6–76.2
5 10	1.78	11 5–12	11	72.1–81.2	10 13–12	5	69.4–78.5
5 11	1.80	11 10–13	1	74.4–83.5			
6 0	1.83	12 0–13	7	76.2–85.7			
6 1	1.85	12 5–13	12	78.5–88			
6 2	1.88	12 10–14	3	80.7–90.3			
6 3	1.91	13 0–14	8	82.6–92.5			

Daily Calories for maintenance of desirable weight

Calculated for a moderately active life. If you are very active add 50 Calories; if your life is sedentary take away 75 Calories.

Weight			Age 18–35		Age 35–55		Age 55–75	
st	lb	kgs	Men	Women	Men	Women	Men	Women
7	1	44.9		1700		1500		1300
7	12	49.9	2200	1850	1950	1650	1650	1400
8	9	54.9	2400	2000	2150	1750	1850	1550
9	2	58.1		2100		1900		1600
9	6	59.9	2550	2150	2300	1950	1950	1650
10	3	64.9	2700	2300	2400	2050	2050	1800
11	0	69.9	2900	2400	2600	2150	2200	1850
11	11	74.8	3100	2550	2800	2300	2400	1950
12	8	79.8	3250		2950		2500	
13	5	84.8	3300		3100		2600	

Product	Brand	Calories per 100g/ 100ml	Calories per oz/ pack/ portion
Abalone, canned, drained		145	41
ABC letters	Bassett's	351	100
Aberdeen rolls	St Michael	423	120
Acid drops	Boots	363	103
	Trebor	349	per sweet 22
Ackee, canned		151	43
Aduki beans, dried	Holland and Barrett	250	71
Advocaat		272	77
Adzuki beans, dried	Boots	319	90
Aero:			
milk chocolate	Rowntree Mackintosh	520	per 40g bar 210
orange	Rowntree Mackintosh	530	per 40g bar 210
peppermint	Rowntree Mackintosh	530	per 40g bar 210
After Dinner mints	Tesco	463	131
After Eight mints	Rowntree Mackintosh	410	per mint 35
Agar, dried		312	88
Alfalfa and radish, fresh	Tesco	79	22
All beef quarter pounders	Findus	283	80
All-bran		273	77
All-Bran	Kellogg's	249	71
All butter biscuits	St Michael	481	136
	Tesco	482	137
All butter cherry cake	Safeway	311	88

Product	Brand	Calories per 100g/ 100ml	Calories per oz/ pack/ portion
All butter cherry genoa cake	St Michael	327	93
All butter coconut cake	Safeway	417	118
All butter iced top Christmas cake	Tesco	351	100
All butter Madeira cake	Safeway	376	107
All butter shortbread assortment	St Michael	517	147
All butter shortbread fingers	St Michael	525	149
	Tesco	510	145
All butter sultana cookies	St Michael	442	125
All butter thins	Tesco	509	144
All butter thistle shortbread	St Michael	517	147
All butter wholemeal fruit cake	Safeway	348	99
Allinson 100% wholemeal bread	Sunblest	226	per slice 75
stoneground	Sunblest	210	per slice 69
toaster	Sunblest	226	per slice 90
Allinson wholemeal malt loaf	Allinson	247	70
Allspice		263	75
Almond biscuits	Littlewoods	510	145
	Safeway	506	143
	St Michael	506	143
Almond rondo cake	Tesco	413	117
Almond shorties	Tesco	508	144

Product	Brand	Calories per 100g/ 100ml	Calories per oz/ pack/ portion
Almond slice mix (as sold)	Green's	432	made up per portion 164
Almonds (Badam)		565	160
with shells		210	60
Almonds	Holland and Barrett	560	159
cooking	Tesco	625	177
flakes	Whitworths	565	160
ground	Safeway	622	176
	Whitworths	565	160
kernels	Littlewoods	565	160
Marcona	St Michael	565	160
smoked	Tesco	630	179
sweet	Whitworths	566	160
whole	Safeway	565	160
whole blanched	Whitworths	565	160
Almonds, sugared	Littlewoods	417	118
	St Michael	460	130
Alpen	Weetabix	366	104
with tropical fruit	Weetabix	377	107
Alphabetti spaghetti in tomato sauce	Crosse & Blackwell	61	17
Alphabites:			
baked or grilled	Birds Eye	212	60
deep-fried	Birds Eye	229	65
shallow-fried	Birds Eye	300	85
Alpine ice cream			per 1/10 of pack
chocolate	Wall's		125
lemon sorbet	Wall's		per 1/10 of pack 85
orange sorbet	Wall's		per 1/10 of pack 85

4

Product	Brand	Calories per 100g/ 100ml	Calories per oz/ pack/ portion
Alpine ice cream			
strawberry	Wall's		per 1/10 of pack 120
vanilla	Wall's		per 1/10 of pack 125
Amaranth: see Chinese leaves			
Ambrosia products: see Rice, Sago, etc.			
American barbecue marinade	Knorr	328	93
American fries	Bejam	236	per 170g portion deep-fried 402
American ginger low calorie	Safeway Safeway	36 4	11 1
American ginger ale	Hunts Safeway Schweppes Tesco	36 36 21 28	11 11 6 8
low calorie	Diet Hunts Schweppes Slimline Tesco	1 1 6	2
American hard gums	Bassett's Bassett's Littlewoods Tesco	327 327 325 377	93 93 92 107
American mustard	Colman's	110	31
American rice, parboiled	Whitworths	364	103
American salad	Eden Vale	142	40
American style chocolate brownie mix (as sold)	Green's	453	made up per portion 79

Product	Brand	Calories per 100g/ 100ml	Calories per oz/ pack/ portion
American style pizza with cheese and tomato	Tesco	233	66
	St Michael	212	60
with pepper and mushroom	St Michael	209	59
American style toffee almond ice cream	St Michael	225	64
Anchovies in oil, canned, fish only		280	79
Anchovy paste	Shippams	176	per 35g pack 62
Angel cake	St Michael	574	163
	Tesco	384	109
Animal biscuits	Cadbury's	480	per biscuit 30
Anise seeds		337	96
Aniseed balls	Barratt	376	107
Aniseed drops	Boots	363	103
Apple and almond slice	Lyons	420	119
Apple and apricot	Heinz Baby Foods	48	per 128g can or jar 61
Apple and apricot farmhouse bran	Weetabix	326	92
Apple and banana	Heinz Baby Foods	53	per 128g can or jar 68
Apple and banana dessert	Cow and Gate	55	per 110g jar 61, 150g jar 83
Apple and banana fruity juice dessert	Heinz Baby Foods	53	per 128g jar 68
Apple and blackberry drink			
low calorie	Boots Shapers	6	2
undiluted	Quosh	104	31
Apple and blackberry dumplings	Ross	250	71

Product	Brand	Calories per 100g/ 100ml	Calories per oz/ pack/ portion
Apple and blackberry fruit filling	Morton	62	18
Apple and blackberry fruit harvest ice cream	Lyons Maid	175	50
Apple and blackberry fruit pie filling	Tesco	92	26
Apple and blackberry Pack-A-Pie	Batchelors	63	18
Apple and blackberry sponge pudding	Heinz	265	75
Apple and blackberry treat	Boots Baby Foods	400	113
Apple and blackcurrant crunch bar mix (as sold)	Green's	408	made up per portion 220
Apple and blackcurrant drink	Boots Baby Drinks	298	84
Apple and blackcurrant drink	Tesco	45	13
Apple and blackcurrant fruity juice dessert	Heinz Baby Foods	62	per 128g jar 79
Apple and blackcurrant juice	Baby Ribena	19	6
	Robinsons	45	13
Apple and blackcurrant pie	Littlewoods	340	96
popular	Lyons	353	100
Apple and blackcurrant pure juice	Cow and Gate	40	per 125g jar 50
concentrated	Cow and Gate	227	per 130ml jar 295

Product	Brand	Calories per 100g/ 100ml	Calories per oz/ pack/ portion
Apple and blackcurrant whole fruit drink	Robinsons	100	30
Apple and blackcurrant yogurt dessert	Cow and Gate	63	per 110g jar 69
Apple and bran original crunchy bar	Jordans	394	per bar 132
Apple and cherry juice	Baby Ribena	19	6
	Prewetts	46	14
Apple and hazelnut bar	Holly Mill		per bar 147
Apple and hazelnut cluster	Lyons	381	108
Apple and honey juice drink (undiluted)	Baby Ribena	316	94
Apple and mango juice	St Michael	42	12
Apple and orange	Heinz Baby Foods	47	per 128g can or jar 60
Apple and orange dessert	Cow and Gate	61	per 110g jar 67; 150g jar 92
Apple and orange fruity juice dessert	Heinz Baby Foods	60	per 128g jar 77
Apple and orange pure juice	Cow and Gate	40	per 125g jar 50
concentrated	Cow and Gate	227	per 130ml jar 295
Apple and pear	Heinz Baby Foods	45	per 128g can or jar 58
Apple and pear pure juice	Cow and Gate	40	per 125g jar 50

Product	Brand	Calories per 100g/ 100ml	Calories per oz/ pack/ portion
Apple and raspberry fruit filling	Morton	63	18
Apple and raspberry fruit pie filling	Tesco	66	19
Apple and raspberry juice	Robinsons	45	13
Apple and raspberry Pack-A-Pie	Batchelors	65	18
Apple and rhubarb drink	Safeway	140	41
Apple and rhubarb whole milk yogurt	Safeway	55	per 150g pack 83
Apple and rosehip pure juice	Cow and Gate	227	per 130ml jar 295
Apple and sultana coleslaw	Safeway	202	57
Apple and sultana dessert	Boots Baby Foods	380	108
Apple biscuits	Boots Second Nature	443	126
Apple 'C'	Libby	45	13
Apple cheesecake	St Michael	220	62
Apple chutney		193	55
Apple coleslaw	Tesco	157	45
Apple crumble		208	59
Apple crunch bar mix (as sold)	Green's	355	per portion made up 224
Apple crush, low calorie	Slimsta	4	per 180ml bottle 7
Apple dessert	Boots Baby Foods	58	16

Product	Brand	Calories per 100g/ 100ml	Calories per oz/ pack/ portion
Apple dessert	Cow and Gate	59	per 110g jar 65; 150g jar 89
	Heinz Baby Foods	63	per 128g can 81
Apple dessert pie	Lyons	349	99
Apple drink, sparkling	Tango	36	11
Apple drops	Boots	363	103
Apple dumplings	Ross	250	71
Apple fruit filling	Morton	76	22
Apple fruit juice	Del Monte	44	13
Apple fruit pie	Lyons	376	107
Apple fruit pie filling	Tesco	64	18
Apple fruity juice dessert	Heinz Baby Foods	74	per 128g jar 95
Apple, jam and nut dessert cake	Tesco	424	120
Apple juice	Appella	38	per 250ml pack 96
	Aspall	40	12
	Boots	39	12
	Britvic	43	per 170ml can 72
	Copella	30	9
	Prewetts	47	14
	Robinsons	40	12
	St Ivel Mr Juicy	39	12
	St Ivel Real	42	12
	Tesco	45	13
concentrated longlife	Marlet	207	61
	Safeway	42	12
	Tesco	45	13
longlife sparkling sparkling	Safeway	45	13
	Kiri	38	per half pint 109

Product	Brand	Calories per 100g/ 100ml	Calories per oz/ pack/ portion
Apple juice	Schloer	35	10
Apple juice drink	Schloer	35	10
Apple juice, English	Boots	47	14
	Safeway	45	13
	St Michael	39	12
longlife	Safeway	41	12
	Tesco	46	14
Apple muesli bar	Granose	416	per 25g bar 104
Apple Pack-A-Pie	Batchelors	65	18
Apple, peach and nut salad	Littlewoods	170	48
Apple pie	Bejam		per pie, as sold 162
	Littlewoods	352	100
	St Michael	220	62
popular	Lyons	349	99
Apple pie ice cream	Safeway	228	67
Apple pies	St Michael	323	92
Apple puffs	St Michael	262	74
Apple rings, dried	Tesco	254	72
Apple sauce	Heinz	65	18
	O.K.	80	23
Apple sauce mix	Knorr	349	99
	Safeway	365	per 24g pack 88
Pour Over	Colman's	380	108
Apple slice cake, fresh cream	Tesco	312	88
Apple sparkle	St Michael	46	14
Apple Splitz	Canada Dry	47	per 250ml bottle 118

Product	Brand	Calories per 100g/ 100ml	Calories per oz/ pack/ portion
Apple strudel cake, fresh cream	Tesco	156	44
Apple whole fruit drink	Robinsons	100	30
Apple yogurt	Eden Vale Munch Brunch	102	per 125g pack 128
Apple yogurt dessert	Cow and Gate	65	per 110g jar 72
	Heinz Baby Foods	76	per 128g jar 97
Apples, cooking			
baked (with skin)		31	9
baked without sugar		39	11
raw		37	10
stewed with sugar		66	19
stewed without sugar		32	9
Apples, cooking	Littlewoods	37	10
Bramley, baked	Tesco	31	9
stewed, no sugar	Tesco	32	9
Apples, eating		46	13
with skin and core		35	10
Apples, eating	Littlewoods	35	10
	Tesco	46	13
Apples with vitamin C	Heinz Baby Foods	66	per 128g can 84
Appletise	Schweppes	43	13
Applewood smoked Cheddar cheese	Tesco	419	119
Apricot and apple cake, fresh cream	Tesco	148	42
Apricot and apple cottage cheese	Eden Vale	92	26

Product	Brand	Calories per 100g/ 100ml	Calories per oz/ pack/ portion
Apricot and chocolate chip cluster	Lyons	384	109
Apricot and date carob bar	Newform Foods		per bar 119
Apricot and guava yogurt	Gold Ski	114	per 150g pack 171
	St Michael	109	31
Apricot and mango yogurt	Raines	97	27
	Safeway	86	per 150g pack 129
Apricot and passionfruit yogurt	St Michael	100	28
Apricot and sultana stuffing mix	Knorr	326	92
Apricot brulee	Young's	280	79
Apricot cheesecake	St Michael	189	54
Apricot chutney	Sharwood	148	42
	Tesco	147	42
Apricot conserve	Safeway	248	per 340g jar 840
	St Michael	240	68
	Tesco	268	76
Apricot custard	Heinz Baby Foods	63	per 128g can 81
Apricot date bar	Granose	283	per 30g bar 85
Apricot dessert with rice	Heinz Baby Foods	71	per 128g can 91
Apricot flavour rusk, low sugar	Boots Baby Foods	400	113
Apricot fruit filling	Morton	64	18
Apricot Fruit For-All	Chivers	115	per portion 85
Apricot Fruit Softy	Eden Vale	129	37
Apricot halves in syrup	Del Monte	70	20

Product	Brand	Calories per 100g/ 100ml	Calories per oz/ pack/ portion
Apricot jam	Robertson's	251	71
	Safeway	251	71
diabetic	Boots	236	67
	Dietade	233	66
no added sugar	Safeway	139	per 227g jar 316
reduced sugar	Boots	146	41
	Heinz Weight Watchers	124	35
Apricot jam Swiss roll	Tesco	409	116
Apricot lunchpack	Limmits		per pack 210
Apricot madeleines	Lyons	335	95
Apricot popular pie	Lyons	361	102
Apricot preserve	Baxters	241	per 340g jar 819
	Tesco	255	72
reduced sugar	Robertson's	150	43
Apricot pure fruit spread	Robertson's	120	34
Apricot sponge roll	St Michael	352	100
Apricot sundae	Lyons	396	112
Apricot yogurt	St Michael	39	11
French style	Littlewoods	102	per 150g pack 153
low fat	Littlewoods	83	per 150g pack 125
	Tesco	99	28
Apricot yogurt dessert	Heinz Baby Foods	82	per 128g jar 105
Apricots			
raw		28	8
raw (with stones)		25	7
stewed with sugar		60	17
stewed with sugar (with stones)		57	16
stewed without sugar		23	7
stewed without sugar (with stones)		21	6

Product	Brand	Calories per 100g/ 100ml	Calories per oz/ pack/ portion
Apricots, canned		106	30
Apricots, canned	Libby	69	20
in natural juice	Tesco	40	11
in syrup	Tesco	71	20
in water, low calorie	Dietade	16	5
Apricots, dried			
raw		182	52
stewed without sugar		66	19
stewed with sugar		81	23
Apricots, dried	Holland and Barrett	180	51
	Tesco	234	66
	Whitworths	138	39
hunza	Holland and Barrett	160	45
Arctic circles			
double choc	Birds Eye		per piece 165
vanilla	Birds Eye		per piece 155
Arctic cup	Birds Eye		per tub 185
Arctic gateau			
choc 'n' cherry	Birds Eye		per 1/5 gateau 100
strawberry	Birds Eye		per 1/5 gateau 105
Arctic log	Birds Eye		per 1/6 log 100
Arctic roll	Birds Eye		per 1/6 small roll
Areca nuts: see *Betel nuts*			
Aromat	Knorr	176	50
Arrowhead, raw		107	30
Arrowmint chewing gum	PK		per pellet 6
Arrowroot, raw		355	raw
Arrowroot	Boots	355	101

Product	Brand	Calories per 100g/ 100ml	Calories per oz/ pack/ portion
Artichoke, globe			
raw		73	21
boiled		15	4
boiled (as served)		7	2
Artichoke, globe, fresh, cooked	Tesco	44	12
Artichoke, Jerusalem (boiled)		18	5
Arvi (colocasia) root, raw		85	24
Asafoetida (Hing)		297	84
Asparagus, boiled		18	5
boiled (as served)		9	3
Asparagus cream soup	Knorr "No Simmer"	497	141
Asparagus soup	Heinz Weight Watchers	22	per 295g can 65
condensed	Campbell's	62	18
dried	Batchelors Cup-a-Soup	412	per 25g sachet as sold 103
	Safeway	373	106
	Tesco	365	103
Asparagus soup mix	St Michael	360	102
Asparagus with ham crepes	Findus	141	40
Assorted Tools	Trebor	600	per sweet 48
Aubergine (brinjal, eggplant), raw		14	4
Aubergines, fresh			
	Littlewoods	14	4
fresh, fried	Tesco	175	50
sliced (frozen)	Ross	15	4
Austrian smoked cheese	St Ivel	315	89

Product	Brand	Calories per 100g/ 100ml	Calories per oz/ pack/ portion
Austrian style coffee cake mix (as sold)	Green's	388	made up per portion 292
Autumn Gold cider			
bottle or can	Taunton	30	per pint 170
keg	Taunton	40	per pint 230
Avocado dressing	Duchesse	33	10
Avocado pear, fresh, raw		*223*	*63*
BA ice cream	Wall's		per portion 45
Baby carrots: see Carrots, baby			
Baby muesli with fruit, cereal and yogurt	Heinz Baby Foods	63	per 128g jar 81
Baby orange juice, sweetened, concentrated	Boots Baby Foods	203	58
Baby Ribena juice			
apple and blackcurrant	Beecham	19	6
apple and cherry	Beecham	19	6
blackcurrant	Beecham	19	6
Baby Ribena juice drink, undiluted			
apple and honey	Beecham	316	94
blackcurrant	Beecham	316	94
blackcurrant and apple	Beecham	316	94
Baby Ribena, undiluted	Beecham	316	94
Baby rice	Boots Baby Foods	370	105
Bacon			
collar joint, lean and fat, raw		*319*	*90*
collar joint, lean and fat, boiled		*325*	*92*
collar joint, lean only		*191*	*54*

Product	Brand	Calories per 100g/ 100ml	Calories per oz/ pack/ portion
Bacon			
dressed carcase, raw		352	100
fat, raw (average)		747	212
lean, raw (average)		147	42
rashers, lean only, fried (average)		332	94
rashers, lean only, grilled (average)		292	83
fat, cooked		692	196
cooked shoulder, sliced	Tesco	123	35
cured sweet Dutch	Littlewoods	230	65
half gammon, unsmoked, British	St Michael	350	99
joints	Littlewoods	120	34
loin	Littlewoods	160	45
shoulder joint, unsmoked, British	St Michael	390	111
steaks	Littlewoods	246	70
	Safeway	455	129
	Tesco	88	25
steaks, sweetcure	Tesco	246	70
Bacon, back			
rashers, raw		428	121
rashers, lean and fat, fried		465	132
rashers, lean and fat, grilled		405	115
Canadian style	St Michael	390	111
extra lean, British	St Michael	195	55
green	Littlewoods	246	70
green, Dutch	Littlewoods	226	64
rashers	Tesco	312	88
smoked, British	St Michael	390	111
smoked, Danish	St Michael	350	99
smoked, Dutch	Littlewoods	239	68
smoked, grilled	Bejam	314	89

Product	Brand	Calories per 100g/ 100ml	Calories per oz/ pack/ portion
Bacon, back			
unsmoked, Danish	St Michael	350	99
unsmoked, Dutch	St Michael	350	99
unsmoked, grilled	Bejam	229	65
Bacon, gammon			
joint, lean and fat, raw		236	67
joint, lean and fat, boiled		269	76
joint, lean only		167	47
rashers, lean and fat, grilled		228	65
rashers, lean only		172	49
steaks, unsmoked, grilled	Bejam	138	39
Bacon, middle			
rashers, raw		425	120
rashers, lean and fat, fried		477	135
rashers, lean and fat, grilled		416	118
green, Dutch	Littlewoods	217	62
rashers	Tesco	269	76
smoked	Littlewoods	420	119
smoked, Dutch	Littlewoods	230	65
smoked, grilled	Bejam	349	99
unsmoked, grilled	Bejam	286	81
Bacon, middle back, unsmoked, Ayrshire	St Michael	350	99
Bacon, streaky			
rashers, raw		414	117
rashers, lean and fat, fried		496	141
rashers, lean and fat, grilled		422	120
Canadian style	St Michael	390	111
green, Dutch	Littlewoods	281	80
rashers	Tesco	286	81
smoked, Dutch	Littlewoods	294	83
smoked, grilled	Bejam	325	92
unsmoked, British	St Michael	375	106

Product	Brand	Calories per 100g/ 100ml	Calories per oz/ pack/ portion
Bacon, streaky unsmoked, grilled	Bejam	325	92
Bacon and cheese burgers, breaded	St Michael	350	99
Bacon and cheese flan (as sold)	Bejam		per flan 316
Bacon and egg savoury toasts	Findus	198	56
Bacon and mushroom soup with croutons	Knorr Quick Soup	401	114
Bacon bites	Tesco	450	128
Bacon misshapes, grilled	Bejam	286	81
Bacon puffs	Tesco	497	141
Bacon sandwich	St Michael	95	27
Bacon snacks	Waitrose	490	139
Bacon, egg and sausage flan	St Michael	285	81
Bacon, egg and tomato breakfast	Cow and Gate	53	per 150g jar 80
Bacon, lettuce and tomato sandwich	St Michael Waitrose	314 209	89 59
Bacon, peppers and mushroom French bread pizza	Findus	192	54
Badam: see Almonds			
Baked bean jackets	St Michael	138	39
Baked beans, in tomato sauce		64	18
Baked beans	Hartley's	65	18
	Safeway	73	21
	Whole Earth	18	5
in barbecue sauce	Heinz	72	20

Product	Brand	Calories per 100g/ 100ml	Calories per oz/ pack/ portion
Baked beans			
in barbecue sauce	Waitrose	91	26
in curry sauce	Waitrose	101	29
in tomato sauce	Crosse & Blackwell	73	21
in tomato sauce	St Michael	96	27
in tomato sauce	Waitrose	64	18
in tomato sauce, no added sugar/starch	Waitrose	81	23
no added sugar	Heinz Weight Watchers	54	per 225g can 122
with hamburgers	Chef	122	35
with pork sausages	Chef	124	35
with pork sausages in tomato sauce	Heinz	124	35
with tomato sauce	Armour	64	18
with tomato sauce	Heinz	72	20
Baked beans and bacon	Heinz Baby Foods	54	per 128g can 69
Baked potato with cheese	St Michael	188	53
Baked potatoes, old		105	30
old (with skins)		85	24
Baked raspberry jam roll	Safeway	408	116
Bakewell cake, cherry	Littlewoods	409	116
Bakewell cream biscuits	Tesco	482	137
Bakewell slice mix (as sold)	Green's	432	made up per portion 202
Bakewell tart	Lyons	420	119
Bakewell tart mix (as sold)	Green's	422	made up per portion 216

Product	Brand	Calories per 100g/ 100ml	Calories per oz/ pack/ portion
Baking powder		163	46
	Boots	167	47
	Tesco	130	37
Balor (valor) beans			
fresh, raw		23	7
canned, drained		19	5
Bamboo shoots, canned		27	8
Banana and brazil muesli tubs	Jordans	430	122
Banana and chocolate Megabite	Wall's		each 120
Banana and chocolate yogurt dessert	Boots Baby Foods	390	111
Banana and oatmeal cake	St Michael	364	103
Banana blancmange	Brown and Polson	327	93
Banana chips, dried	Tesco	529	150
	Whitworths	517	147
Banana dessert	Waitrose	444	per 69g pack 138
Banana dessert with vitamin C	Heinz Baby Foods	50	per 128g can 64
Banana flavour drink, sparkling	Corona	24	7
Banana fruit bar	Prewetts	179	per 42g bar 75
Banana hazelnut treat	Boots Baby Foods	395	112
Banana in custard	St Michael	91	26
Banana Liga rusks	Cow and Gate	381	per rusk 27
Banana mousse	Bejam		per tub as sold 77

Product	Brand	Calories per 100g/ 100ml	Calories per oz/ pack/ portion
Banana snack bar, yogurt coated	Sunwheel Kalibu	323	per 30g bar 97
Banana soft scoop ice cream	Safeway	169	50
Banana Split chews	Trebor	385	per chew 15
Banana supershake	Eden Vale	75	per 194g pack 146
Banana supreme	Eden Vale	105	per 125g pack 131
Banana Supreme Delight	Safeway	431	122
Banana yogurt	Munch Bunch	99	per 125g pack 124
	Mr Men	96	27
	Safeway	95	per 150g pack 143
	Safeway Funtime	92	per 150g pack 138
	St Ivel Real	84	24
	St Ivel Shape	43	12
	Ski	83	per 150g pack 125
low fat	Littlewoods	96	per 150g pack 144
	Tesco	96	27
	Waitrose	90	per 150g pack 135
Banana yogurt dessert	Cow and Gate	65	per 110g jar 72
	Heinz Baby Foods	79	per 128g jar 101
Banana, rice and rosehip dessert	Heinz Baby Foods	63	per 128g can 81
Bananarama	Wall's		per 1/5 500ml pack 80
Bananas			
raw		79	22
raw (with skin)		47	13
fresh, without skin	Littlewoods	79	22
Baps: *see Bread rolls*			

Product	Brand	Calories per 100g/ 100ml	Calories per oz/ pack/ portion
Bar six	Cadbury's	550	per bar 220
Barbecue beef and onion crisps	St Michael	533	151
Barbecue chicken	Tesco	222	63
Barbecue Dish of the Day, dried	Crosse & Blackwell	382	108
Barbecue marinade, American	Knorr	328	93
Barbecue pork spare ribs	St Michael	239	68
Barbecue ribs, cooked	Tesco	314	89
Barbecue sauce		75	21
Coat and Cook	Homepride	170	per 43g pack 73
Cook In	Homepride	77	per 376g pack 290
Cooking-in	Baxters	68	per 425g jar 289
Barbecue sauce mix			
Cook In	Colman's	310	88
Pour Over	Colman's	310	88
Barbecue spare rib crisps	Christies	520	per 26g bag 130
	Hunters	520	per 26g bag 130
	St Michael	520	147
Barbecue spare ribs	Waitrose	165	47
Barbecue Super Noodles (as sold)	Batchelors	465	per pack 460
Barbecue tomato Saucy Noodles (as sold)	Batchelors	345	per 199g pack 411
Barbican	Britvic	14	per 275ml can 39, 440ml bottle 62
Barcelona nuts		639	181
with shells		396	112

Product	Brand	Calories per 100g/ 100ml	Calories per oz/ pack/ portion
Barley			
boiled		120	34
whole grain, raw		327	93
Barley, pearl	Waitrose	360	102
Barley, pot	Boots	360	102
	Holland and Barrett	360	102
Barley flakes	Holland and Barrett	313	89
Barley kernels muesli	Sunwheel	366	104
Barley sugar	Littlewoods	365	103
	Trebor	365	per sweet 23
Barley sugar drops	Boots	363	per 33g stick 120
	Needlers	350	99
Barley, pearl	Safeway	360	102
	Whitworths	360	102
boiled	Whitworths	120	34
Barley, pearl, raw		360	102
Barlotti beans	Boots	105	30
Barmy banana	Lyons Maid		each 78
Basmati rice: *see Rice, Basmati*			
Bassetti	Barratt	310	88
Bath buns	St Michael	420	119
	Tesco	290	82
Bath Oliver biscuits	Fortts	375	per biscuit 45
	Safeway	375	per biscuit 12
Battenburg cake	Littlewoods	433	123
	Lyons	358	101
	St Michael	361	102
	Waitrose	362	103

Product	Brand	Calories per 100g/ 100ml	Calories per oz/ pack/ portion
Batter mix	Tesco	209	59
Complete	Green's	359	102
crispy	Green's	341	97
fish	Green's	341	97
pouch	Green's	348	99
quick	Whitworths	338	96
Battercrisp prawns, deep fried	Dan Maid	240	68
Bavarian ham, joints or slices	St Michael	161	46
Bavarian meatball casserole	Findus Lean Cuisine	81	23
Bavarian smoked cheese	St Michael	305	86
plain	Waitrose	272	77
Bavarian style sandwich cake mix (as sold)	Green's	397	made up per portion 258
Bean and mushroom stew	Granose	78	22
Bean and potato salad	Littlewoods	210	60
Bean mix, de luxe, dried	Holland and Barrett	265	75
Bean salad	Tesco	104	29
in wine vinegar	Tesco	63	18
Bean stew, Mexican	Granose	130	37
Beanmilk	Itona	130	per 425g can 552
Beans and pork sausages in tomato sauce	Tesco	113	32
Beans and sausage	Littlewoods	100	28
Beans in tomato sauce	Tesco	94	27

Product	Brand	Calories per 100g/ 100ml	Calories per oz/ pack/ portion
Beans soup mix, dried	Holland and Barrett	285	81
Beans stew mix, dried	Holland and Barrett	262	74
Beans, refried	Old El Paso	92	per 453g can 417
Beansprout salad with water chestnuts	Tesco	44	12
	Haywards New Seasons	33	9
Beansprouts			
canned		9	3
mung (moong), fresh, raw		35	10
mung (moong), canned		9	3
fresh	Tesco	40	11
with pineapple	Haywards New Seasons	42	12
Beatall lollies	Trebor	356	per lolly 32
Beef			
dressed carcase, raw		282	80
fat, cooked		613	174
fat, raw (average)		637	181
lean, raw		123	35
lean (average)		123	35
mince, raw		221	63
mince, stewed		229	65
salted, dried, raw		250	71
salted, fat removed, raw		119	34
braised steak	St Michael	100	28
	St Michael	128	36
braising steak, casseroled	Bejam	208	59
cooked	Littlewoods	155	44

Product	Brand	Calories per 100g/ 100ml	Calories per oz/ pack/ portion
Beef			
diced steak, casseroled	Bejam	208	59
diced, economy, casseroled	Bejam	176	50
fillet steak, grilled	Bejam	159	45
ground	St Michael	128	36
joint, cooked	Tesco	183	52
joints with beef fat	St Michael	179	51
minced	St Michael	221	63
minced steak, boiled	Bejam	198	56
minute steak, grilled	Bejam	173	49
potted (canned)	St Michael	170	48
roast	Waitrose	189	54
roast with mustard	Waitrose	246	70
T-bone steak, grilled	Bejam	240	68
Beef: brisket			
lean and fat, raw		252	71
lean and fat, boiled		326	92
cooked	Waitrose	140	40
rolled, roasted	Bejam	190	54
Beef: chuck steak			
lean minced, boiled	Bejam	162	46
lean, casseroled	Bejam	173	49
Beef: forerib			
lean and fat, raw		290	82
lean and fat, roast		349	99
lean only		225	64
joint and rib steaks	St Michael	179	51
Beef: rump steak			
lean and fat, raw		197	56
lean and fat, fried		246	70

Product	Brand	Calories per 100g/ 100ml	Calories per oz/ pack/ portion
Beef: rump steak			
lean and fat, grilled		218	62
lean only, fried		246	70
lean only		190	54
lean only, grilled		168	48
and joints	St Michael	116	33
grilled	Bejam	201	57
Beef: silverside			
salted, lean and fat, boiled		242	69
salted, lean only, boiled		173	49
joint, roasted	Bejam	194	55
sliced	Tesco	105	30
Beef: sirloin			
lean and fat, raw		272	77
lean and fat, roast		284	81
lean only, roast		192	54
steak, grilled	Bejam	236	67
steaks	St Michael	116	33
Beef: stewing steak			
lean and fat, raw		176	50
lean and fat, stewed		223	63
	St Michael	128	36
stewed	Bejam	155	44
Beef: topside			
lean and fat, raw		179	51
lean and fat, roast		214	61
lean only		156	44
joint, roasted	Bejam	180	51
roast	Waitrose	140	40
Beef and bone broth	Cow and Gate	62	per 110g jar 68
Beef and bone hotpot	Heinz Baby Foods	70	per 128g can 90

Product	Brand	Calories per 100g/ 100ml	Calories per oz/ pack/ portion
Beef and carrot casserole	Heinz Baby Foods	68	per 128g can 87
Beef and dumplings	Tesco Ready Meal	125	35
Beef and ham paste	Littlewoods	239	per 35g pack 84
Beef and kidney diced, economy, casseroled	Tyne Brand	111	31
	Bejam	198	56
Beef and kidney dinner	Cow and Gate	64	per 150g jar 96
Beef and kidney pie	Tesco	367	104
	Tyne Brand	179	51
Beef and kidney stewpot pie, individual	Ross	251	71
Beef and mushroom pasties	St Michael	258	73
Beef and mushroom pie	Tyne Brand	195	55
Beef and onion	Tyne Brand	119	34
Beef and onion pasties	St Michael	262	74
Beef and onion sandwichmaker	Shippams	131	per 95g can 124
Beef and onion soup, low calorie	Knorr Quick Soup	315	89
Beef and oxtail dinner	Heinz Baby Foods	69	per 128g can 88
Beef and oxtail hotpot	Heinz Baby Foods	65	per 128g jar 83
Beef and pork cannelloni	Findus Lean Cuisine	86	24

Product	Brand	Calories per 100g/ 100ml	Calories per oz/ pack/ portion
Beef and tomato soup,	Batchelors Cup-		
dried (as sold)	a-Soup	333	per 21g sachet 70
	Batchelors	307	per 58g pint pack 178
instant	Safeway	354	100
low calorie	Batchelors Slim-		
	a-Soup	292	per 13g sachet 38
with croutons	Batchelors Cup-		
	a-Soup Special	367	per 27.5g pack 101
Beef and vegetable casserole	Boots Baby Foods	63	18
Beef and vegetable soup	Campbell's Main Course	55	16
	Heinz Big Soups	36	10
	St Michael	76	22
homestyle	Heinz Ready to Serve	39	11
Beef 'n' vegetable soup with croutons (as sold)	Batchelors Snack-a-Soup	314	per 31.5g sachet 99
Beef bourguignon cooking mix	Colman's	350	99
Beef brochettes	Waitrose	150	43
Beef broth	Heinz Big Soups	29	8
	Heinz Ready to Serve	39	11
	Waitrose	40	11
condensed (undiluted)	Campbell's	67	19
Beef broth with vegetables, 3-9 months	Heinz Baby Foods	67	per 128g jar 86

Product	Brand	Calories per 100g/ 100ml	Calories per oz/ pack/ portion
Beef broth with vegetables 7-15 months	Heinz Baby Foods	75	per 170g jar 128
Beef burgundy crepes	Findus	140	40
Beef casserole	Boots Baby Foods	390	111
Beef casserole	St Michael	128	36
	Tyne Brand	87	25
Beef casserole cooking mix, traditional	Colman's	320	91
Beef chop suey ready meal	Bejam		per serving baked 105
Beef cobbler	Waitrose	139	39
Beef consomme	Waitrose	14	per 425g can 60
Beef crisps	Tesco	523	148
lower-fat	St Michael	476	135
Beef croquettes	Safeway	250	per croquette 142
Beef cubes	Knorr	332	94
	Waitrose	296	84
Beef curry	Campbell's Quick Snack	103	29
	Findus	113	32
	Tesco	121	34
	Tyne Brand	93	26
	Vesta	374	per 253g pack for 2 as served 947
and rice	Bejam		per serving baked 472
	Tyne Brand	119	per 369g pack 440
with rice	Birds Eye MenuMaster		per meal 380
with separate rice	Crosse & Blackwell	135	38

Product	Brand	Calories per 100g/ 100ml	Calories per oz/ pack/ portion
Beef dinner	Boots Baby Foods	385	109
	Cow and Gate	70	per 110g jar 77; 150g jar 105
Beef drink	Knorr	278	79
	Oxo	100	28
Beef dripping		891	253
	Tesco	875	248
	Waitrose	900	255
Beef en croute	Waitrose	207	per 206 pack 427
Beef fingers snack	Bejam		per finger baked 37
Beef flavour and vegetable soup, dried (made up)	Chef Box	25	7
Beef flavour rice, frozen (cooked)	Uncle Ben's	115	33
Beef flavour savoury rice (as sold)	Whitworths	323	92
Beef flavour vegetarian chunks	Direct Foods	273	77
Beef flavour vegetarian mince	Direct Foods	273	77
Beef goulash	Campbell's Quick Snack	80	23
Beef goulash Cook in the Pot	Crosse & Blackwell	380	108
Beef goulash cooking mix	Colman's	275	78
Beef grill steaks	Findus	233	66

Product	Brand	Calories per 100g/ 100ml	Calories per oz/ pack/ portion
Beef grills	Birds Eye Steakhouse		each grilled or fried, 185
low fat	Birds Eye Steakhouse		each grilled or baked, 155
Beef grillsteak joint, cooked	Tesco	284	81
Beef grillsteaks	St Michael	279	79
Beef julienne	Findus Lean Cuisine	99	28
Beef kheema		411	117
Beef koftas		350	99
Beef Madras	Vesta	366	per 252g pack for 2 as served 923
Beef meatballs with a provencal sauce	Waitrose	269	76
Beef noodle soup	Heinz Weight Watchers	18	per 306g can 55
Beef oriental	Birds Eye MenuMaster		per meal 310
	Findus	106	30
Beef paste	Safeway	205	58
	Shippams	205	per 35g pack 72
	Tesco	200	57
Beef pasty pies	Tesco	323	92
Beef provencale	Birds Eye MenuMaster		per meal 340
	Findus Lean Cuisine	100	28
Beef risotto	Tyne Brand	124	per 369g pack 460
	Vesta	403	per 187g pack for 2 as served 753

Product	Brand	Calories per 100g/ 100ml	Calories per oz/ pack/ portion
Beef risotto			
low calorie	Batchelors Slim-a-Meal	369	per 67.5g pack 249
Beef sausage	St Michael	375	106
Oxford	Waitrose	169	48
Beef sausages			
fried		269	76
grilled		265	75
	Waitrose	229	65
butcher's	Littlewoods	258	73
premium	Tesco	307	87
	Waitrose	229	65
thick	Bejam		per sausage, grilled 144
thick	Littlewoods	265	per sausage 150
thin	Littlewoods	265	per sausage 75
Beef sausages, raw		299	85
Beef savoury rice (as sold)	Batchelors	330	94
Beef seasoning sauce mix	Colman's Cook In	315	89
	Colman's Pour Over	315	89
Beef slices	Soyapro	210	60
Beef soup	Heinz Ready to Serve	37	10
Beef spread	Littlewoods	168	per 35g pack 59
Beef steak pie	Birds Eye		per pie for one 370
Beef steak pudding, cooked		223	63
Beef stew, cooked		119	34
Beef stew	Campbell's	70	20
	Tyne Brand	75	21

Product	Brand	Calories per 100g/ 100ml	Calories per oz/ pack/ portion
Beef stew			
and dumplings	Birds Eye MenuMaster		per pack 240
	St Michael	147	42
and dumplings (baked)	Bejam		per serving 446
and dumplings (canned)	St Michael	110	31
Beef stock cubes	Safeway	273	per 11.5g cube 31
Beef stock drink	Waitrose	199	per 227g pack 452
Beef stock powder	Knorr	197	56
Beef stroganoff	St Michael	167	47
and rice (baked)	Bejam		per serving 444
Beef stroganoff mix (as sold)	Tesco	328	93
Cook in the Pot	Crosse & Blackwell	418	119
Beef stroganoff sauce	Homepride Cook in	93	per 376g can 350
Beef strognoff cooking mix (as sold)	Colman's	320	91
Beef suet, shredded	Tesco	797	226
Beef taco filling	Old El Paso	176	per 205g can 361
Beef teriyaki	Findus	104	29
Beef, tomato and coleslaw sandwich	Waitrose	285	81
Beef vindaloo	Waitrose	181	per 320g pack 579
Beefburger and tomato corn puffs	Hunters	549	per 23g pack 126
Beefburgers			
frozen, raw		265	75
fried		264	75

Product	Brand	Calories per 100g/ 100ml	Calories per oz/ pack/ portion
Beefburgers	Safeway	298	per beefburger 168
	St Michael	260	74
	Waitrose	246	per beefburger 140
best	Ross	260	74
economy	Ross	270	77
80%	Bejam		per burger, grilled 88
extra lean in brown sauce	St Michael	560	159
(canned)	St Michael	102	29
in gravy (canned)	Tesco	145	41
low fat	Birds Eye Steakhouse		per burger, grilled 85, fried 90
	Bejam		per burger, grilled 95
90%	Findus	283	80
100%	Bejam		per burger, grilled 100
100%	Birds Eye Steakhouse		per burger, grilled 120
	Ross	330	94
original	Birds Eye Steakhouse		per burger, grilled or fried 130
premium, grilled	Tesco	270	77
premium, raw	Tesco	290	82
prime	Ross	252	71
quarter pound	Bejam		per burger, grilled 209
quarter pounder	Waitrose	338	96
top quality	St Michael	260	74
with onion	Bejam		per burger, grilled 125

Product	Brand	Calories per 100g/ 100ml	Calories per oz/ pack/ portion
Beefburgers			
with onion	St Michael	260	74
Beefy beverage	Boots	205	61
Beefy drink	Safeway	181	per 113g pack 204
Beer			
bitter, canned		32	9
bitter, keg		31	9
bitter, draught		32	9
mild, draught		25	7
Beer shandy	Corona	25	7
Beetroot, raw		28	8
boiled		44	12
Beetroot	Tesco	44	12
baby	Safeway	26	per 327g pack 85
baby, sweet	Tesco	48	14
in redcurrant jelly	Baxters	162	per 305g jar 494
Beetroot, pickled			
all varieties	Haywards	40	11
baby	Waitrose	26	per 340g jar 88
	Safeway	26	per 327g jar 85
sliced or whole	Tesco	37	10
sliced	Littlewoods	37	per 340g pack 126
	St Michael	55	16
	Waitrose	37	per 340g jar 126
sliced, in sweet vinegar	Waitrose	55	per 340g jar 187
small whole	St Michael	55	16
Belgian buns	Tesco	343	97
Belle des champs cheese	Waitrose	300	85
Bemax		347	98
	Beecham	300	85
crunchy	Beecham	310	88

Product	Brand	Calories per 100g/ 100ml	Calories per oz/ pack/ portion
Bengal gram: see Chickpeas			
Bengal hot chutney	Sharwood	217	62
Besan flour: see Chickpeas			
Betel (Areca) nuts		394	112
Betel leaves (Pan)		61	17
Bierwurst oval	Waitrose	290	82
Bierwurst sausage, sliced	Tesco	254	72
Big Squeeze	Lyons Maid		each 109
Bilberries, raw		56	16
Bircher muesli	Granose	379	107
Biscuits			
home made		469	133
sandwich		513	145
semi-sweet		457	130
short-sweet		469	133
Bitter lemon	Schweppes	33	10
	Waitrose	34	10
low calorie	Schweppes		
	Slimline	2	1
	Tesco	6	2
	Waitrose	3	1
Bitter lemon drink	Canada Dry	40	11
	Safeway	55	16
	Tesco	33	10
	Waitrose	34	10
	Hunts	34	10
low calorie	Canada Dry		
	Slim	2	1
	Safeway	5	1
	Diet Hunts	1	0.5 per 100ml

Product	Brand	Calories per 100g/ 100ml	Calories per oz/ pack/ portion
Bitter lemon drops	Boots	363	103
Bitter lemon roll	Trebor	342	per sweet 14
Bitter orange, sparkling	Schweppes	45	13
Bitter orange drink low calorie	Diet Hunts	3	1
Bitter orange fruit spread	Waitrose	560	159
Bitter orange roll	Trebor	342	per sweet 14
Bitter sweet drink, low calorie, sparkling			
lemon/lime	Beecham	4	1
orange	Beecham	5	1
Black 'n' white chews	Trebor	379	per sweet 36
Black cherry and kirsch ice cream	Bejam	169	48
Black cherry conserve	Tesco	268	76
	Waitrose	250	71
Black cherry double decker	St Michael	124	35
Black cherry flavour jelly	Waitrose	272	77
Black cherry fruit filling	Morton	70	20
	Waitrose	70	20
Black cherry fruit harvest ice cream	Lyons Maid	180	51
Black cherry jelly	Safeway	268	76
	Tesco	57	16
Black cherry luxury cheesecake mix (as sold)	Green's	283	made up per portion 253

Product	Brand	Calories per 100g/ 100ml	Calories per oz/ pack/ portion
Black cherry preserve	Baxters	244	69
	Tesco	255	72
Black cherry Regale dessert	St Ivel	142	40
Black cherry ripple ice cream	Tesco	176	50
Black cherry spreading cheese	Medley	321	per 75g pack 241
Black cherry tartlets	St Michael	386	109
Black cherry yogurt	Mr Men	95	27
	Raines	96	27
	Safeway	95	per 150g pack 143
	St Ivel Rainbow	71	20
	St Ivel Real	82	23
	Ski	82	per 150g pack 123
low fat	Diet Ski	55	per 150g pack 83
	St Ivel Shape	42	12
	St Michael	40	11
	Littlewoods	84	per 150g pack 126
	Tesco	103	29
	Waitrose	95	per 150g pack 143
whole milk	Waitrose	115	per 150g pack 173
Black Forest cake	Birds Eye		per 1/6 cake 150
Black Forest Cornetto	Wall's		per super cone 230
Black Forest gateau	Bejam		per 1/8 gateau 235;1/14 party gateau 193
	Birds Eye		per 1/6 cake 250
	Safeway	319	90
	St Ivel	199	56
	St Michael	247	70
	Tesco	335	95

Product	Brand	Calories per 100g/ 100ml	Calories per oz/ pack/ portion
Black Forest gateau	Waitrose	244	69
Black Forest slice	Waitrose	240	68
Black Forest sponge	Birds Eye		per 1/6 sponge 120
Black Forest trifle	Eden Vale	152	43
Black Forest tub dessert	Birds Eye		per tub 155
Black gram (Urad dahl), raw		347	98
Black Jack chews	Trebor	385	per sweet 15
Black Magic Assortment			
brandy flavoured truffle	Rowntree Mackintosh		per sweet 45
butterscotch	Rowntree Mackintosh		per sweet 30
caramel	Rowntree Mackintosh		per sweet 40
chocolate Brazil	Rowntree Mackintosh		per sweet 35
coffee cream	Rowntree Mackintosh		per sweet 30
hazelnut cluster	Rowntree Mackintosh		per sweet 45
liquid cherry	Rowntree Mackintosh		per sweet 30
montelimar	Rowntree Mackintosh		per sweet 45
orange cream	Rowntree Mackintosh		per sweet 45
strawberry cup	Rowntree Mackintosh		per sweet 45
toffee and mallow	Rowntree Mackintosh		per sweet 45

Product	Brand	Calories per 100g/ 100ml	Calories per oz/ pack/ portion
Black Magic Assortment			
truffle and nougat	Rowntree Mackintosh		per sweet 50
Black pepper			
ground	Safeway	405	115
	Tesco	275	78
whole	Safeway	405	115
	Tesco	275	78
Black pudding, fried		305	86
Black pudding			
sliced	Tesco	341	97
ring	Waitrose	226	64
Blackberries, raw		29	8
stewed without sugar		25	7
stewed with sugar		60	17
Blackberry and apple pie	St Michael	263	75
Blackberry and apple yogurt, low fat	Tesco	97	27
	Waitrose	89	per 150g pack 134
Blackberry bar	Granose	376	per 50g bar 188
Blackberry cheesecake mix (made up)	Lyons	235	67
Blackberry luxury cheesecake mix (as sold)	Green's	287	made up per portion 247
Blackberry yogurt	Munch Bunch	95	per 125g pack 119
Blackcurrant and aniseed twists	Trebor	356	per sweet 26
Blackcurrant and apple drink, low calorie	Boots Shapers		per 330ml bottle 2

Product	Brand	Calories per 100g/ 100ml	Calories per oz/ pack/ portion
Blackcurrant and apple fruit pie	Lyons	387	110
Blackcurrant and apple juice	Appella	40	12
	Copella	50	15
Blackcurrant and apple juice drink	Ribena	56	17
concentrated	Ribena	278	82
undiluted	Baby Ribena	316	94
Blackcurrant and apple lattice pie	Lyons	324	92
Blackcurrant and apple pie	St Michael	271	77
Blackcurrant and apple sundae	Lyons	389	110
Blackcurrant and cream cheesecake	Young's	240	68
Blackcurrant and lemon barley drink, undiluted	C-Vit	192	57
Blackcurrant and lime juice drink	Ribena	56	17
Blackcurrant and liquorice	Needlers	356	101
Blackcurrant and rose hip creamy yoghurt	Waitrose	146	per 125g pack 183
Blackcurrant and rosehip drink	Boots Baby Drinks	281	80
Blackcurrant and rum yogurt	St Ivel Cabaret	110	31
Blackcurrant 'C'	Libby	42	12

Product	Brand	Calories per 100g/ 100ml	Calories per oz/ pack/ portion
Blackcurrant cheesecake	Eden Vale	207	59
	St Michael	263	75
	Young's	250	71
individual	Young's	245	69
Blackcurrant cheesecake mix (made up)	Lyons	234	66
Blackcurrant conserve	Safeway	248	70
	St Michael	240	68
	Tesco	268	76
	Waitrose	250	71
Blackcurrant crush, low calorie	Slimsta	3	1
Blackcurrant delice	St Michael	240	68
Blackcurrant Devonshire cheesecake	St Ivel	250	71
Blackcurrant drink	Boots	57	17
	Lanes	152	45
	St Michael	56	17
concentrated	Boots	205	61
	Kia-Ora	289	86
	Safeway	227	67
	Tesco	285	84
	Waitrose	229	68
Blackcurrant drops with vitamin C	Boots	363	103
Blackcurrant flan filling	Armour	100	28
Blackcurrant flavour cordial	Britvic	24	7
concentrated	Schweppes	135	40
	Britvic	122	35

Product	Brand	Calories per 100g/ 100ml	Calories per oz/ pack/ portion
Blackcurrant flavour cordial			
concentrated	Corona	100	30
Blackcurrant flavour dessert mix, low calorie	Dietade	264	75
Blackcurrant flavour jelly	Waitrose	272	77
Blackcurrant fruit filling	Morton	78	22
	Waitrose	78	22
Blackcurrant fruit fool	St Michael	165	47
Blackcurrant Fruit For-All	Chivers	110	per portion 85
Blackcurrant fruit harvest ice cream	Lyons Maid	174	49
Blackcurrant fruit spread	Waitrose	124	35
Blackcurrant health drink	Lanes	130	37
Blackcurrant ice cream	Tesco	187	53
Blackcurrant jam	Robertson's	251	71
	Safeway	251	71
	Waitrose	248	70
diabetic	Boots	236	67
no added sugar	Safeway	141	40
reduced sugar	Boots	156	44
	Heinz Weight Watchers	124	35
	Waitrose	124	35
Blackcurrant jam Swiss roll	Tesco	354	100

Product	Brand	Calories per 100g/ 100ml	Calories per oz/ pack/ portion
Blackcurrant jelly	Safeway	268	76
	Tesco	57	16
	Waitrose	248	70
Blackcurrant juice	Baby Ribena	19	6
	Copella	50	14
	Hycal	243	72
concentrated	Western Isles	325	96
Blackcurrant juice drink	Ribena	59	17
sparkling	Ribena	53	16
concentrated	Ribena	293	87
	Baby Ribena	316	94
Blackcurrant, lemon and honey drink, fresh	Safeway	44	13
Blackcurrant luxury cheesecake mix (as sold)	Green's	274	made up per portion 240
Blackcurrant Pack-A-Pie	Batchelors	68	19
Blackcurrant pastilles, diabetic	Boots	100	28
Blackcurrant pies, mini	Waitrose	374	106
wholemeal	Waitrose	374	106
Blackcurrant preserve	Baxters	240	68
	Tesco	255	72
reduced sugar	Robertson's	150	43
Blackcurrant puffs	Lyons	453	128
Blackcurrant pure fruit spread	Robertson's	120	34
Blackcurrant sorbet	Waitrose	132	39

Product	Brand	Calories per 100g/ 100ml	Calories per oz/ pack/ portion
Blackcurrant sponge with buttercream	Safeway	380	108
Blackcurrant syrup	Boots	272	81
Blackcurrant table jelly	Littlewoods	260	74
Blackcurrant Topsy Turvy	Ambrosia	103	29
Blackcurrant vitamin C drink, undiluted	C-Vit	210	62
Blackcurrant yogurt	Safeway	93	
	Safeway Funtime	92	per 150g pack 140 per 150g pack 138
	Ski	81	per 150g pack 122
low fat	Tesco	100	28
	Waitrose	90	per 150g pack 135
Blackcurrantade, sparkling	Corona	24	7
Blackcurrants, raw		28	8
stewed without sugar		24	7
stewed with sugar		59	17
Blackcurrants, canned	Hartley's	60	per 117g can
Blackeye beans (Cow peas), dried		340	96
Blackeye beans			
dried	Boots	340	96
cooked	Tesco	132	37
raw	Tesco	338	96
Blackeye peas, dried	Holland and Barrett	340	96
Blackthorn cider	Taunton	34	per pint 200
Bloater, grilled		251	71
(with bones)		186	53

Product	Brand	Calories per 100g/ 100ml	Calories per oz/ pack/ portion
Bloater paste	Shippams	183	per 35g pack 64
Blue Band margarine	Van den Berghs	740	per 250g pack 1850
Blue cheese dressing	Kraft	482	143
	Safeway	260	74
Blue cheese flavour bite biscuits	Tesco	475	135
Blue cheese Prawnaise	Lyons Seafoods	200	57
Blue Hawaiian cocktail	Lyons Maid		each 34
Blue Riband	Rowntree Mackintosh	510	per biscuit 100
Blue ribbon vanilla ice cream	Wall's	90	per tub 105
cream of Cornish	Wall's	95	37
raspberry ripple	Wall's	100	per 1/20 2-litre 100
rum and raisin	Wall's	100	per 1/20 2-litre pack 100
Blue ribbon vanilla ice cream bar	Wall's		per bar 85
Blue Stilton cheese	Dairy Crest	405	115
	St Ivel	405	115
	St Michael	405	115
Blue Tendale cheese	Dairy Crest	252	71
Bobby beans, fresh, cooked	Tesco	35	10
Bobo chews	Trebor	385	per sweet 15
Boeuf bourgignon	Baxters	89	per 440g can 378
Boiled sweets		327	93
	Barratt	368	104

Product	Brand	Calories per 100g/ 100ml	Calories per oz/ pack/ portion
Bologna/Vegelinks	Granose	167	47
Bolognaise lattice pie	St Michael	245	69
Bolognaise Pour Over sauce	Crosse & Blackwell	70	20
Bolognese Dish of the Day	Crosse & Blackwell	353	100
Bolognese mix (soya)	Protoveg Menu	275	78
Bolognese sauce, cooked		139	39
Bolognese sauce	Buitoni	51	14
	Campbell's		
	Prego	98	28
	St Michael	73	21
	Signor Rossi	65	18
	Tesco	100	28
	Waitrose	70	20
dried	Beanfeast	291	82
vegetable	Hera	333	94
Bolognese spaghetti sauce	Campbell's	90	26
Bombay Dhansak curry sauce	Sharwood	127	36
Bon Bons, all flavours	Trebor	403	per sweet 27
BonBons, fruit	Cadbury's	380	per sweet standard pack 25
Bone and beef broth with vegetables	Heinz Baby Foods	62	per 128g can 79
Bone and vegetable broth		60	17
Boost	Cadbury's	485	per bar 255
Bounty Bar		473	134
Bounty milk chocolate	Mars	483	137

Product	Brand	Calories per 100g/ 100ml	Calories per oz/ pack/ portion
Bounty			
plain chocolate	Mars	485	137
Bouquet garni (Provencal) crisps	Waitrose	520	per 75g pack 390
Bourbon biscuits	Peek Frean	468	per biscuit 60
	Waitrose	468	133
Bourbon creams	Rakusen	468	133
	Safeway	486	138
	St Michael	487	138
	Tesco	477	135
diabetic	Boots	467	132
Bourneville digestive biscuits	Cadbury's	480	per biscuit 145
Bournville assorted biscuits	Cadbury's	500	per biscuit 60
Bournville chocolate bar, dark	Cadbury's	510	per 50g bar 255
Bournville cocoa	Cadbury's	310	per portion 15
Bournvita		377	107
	Cadbury's	375	per portion 20
Bovril		174	49
	Beecham	174	52
granules	Bovril	186	53
Boy and girl yogurt	St Michael	10	3
Boysenberry and passionfruit yogurt	Gold Ski	118	per 150g pack 177
Brain			
calf, boiled		152	43
calf and lamb, raw		110	31
lamb, boiled		126	36
Braised beef and vegetables	Tyne Brand	121	34
	St Michael	90	26

Product	Brand	Calories per 100g/ 100ml	Calories per oz/ pack/ portion
Braised chicken with vegetables	Heinz Baby Foods	57	per 128g jar 73
Braised kidneys in gravy	Birds Eye MenuMaster		per pack 200
Braised lamb dinner	Heinz Baby Foods	74	per 128g can 95
Braised liver and bacon lunch	Heinz Baby Foods	61	per 170g jar 104
Braised steak	St Michael	100	28
Braised steak and kidney dinner	Heinz Baby Foods	72	per 128g can 92
Braised steak dinner	Heinz Baby Foods	70	per 128g jar 90
Bramble jelly	Safeway	248	70
	Waitrose	248	70
Bramble jelly preserve	Tesco	255	72
Bramley apple pies	Safeway	338	per 283g pack 957
Bramley apple sauce	Pan Yan	121	34
	Tesco	92	26
Bramley apple trellis tart	St Michael	223	63
Bramley apples, cooking (baked)	Tesco	31	9
Bran			
crunchy	Allinson	360	102
natural	Boots Second Nature	166	47
natural country	Jordans	167	47
toasted	Meadow Farm	360	102

Product	Brand	Calories per 100g/ 100ml	Calories per oz/ pack/ portion
Bran and apple original crunchy	Jordans	369	105
Bran biscuits	Boots Second Nature	433	123
	Holland and Barrett		per biscuit 65
wholemeal	St Michael	433	123
Bran bread: see Bread, brown			
Bran breakfast with apple and banana	Holly Mill	440	125
	Holly Mill	440	125
Bran Buds	Kellogg's	271	77
Bran cakes	La Source de Vie	374	106
Bran cereal fruit and nuts	St Michael	250	71
Bran cereal muesli	St Michael	350	99
Bran crispbread			
Ideal	Holland and Barrett		per biscuit 20
Scan	Holland and Barrett		per biscuit 10
Bran crunch			
with apple	Tesco	440	125
with banana	Tesco	420	119
Bran Fare	Weetabix	228	65
Bran flakes	Kellogg's	302	86
	Tesco	325	92
	Waitrose	340	96
crunchy	St Michael	308	87
with sultana	Tesco	350	99
Bran germ	Just Naturally	260	74

Product	Brand	Calories per 100g/ 100ml	Calories per oz/ pack/ portion
Bran muesli	Prewetts	320	91
	Waitrose	363	103
unsweetened	St Michael	332	94
Bran oat crunch	Boots Second Nature	335	95
Bran oatcakes	Allinson		per biscuit 50
Bran sunnywheat crackers	St Michael	380	108
Bran wheat		206	58
Brandy Alexander cocktail	Lyons Maid		each 81
Brandy butter	Waitrose	530	150
Brandy cream	Waitrose	443	131
Branston fruity sauce	Crosse & Blackwell	90	26
Branston spicy sauce	Crosse & Blackwell	112	32
Branston sweet pickle	Crosse & Blackwell	131	37
Brawn		153	43
	Waitrose	153	43
Hungarian style	Waitrose	224	64
Brazil nut chocolate bar	Cadbury's	550	156
Brazil nut fudge sweets	Littlewoods	1629	462
Brazil nut toffees	Trebor	412	per sweet 28
Brazil nuts *with shells*		619 277	175 79
Brazil nuts	Holland and Barrett	600	170

Product	Brand	Calories per 100g/ 100ml	Calories per oz/ pack/ portion
Brazil nuts	Whitworths	619	175
	Tesco	637	181
kernels	Littlewoods	619	175
Bread, brown		223	63
	Littlewoods	223	63
bran loaf, sliced	Tesco	221	63
hi-bran	St Michael	203	58
Hibran medium sliced	Vitbe	201	per slice 66
Hibran thick sliced	Vitbe	201	per slice 80
mixed grain	St Michael	226	64
multi-grain	St Michael	226	64
original Allinson	St Michael	215	61
sliced	Tesco	249	71
Vitbe-wheatgerm	St Michael	241	68
Bread, currant		250	71
Bread, garlic	Bejam		per baguette baked, 690
Bread, Hovis		228	65
	Littlewoods	228	65
original	Tesco	239	68
sliced	Tesco	233	66
small	St Michael	232	66
Bread, malt		248	70
Bread, soda		264	75
Bread, West Indian		284	81
Bread, wheatgerm			
sliced	Tesco	254	72
sliced	Vitbe	230	per slice 76
Bread, white		233	66
dried crumbs		354	100
fried		558	158

Product	Brand	Calories per 100g/ 100ml	Calories per oz/ pack/ portion
Bread, white			
large		218	62
pitta		265	75
toasted		297	84
	Littlewoods	233	66
batched	St Michael	251	71
Big Country	St Michael	259	73
crusty	St Michael	251	71
crusty bloomer	Tesco	260	74
crusty farmhouse	Tesco	238	67
crusty French stick	Tesco	304	86
crusty split tin	Tesco	234	66
Danish loaf, sliced	Tesco	232	66
Danish loaf, toaster	Tesco	244	69
medium, long loaf	Sunblest	230	per slice 76
Mighty, medium	Sunblest	237	per slice 78
Mighty, thick	Sunblest	237	per slice 95
natural	Tesco	276	78
Old English small	St Michael	242	69
pitta	Tesco	242	69
sliced	Tesco	233	66
soft, batch	Tesco	251	71
thick, long loaf	Sunblest	230	per slice 92
thin, long loaf	Sunblest	230	per slice 64
toasting	St Michael	270	77
Bread, wholemeal		216	61
	Littlewoods	216	61
	Tesco	239	68
100%	Allinson	226	per slice 75
sandwich	St Michael	211	60
sliced	Tesco	242	69
stoneground 100%	Allinson	210	per slice 69
toaster 100%	Allinson	226	per slice 90

Product	Brand	Calories per 100g/ 100ml	Calories per oz/ pack/ portion
Bread, wholemeal/ wholewheat 100%	Holland and Barrett	220	62
Bread and butter pudding		159	45
Bread mix			
country harvest			per 455g pack
brown	Granny Smiths	225	made up 1024
white	Granny Smiths	248	per 480g pack
			made up 1190
Bread rolls			
starch reduced		384	109
Big Country sesame	St Michael	270	77
breakfast/morning	St Michael	255	72
burger buns	Bejam		per bun as sold 128
croissants	St Michael	383	109
croissants	Tesco	424	120
crusty cob	St Michael	282	80
farmhouse baps	St Michael	268	76
French half baguettes	Bejam		per half baguette baked 263
French rolls	Bejam		per roll baked 130
Old English and Scottish	St Michael	280	79
Scottish buns	Tesco	316	90
Bread rolls, brown			
crusty		289	82
soft		282	80
Big Country	St Michael	262	74
bran baps	Tesco	239	68
harvest bran	Bejam		per roll baked 97
harvest bran French roll	Bejam		per roll baked 120
mini Hovis loaves	St Michael	250	71

Product	Brand	Calories per 100g/ 100ml	Calories per oz/ pack/ portion
Bread rolls, brown			
morning	Tesco	272	77
snack	Tesco	251	71
soft	St Michael	249	71
wheaten	Tesco	280	79
Bread rolls, white			
crusty		290	82
soft		305	86
baps	Tesco	248	70
crusty	Bejam		per roll baked 105
crusty	Tesco	277	79
finger	Tesco	270	77
morning	Tesco	275	78
seeded burger buns	Tesco	271	77
snack	Tesco	246	70
Bread rolls, wholemeal			
baps for salad	Tesco	238	67
spiced buns	Tesco	293	83
stoneground baps	Tesco	269	76
Bread sauce		110	31
Bread sauce mix	Colman's Pour Over	320	91
	Knorr	368	104
	Safeway	352	100
	Tesco	332	94
	Whitworths	340	96
Breaded scampi, deep fried	Dan Maid	220	62
Breadfruit, canned, drained		64	18
Breadsticks (grissini)	Buitoni	360	102
Break biscuits	St Michael	502	142
Break-In chocolate biscuits	St Michael	590	167

Product	Brand	Calories per 100g/ 100ml	Calories per oz/ pack/ portion
Breakaway			
milk	Rowntree Mackintosh	500	each 105
plain	Rowntree Mackintosh	445	each 90
Breakfast booster	Whitworths	268	76
Breakfast bran	Tesco	349	99
Breakfast cereal			
special	St Michael	347	98
wholewheat	St Michael	333	94
Breakfast porridge oats	Boots Baby Foods	395	112
Brie cheese	Safeway	310	88
	St Ivel	300	85
	St Michael	310	88
baby Peche Mignon	St Michael	388	110
French	Tesco	306	87
	Waitrose	430	122
French Supreme	Waitrose	366	104
German	Waitrose	430	122
German, with mushrooms	Waitrose	430	122
royale	Tesco	356	101
Somerset	Waitrose	305	86
Brie cheese, blue	St Michael	450	128
Bavarian	Tesco	269	76
Bavarian, with herbs	Tesco	371	105
Bavarian, with mushroom	Tesco	371	105
German	Waitrose	430	122
Brie quiche	St Michael	302	86

Product	Brand	Calories per 100g/ 100ml	Calories per oz/ pack/ portion
Brinjal: see Aubergine			
Broad beans, boiled		48	14
Broad beans	Safeway	48	14
	Waitrose	50	14
boiled	Tesco	48	14
Broad beans, canned	Del Monte	94	27
	Hartley's	85	per 112g can 95
	Tesco	66	19
Broad beans, dried		328	93
Broad beans, frozen	Bejam	86	per 57g portion boiled 49
	Birds Eye	53	15
	Findus	53	15
	Ross	55	16
	Safeway	53	15
Broccoli	Littlewoods	23	7
	Waitrose	26	7
Broccoli, raw		23	7
boiled		18	5
Broccoli and Swiss cheese quiche	Waitrose	200	per 397g quiche 798
Broccoli in cream sauce	St Michael	112	32
Broccoli quiche	St Michael	234	66
Broccoli spears, frozen	Bejam	24	per 113g portion 27
	Birds Eye	25	7
	Findus	32	9
	Ross	20	6
	Safeway	32	9

Product	Brand	Calories per 100g/ 100ml	Calories per oz/ pack/ portion
Broccoli with chicken gratin	Findus	149	42
Brown ale, bottled		28	8
Brown bread: *see Bread, brown*			
Brown rice: *see also Rice, brown*			
Brown rice and rye with raisins	Kellogg's Nutrigrain	342	97
Brown rice and vegetables cooked	Whole Earth	135	38
	Tesco	101	29
Brown rice flakes	Holland and Barrett	203	58
Brown rice flour	Holland and Barrett	360	102
Brown sauce, bottled		99	28
	Waitrose	60	per 624g jar 374
Brown sugar: *see Sugar, brown*			
Browning	Crosse & Blackwell	195	55
Brunchies	Birds Eye		each grilled 155, fried 180
Brussels pate	Tesco	410	116
Brussels sprouts, raw		26	7
boiled		18	5
Brussels sprouts	Bejam	46	per 57g portion boiled 26
	Birds Eye	35	10
	Findus	26	7
	Ross	30	9
	Safeway	40	11
button	Waitrose	18	5

Product	Brand	Calories per 100g/ 100ml	Calories per oz/ pack/ portion
Brussels sprouts fresh	Littlewoods	26	7
Bubble and squeak	Ross	60	17
Bubble gum	Wrigley Hubba Bubba		per chunk 15/24
Bubble-O-Bill ice cream	Wall's		per portion 110
Bubbly bar	St Michael	552	156
Buckwheat flour	Holland and Barrett	330	94
Buffet pie	Tesco	393	111
Buffet pork pie	Littlewoods	395	per pie 320
Bulgur wheat	Holland and Barrett	370	105
Bumper Harvest soups (Campbell's): *see flavours*			
Bunnytots	Rowntree Mackintosh	420	per 43g bag 180
Buns: *see Bread rolls*			
Burfi, Asian		292	83
Burgamix, vegetarian	Ranch House Meals	538	153
Burger bite corn puffs beefburger and tomato	Hunters	549	per 23g pack 126
cheeseburger	Hunters	549	per 23g pack 126
Burger bites	Littlewoods	549	per 50g pack 275
	St Michael	539	153
Burger buns: *see also Bread rolls*			
Burger buns	Bejam		per bun 128
white seeded	Tesco	271	77
Burger mix	Granose	455	129

Product	Brand	Calories per 100g/ 100ml	Calories per oz/ pack/ portion
Burger mustard, mild	Colman's	110	31
Burgers, economy	Birds Eye Steakhouse		per burger grilled 100, fried 110
Burgersteaks, English	Waitrose	290	per 227g pack of two 656
Burgundy wine sauce	Baxters Cooking-in	59	per 425g can 251
Butter, salted		740	210
Butter	St Ivel	740	210
all types	Tesco	734	208
Cornish	St Michael	740	210
Cornish tub	Safeway	731	207
dairy blend	Waitrose	750	213
Devon	Littlewoods	740	210
Devon Cottage	Dairy Crest	740	210
Devon roll	Safeway	731	207
Devonshire	Waitrose	750	213
English	Safeway	731	207
English roll	St Michael	740	210
garlic	Safeway	695	197
herb (Welsh)	Safeway	704	200
home produced	Waitrose	750	213
Longboat, slighty salted	Dairy Crest	740	210
Scandinavian style, salted	Safeway	740	210
Scottish	Littlewoods	740	210
Shir gar Welsh	St Ivel	720	204
sweet cream	Safeway	749	212
Welsh Cottage	Dairy Crest	740	210
Butter, unsalted	St Ivel	750	213
	St Michael	740	210
Longboat	Dairy Crest	758	215

Product	Brand	Calories per 100g/ 100ml	Calories per oz/ pack/ portion
Butter, unsalted			
Normandy	Waitrose	750	213
Scandinavian style	Safeway	749	212
Butter beans, raw		273	77
boiled		95	27
Butter beans	Safeway	59	17
	Tesco	331	94
	Waitrose	95	27
	Tesco	103	29
Butter beans, canned	Batchelors	79	22
	Boots	95	27
	Del Monte	73	21
	Hartley's	75	per 112g can 85
	Tesco	95	27
Butter beans, dried	Boots	273	77
	Holland and Barrett	270	77
	Safeway	273	77
	Waitrose	273	77
	Whitworths	273	77
(boiled)	Whitworths	95	27
Butter biscuits	Huntley & Palmer	469	per biscuit 48
	Littlewoods	495	per biscuit 43
	Safeway	481	136
	Waitrose	480	136
Butter cherry Genoa cake	Safeway	335	95
Butter crinkles	Safeway	449	127
Butter crunch biscuits	St Michael	463	131
	Waitrose	456	129
Butter crunch creams	Safeway	498	141
	St Michael	503	143

Product	Brand	Calories per 100g/ 100ml	Calories per oz/ pack/ portion
Butter drops	Boots	448	per 33g stick 148
Butter Dundee cake	Safeway	382	108
Butter fruit biscuits	Littlewoods	485	per biscuit 42
Butter iced fruit bar	Safeway	371	105
Butter Madeira cake	Lyons	378	107
	St Michael	405	115
Butter mintoes	Waitrose	394	112
Butter mints	Cadbury's	435	per mint 30
Butter puffs	St Michael	508	144
Butter ring biscuits	Tesco	493	140
Butter shorties	Cadbury's	475	per biscuit 45
	Safeway	487	138
Butter toffee assortment	St Michael	437	124
Butter walnut sandwich cake	St Michael	412	117
Buttered eclairs	Littlewoods	407	115
Buttered kipper fillets	Birds Eye	194	55
Butterfly crackers	St Michael	483	137
Butterfly tops cake mix	Granny Smiths	432	per 363g pack made up 1568
Butterkist popcorn	Tesco	390	111
Buttermilk	Raines	39	11
Buttermints	St Michael	440	125
Butterscotch and fudge milk shake	Waitrose	98	29
Butterscotch Complan (as sold)	Farley	436	124
Butterscotch dessert	Waitrose	442	125

Product	Brand	Calories per 100g/ 100ml	Calories per oz/ pack/ portion
Butterscotch dessert sauce	Lyons Maid	314	89
Butterscotch sensations	Needlers	435	123
Butterscotch Supreme Delight	Safeway	423	120
Butterscotch sweets	Littlewoods	388	110
Button sprouts	Bejam	46	per 57g portion boiled 25
Buttons, chocolate	Cadbury's	530	per 33g standard pack 175
Cabana	Rowntree Mackintosh	440	each 235
Cabanos	Waitrose	387	110
sliced	Tesco	253	72
Cabaret biscuits, chocolate	Cadbury's	470	per biscuit 45
Cabaret yogurt (St Ivel): see flavours			
Cabbage			
Savoy, raw		26	7
spring, boiled		7	2
white, raw		22	6
Savoy, boiled		9	3
winter, boiled		15	4
winter, raw		22	6
Cabbage			
boiled	Tesco	9	3
chopped	Birds Eye	21	6
cut, boiled	Bejam	26	per 113g portion 30
Savoy	Littlewoods	26	7
shredded	Ross	20	6

Product	Brand	Calories per 100g/ 100ml	Calories per oz/ pack/ portion
Cabbage			
white	Littlewoods	22	6
white, shredded	Safeway	62	18
white/red, shredded	Safeway	56	16
winter	Littlewoods	22	6
Cabbage, red, raw		20	6
Cabbage, red	Haywards	10	3
	Littlewoods	20	6
	Tesco	14	4
	Safeway	24	7
with apple	Bejam		per 5 mini portions boiled 61
	Haywards New Seasons	37	10
Cacciatore Prego sauce	Campbell's	37	10
Caerphilly cheese	Dairy Crest	375	106
	Safeway	375	106
	St Ivel	375	106
	Tesco	353	100
farmhouse	Waitrose	390	111
Cafe noir biscuits	Waitrose	391	111
Cake mix			
small (dry)	Tesco	424	120
(made up)	Tesco	388	110
spicy	Granny Smiths	324	per 370g pack made 1199
Calabrese, fresh, boiled	Tesco	19	5
Californian corn chips	St Michael	570	162
Calypso beans (canned)	Batchelors	70	20
Calypso cubes	Trebor	354	per sweet 17

Product	Brand	Calories per 100g/ 100ml	Calories per oz/ pack/ portion
Cambozola cheese	St Ivel	463	131
Camembert cheese	Safeway	310	88
	St Ivel	288	82
	Tesco	302	86
	Waitrose	285	81
Candy foams	Barratt	361	102
Candy sticks	Barratt	378	107
Candytots	Rowntree Mackintosh	400	per 44g bag 175
Cannelloni	St Michael	140	40
canned	Buitoni	97	per 400g can 388
frozen	Findus	119	34
	Buitoni	548	155
vegetarian	Prewetts Ready Meals	103	29
Cantaloupe: *see Melon, musk*			
Cantonese sweet and sour Classic Chinese sauce	Homepride	120	34
Capelletti (as sold)	Signor Rossi	280	79
Capellini	Waitrose	378	107
Caprice biscuits chocolate and orange	Cadbury's	470	per biscuit 60
ginger and hazelnut	Cadbury's	485	per biscuit 65
honey and almond	Cadbury's	470	per biscuit 60
Captain's Fishburgers	Birds Eye		per burger fried 100, grilled/baked 135
Captain's Pie	Birds Eye MenuMaster	116	33

Product	Brand	Calories per 100g/ 100ml	Calories per oz/ pack/ portion
Caramac	Rowntree Mackintosh	545	per 27g bar 145
Caramel bar	Cadbury's	490	per 50g bar 245
Caramel cake	St Michael	425	120
Caramel chocolate roll	Lyons	437	124
Caramel cookie rings	Tesco	481	136
Caramel delight dessert	St Michael	139	39
Caramel filled milk chocolate	Littlewoods	495	140
Caramel Granymels	Itona	390	111
Caramel log	Tunnock's	441	per log 110
Caramel milk chocolate wafers, diabetic	Boots	523	148
Caramel ministicks	St Michael	473	134
Caramel sauce	Tesco	320	91
Caramel supreme	Eden Vale	127	36
Caramel toffee ice cream	Lyons Maid Gold Seal	210	60
Caramel wafers	Littlewoods	470	133
	Rowntree Mackintosh	395	per wafer 75
	Tesco	452	128
	Tunnock's	446	126
coated	Littlewood	490	139
Caraway seeds		333	94
Carbonara sauce	Waitrose	200	57
Cardamom powder		311	88

Product	Brand	Calories per 100g/ 100ml	Calories per oz/ pack/ portion
Cariba	Schweppes	35	10
low calorie	Schweppes Slimline	4	1
Caribbean cocktail	Sooner	503	143
Caribbean crush	St Michael	47	14
Caribbean drink	St Michael	56	17
	Tesco	49	15
	Waitrose	85	25
Caribbean fruit juice	St Michael	55	16
Caribbean mix	Waitrose	465	132
Caribbean slices	Trebor	357	per sweet 15
Caribbean yogurt	St Ivel Real	83	24
Carlton shell biscuits	Tesco	468	133
Carmelle dessert mix (dry)	Green's	315	made up per portion 152
Carob bar (Newform, Sunwheel Kalibu): see flavours			
Carob chip bar	Holly Mill		per bar 147
Carob chip cookies	Prewetts		per biscuit 82
Carob coated bars	Granose	414	per 35g bar 145
Carob coated biscuits	Holland and Barrett		per biscuit 70
Carob coated fruit bar	Granose	414	per 35g bar 145
Carob coated peanuts and raisins	Sunwheel Kalibu	503	143
Carob coated snack bar	Allinson	469	per 32g bar 150
fruit	Sunwheel Kalibu	340	per 30g bar 102
ginger fudge	Sunwheel Kalibu	403	per 30g bar 121
molasses	Sunwheel Kalibu	437	per 30g bar 131

Product	Brand	Calories per 100g/ 100ml	Calories per oz/ pack/ portion
Carob coated snack bar			
muesli	Sunwheel		
	Kalibu	397	per 30g bar 119
raspberry yogurt	Sunwheel		
	Kalibu	410	per 30g bar 123
raw sugar marzipan	Sunwheel		
	Kalibu	433	per 30g bar 130
Trail	Sunwheel		
	Kalibu	417	per 30g bar 125
Carob coated snack bar: *see also flavours*			
Carob flour	Holland and Barrett	180	51
Carob powder	Sunwheel Kalibu	200	57
Carob rice cakes, original	Newform		per cake 133
sugar free	Newform		per cake 130
Carrot and apple juice	Copella	32	9
Carrot and nut salad	St Michael	253	72
Carrot soup, low calorie	Waistline	19	5
Carrots			
old raw		23	7
old boiled		19	5
raw		23	7
young boiled		20	6
young (canned)		19	5
Carrots	Tesco	23	7
(boiled)	Tesco	19	5
	Waitrose	19	5
fingers, raw	Tesco	23	7
fingers, boiled	Tesco	19	5
mini Dutch, raw	Tesco	23	7

Product	Brand	Calories per 100g/ 100ml	Calories per oz/ pack/ portion
Carrots			
mini Dutch, boiled	Tesco	19	5
rings, fluted	Bejam	21	per 57g portion boiled 12
whole	Safeway	19	5
Carrots, canned	Tesco	18	5
sliced	Del Monte	25	7
	Hartley's	10	3
	Littlewoods	25	7
sliced, no salt added	Del Monte	25	7
whole	Del Monte	25	7
	Waitrose	25	7
whole, no salt added	Del Monte	25	7
whole young	Hartley's	10	3
Carrots, frozen	Ross	20	6
baby, whole quality			per 57g portion
choice	Bejam	18	boiled 10
baby	Birds Eye	18	5
	Safeway	25	7
	Tesco	30	9
	Waitrose	25	7
sliced	Safeway	19	5
	Waitrose	25	7
sliced (cooked)	Tesco	24	7
Carrots parisienne, cooked (frozen)	Tesco	34	10
Carte d'or cup ice cream			
dairy elite	Wall's		per portion 155
dark chocolate	Wall's		per portion 160
strawberry royale	Wall's		per portion 155
Cartoons cake mix (dry)			
Disneys	Green's	408	made up per portion 64

Product	Brand	Calories per 100g/ 100ml	Calories per oz/ pack/ portion
Cartoons cake mix (dry)			
Mr Men	Green's	409	made up per portion 64
My Little Pony	Green's	412	made up per portion 64
Snow White	Green's	414	made up per portion 64
Cashew nuts		561	159
Cashew nuts	Holland and Barrett	561	159
	Sooner	560	per 25g pack 140
	Whitworths	561	159
	Tesco	591	168
roast salted	St Michael	572	162
salted	Tesco	621	176
	Waitrose	650	184
Casilan (as sold)	Farley	376	107
Cassata Denise log dessert	Wall's		per 1/6 log 105
Cassata ice cream	Bejam	166	47
Cassava, fresh, raw		135	38
frozen, raw		139	39
Casserole mix			
frozen	Tesco	34	10
vegetarian meal	Hera	351	per 200g pack
Casserole vegetables mix	Birds Eye	35	10
	Ross	20	6
Cassoulet beans (canned)	Batchelors	65	18
Castaway bar, original	Holly Mill		per bar 197
Caster sugar, white	Tate and Lyle	394	112

Product	Brand	Calories per 100g/ 100ml	Calories per oz/ pack/ portion
Castle orange marmalade	Baxters	246	70
Catherine wheels	Barratt	300	85
centres	Tesco	372	105
liquorice	Tesco	334	95
Cauliflower		13	4
boiled		9	3
	Littlewoods	13	4
boiled	Tesco	9	3
frozen	Birds Eye	18	5
	Tesco	25	7
	Safeway	25	7
Cauliflower and sweetcorn pie	St Michael	108	31
Cauliflower bhajia		107	30
Cauliflower cheese		113	32
Cauliflower cheese	Bejam		per serving baked 355
	Birds Eye MenuMaster		per pack 395
	Tesco Ready Meal	129	37
	Waitrose	76	22
individual	St Michael	149	42
Cauliflower cheese	Boots Baby Foods	390	111
	Heinz Baby Foods	80	per 128g can 102
Cauliflower fleurettes (frozen)	Findus	13	4
Cauliflower florets (frozen)	Bejam	19	per 85g portion boiled 16

Product	Brand	Calories per 100g/ 100ml	Calories per oz/ pack/ portion
Cauliflower florets (frozen)			
	Ross	20	6
	Waitrose	26	7
crisp crumb	Bejam	171	per 113g portion baked 194
Cauliflower, peas and carrots (frozen)	Birds Eye	35	10
Cayenne pepper	Safeway	402	114
Celeriac, boiled		14	4
Celery, raw		8	2
boiled		5	1
Celery	Littlewoods	8	2
	Tesco	10	3
hearts	Waitrose	15	4
Celery and blue cheese cottage cheese	Eden Vale	92	26
Celery and nut salad	Tesco	124	35
Celery, corn and apple spread	Heinz	188	53
Celery, nut and sultana salad	Littlewoods	167	47
Celery salad	Littlewoods	102	29
Celery soup, low calorie	Heinz Weight Watchers	21	per 286g can 60
	Waistline	24	7
	Waitrose	20	per 295g pack 59
Cereal biscuits, wholewheat	Waitrose	335	per biscuit 60
Cereal savoury	Bewell Amazing Grains	347	98
Cereals sandwich spread	Granose	225	64

Product	Brand	Calories per 100g/ 100ml	Calories per oz/ pack/ portion
Cervelat	Waitrose	432	122
sliced	Tesco	434	123
Ceylon tea, infused	Safeway	1	
Champagne rhubarb yoghurt, low fat	Waitrose	94	per 150g pack 141
Champs	Sooner		per packet 56
Chapati, paratha and puri mix	Sharwood	345	98
Chapatis, made with fat		328	93
made without fat		202	57
Chapni kaddu: see Gourd, bottle			
Charcoal biscuits	Scott		per biscuit 40
Charlotte russe	St Michael	231	65
Chayote: see Cho cho			
Cheddar and blue cheese spread	Kraft	273	77
Cheddar and herb cheese	Safeway	406	115
Cheddar and mustard cheese	Safeway	406	115
Cheddar and onion cottage cheese	Eden Vale	121	34
	Safeway	127	36
	Tesco	121	34
	Waitrose	113	32
Cheddar cheese		406	115
Cheddar cheese	Dairy Crest	410	116
	St Ivel	410	116
	Tesco	384	109
Applewood smoked	Tesco	419	119
Canadian	Waitrose	406	115
Canadian mature, white	Safeway	406	115

Product	Brand	Calories per 100g/ 100ml	Calories per oz/ pack/ portion
Cheddar cheese			
Cracker barrel	Kraft	406	115
English	Waitrose	410	116
English mature, coloured	Safeway	410	116
English mature, white	Safeway	410	116
English matured	Waitrose	406	115
English red	Waitrose	406	115
English white	Safeway	410	116
English with walnuts	Waitrose	416	118
English, coloured	Safeway	410	116
extra mature	Waitrose	410	116
extra mild	Waitrose	410	116
farmhouse	Waitrose	406	115
farmhouse mature (black waxed)	Waitrose	406	115
farmhouse mature, mini	Waitrose	406	115
farmhouse mature, white	Safeway	410	116
home produced	Waitrose	410	116
home produced coloured	Safeway	406	115
home produced white	Safeway	406	115
Irish	Waitrose	410	116
Irish white	Safeway	410	116
mature farmhouse traditional	St Michael	405	115
medium grated	St Michael	410	116
red	St Michael	406	115
red vein	Waitrose	390	111

Product	Brand	Calories per 100g/ 100ml	Calories per oz/ pack/ portion
Cheddar cheese			
red veined	St Ivel	390	111
Scottish coloured	Safeway	410	116
Scottish white	Safeway	410	116
vegetarian	Safeway	410	116
	Waitrose	406	115
white grated	St Michael	400	113
with beer, garlic and parsley	Tesco	410	116
with ham and mustard	St Ivel	385	109
with herbs and garlic	St Ivel	410	116
with pizza herbs	Waitrose	390	111
with port wine	Tesco	410	116
with sweet pickle	Tesco	361	102
with walnuts	St Ivel	420	119
Cheddar cheese and tomato sandwich	Waitrose	155	44
Cheddar cheese pancakes (frozen)	Findus	191	54
Cheddar cheese Potato Saucery	Batchelors	334	per 94g pack as sold 314
Cheddar cheese Pour Over sauce mix	Colman's	415	118
Cheddar cheese slices	Littlewoods	301	per slice 60
	St Michael	340	96
processed	Kraft	326	92
Cheddar cheese spread	Kraft	277	79
	Waitrose	260	74
with ham	Waitrose	260	74
with prawn	Waitrose	260	74

Product	Brand	Calories per 100g/ 100ml	Calories per oz/ pack/ portion
Cheddar-like Tendale cheese	Dairy Crest	253	72
Cheddar spread	Sun-Pat	285	81
Cheddar with onion and chives	St Michael	372	105
Cheese, hard	Holland and Barrett	410	116
soft, full fat	Waitrose	296	84
soft, low fat	St Ivel Shape	135	38
Cheese and asparagus potato pancakes	Waitrose	156	per 283g pack of two 440
Cheese and broccoli flan	Tesco	237	67
Cheese and celery sandwich	St Michael	270	77
Cheese and chive flavour food snack	Boots Shapers	127	36
Cheese and grape Chef's salad meal	St Michael	156	44
Cheese and ham bites	Tesco	486	138
Cheese and ham flavour food snack	Boots Shapers	127	36
Cheese and ham pancakes	Birds Eye Snacks		per pancake shallow-fried 160
in beer batter	St Michael	221	63
Cheese and mushroom pizza	Tesco	228	65
Cheese and onion crisps	Christies	520	per 26g bag 130
	Hunters	520	per 26g bag 130
	Safeway	500	per 25g pack 125
	Tesco	520	147
	Waitrose	520	per 75g pack 390

Product	Brand	Calories per 100g/ 100ml	Calories per oz/ pack/ portion
Cheese and onion crisps **lower-fat**	St Michael	480	136
Cheese and onion flan	Tesco	326	92
Cheese and onion fries (frozen)	Ross	140	40
Cheese and onion pie (frozen)	Littlewoods	284	per 283g pack of 2 402
Cheese and onion pizza (frozen)	Ross	210	60
	Safeway	233	66
	Tesco	229	65
(pack of 4)	Safeway	230	65
Cheese and onion puffs	Tesco	509	144
Cheese and onion quiche	Tesco	230	65
individual	Ross	260	74
Cheese and onion sandwich biscuits	Nabisco	522	per biscuit 47
Cheese and onion spread	Tesco	293	83
Cheese and onion sticks	Peek Frean	538	per biscuit 22
Cheese and peach chutney sandwich	Waitrose	211	60
Cheese and potato bake	Tesco Ready Meal	117	33
Cheese and prawn spread	Tesco	264	75
Cheese and salad poppy seeded bap	Waitrose	263	75

Product	Brand	Calories per 100g/ 100ml	Calories per oz/ pack/ portion
Cheese and tomato crisps, natural	Hedgehog	407	per 27g pack 110
Cheese and tomato crispy base pizza	Findus	208	59
Cheese and tomato pizza		234	66
Cheese and tomato pizza	Safeway	247	70
	Tesco	246	70
	Waitrose	222	63
5 inch	Bejam		per pizza grilled 234
French bread	Safeway	207	59
	Tesco	245	69
pack of 4	Safeway	230	65
Cheese and tomato sandwich	Tesco	243	69
Cheese and tomato savoury	Boots Baby Foods	415	118
	Cow and Gate	60	per 110g jar 66, 150g jar 90
Cheese and tomato sticks	Peek Frean	517	per biscuit 22
Cheese, bacon and egg supper	Heinz Baby Foods	68	per 128g can 87
Cheese, egg and bacon flan	Birds Eye MenuMaster	325	per flan 460
	Birds Eye MenuMaster	273	per flan 850
Cheese, egg and onion flan	Birds Eye MenuMaster	325	per flan 460
	Birds Eye MenuMaster	273	per flan 850

Product	Brand	Calories per 100g/ 100ml	Calories per oz/ pack/ portion
Cheese flavour food snack	Boots Shapers	128	36
Cheese flavoured savoury puffs	Waitrose	526	149
Cheese, gammon and salad granary bap	Waitrose	226	64
Cheese, ham and mushroom pancakes	Waitrose	160	per 180g pack of two 288
Cheese, ham and tomato club sandwich	Waitrose	209	59
Cheese, mushroom and prawn pancakes	Waitrose	156	per 180g pack of two 281
Cheese Pasta Choice	Crosse & Blackwell	344	98
Cheese pudding		170	48
Cheese puffs	Tesco	537	152
Cheese sandwich biscuits	Nabisco	528	per biscuit 48
	St Michael	520	147
	Tesco	418	119
	Waitrose	528	150
Cheese sauce		198	56
Cheese sauce mix (as sold)	Knorr	434	123
	Safeway	418	119
	Tesco	401	114
with chives	Colman's Pour Over	370	105
Cheese sauce, Pour Over	Crosse & Blackwell	106	30
Cheese savouries	Tesco	511	145
	Waitrose	517	147

Product	Brand	Calories per 100g/ 100ml	Calories per oz/ pack/ portion
Cheese savoury	Boots Baby Foods	60	17
Cheese singles	Kraft	302	86
Cheese snaps	St Michael	517	147
Cheese souffle		252	71
Cheese spread	Littlewoods	247	70
	Safeway	285	81
	Tesco	264	75
natural	Tesco	265	75
with blue cheese	Littlewoods	248	70
with butter, soft	St Michael	360	102
with celery flavour	Littlewoods	234	66
with chives	Littlewoods	230	65
with ham	Littlewoods	236	67
with ham and onion	Littlewoods	239	68
with onion	Littlewoods	236	67
with shrimp	Littlewoods	201	57
Cheese sticks	Peek Frean	539	per biscuit 22
	Tesco	602	171
	Safeway	539	153
Cheese supper	Boots Baby Foods	60	17
Cheese tasters	St Michael	517	147
Cheese thins	St Michael	533	151
Cheese twists	Waitrose	465	132
Cheese wedge	St Ivel Shape	260	74
Cheese with walnut, processed	Tesco	344	98
Cheeseburger	Bejam		per burger baked 251

Product	Brand	Calories per 100g/ 100ml	Calories per oz/ pack/ portion
Cheeseburger corn puffs	Hunters	549	per 23g pack 126
Cheesecake: see also flavours			
Cheesecake		421	119
fresh cream	Tesco	275	78
New York style	St Michael	399	113
Cheesecake mix: see also flavours			
Cheesecake mix (as sold)	Granny Smiths	220	per 485g pack made up 1068
	Royal	337	per 500g pack made up 1686
	Safeway	315	89
	Tesco	297	84
	Waitrose	220	62
original	Green's	425	made up per portion 236
plain, luxury recipe	Green's	430	made up per portion 236
Cheeselets	Peek Frean	345	per biscuit 3
Cheesies	Birds Eye Snacks		per Cheesie grilled 75, fried 85
Chelsea buns	Tesco	320	91
Cherries, cooking			
raw		46	13
raw (with stones)		39	11
stewed with sugar		77	22
stewed with sugar (with stones)		67	19
stewed without sugar		39	11
stewed without sugar (with stones)		33	9
Cherries, cocktail, in syrup	Tesco	203	58

Product	Brand	Calories per 100g/ 100ml	Calories per oz/ pack/ portion
Cherries, glace	Safeway	218	62
	Waitrose	212	60
Cherry and apple lattice pie	Lyons	314	89
Cherry and chocolate cheesecake	St Michael	227	64
Cherry bakewell cake	Littlewoods	409	116
Cherry bar	Granose	374	per 50g bar 187
Cherry brandy		255	72
Cherry cake, all butter	Safeway	311	88
Cherry cheesecake	St Michael	258	73
Cherry cheesecake mix (made up)	Lyons	239	68
Cherry Drops roll	Trebor	349	per sweet 14
Cherry flan filling	Armour	115	33
Cherry fruit pie filling	Tesco	105	30
Cherry Genoa cake	Waitrose	372	105
cut	Safeway	318	90
large	Safeway	318	90
Cherry Madeira cake	Tesco	350	99
cut	St Michael	403	114
Cherry Menthol	Boots	363	per 33g stick 120
Cherry Napoli dairy ice cream	Lyons Maid	170	48
Cherry Pack-A-Pie	Batchelors	69	20
Cherry pie	St Michael	266	75
Cherry Red sweets	Trebor	359	per sweet 23
Cherry rondo cake	Tesco	405	115
Cherry sultana biscuits	Peek Frean	304	86

Product	Brand	Calories per 100g/ 100ml	Calories per oz/ pack/ portion
Cherry treat dessert	Cow and Gate	53	per 110g jar 58, 150g jar 80
Cherry truffles, diabetic	Boots	420	119
Cherry yogurt dessert	Cow and Gate	62	per 110g jar 68
Cherry yogurt snack bar, carob coated	Sunwheel Kalibu	383	per 30g bar 115
Cherryade	Corona	25	7
	Safeway	28	8
	Tesco	23	7
	R. Whites	20	6
Cheshire cheese	Dairy Crest	380	108
	St Ivel	380	108
coloured	Safeway	380	108
red	Tesco	415	118
	Waitrose	380	108
slices, processed	Kraft	335	95
white	Safeway	380	108
	Tesco	415	118
	Waitrose	380	108
white, mini	Waitrose	380	108
Cheshire-like Tendale cheese	Dairy Crest	246	70
Chestnut stuffing sausages	St Michael	358	101
Chestnuts		170	48
with shells		140	40
Chevda (chewra, chewra), Asian		396	112
Chevra and chana chur, Asian		539	153
Chevre (goat) cheese	Waitrose	315	89
Chewing gum	Wrigley Doublemint		per stick 9

Product	Brand	Calories per 100g/ 100ml	Calories per oz/ pack/ portion
Chewing gum	Wrigley Juicy Fruit		per stick 9
Chews			
banana splits	Trebor	385	per sweet 15
black 'n' white	Trebor	379	per sweet 36
black jacks	Trebor	385	per sweet 15
bobo	Trebor	385	per sweet 15
cola	Trebor	385	per sweet 15
fizza	Trebor	359	per sweet 14
fruit salad	Trebor	385	per sweet 15
knock knock	Trebor	364	per sweet 16
pear	Trebor	375	per sweet 15
raspbree	Trebor	373	per sweet 28
splits	Trebor	385	per sweet 15
supa 5	Trebor	364	per sweet 16
terror curses	Trebor	364	per sweet 16
tutti frutti	Trebor	379	per sweet 36
Chewy Fruit	Tesco	390	111
Chewy mints	Littlewoods	370	105
Chewy sherbets	Littlewoods	364	103
Chickpea spread: see *Hummus*			
Chickpeas (Bengal gram), raw		320	91
besan flour		326	92
Chick peas	Holland and Barrett	300	85
	Tesco	356	101
(cooked)	Tesco	154	44
canned	Boots	82	23
	Waitrose	75	21
Chicken			
dark meat, boiled		204	58
dark meat, raw		126	36
dark meat, roasted		155	44

Product	Brand	Calories per 100g/ 100ml	Calories per oz/ pack/ portion
Chicken			
light meat, boiled		163	46
light meat, raw		116	33
light meat, roasted		142	40
leg quarter (with bone)		92	26
meat and skin, raw		230	65
meat and skin, roasted		216	61
meat only, boiled		183	52
meat only, raw		121	34
meat only, roasted		148	42
Chicken	Tesco	225	64
	Waitrose	232	66
barbecue	Tesco	222	63
basted, raw	Tesco	225	64
basted, roasted	Tesco	228	65
Chinese style	St Michael	229	65
Chinese style, raw	Tesco	272	77
cornfed, raw	Tesco	208	59
cornfed, roasted	Tesco	264	75
fillets	Waitrose	158	45
frozen, raw	Tesco	137	39
frozen, roasted	Tesco	228	65
oven bake (frozen)	Ross	215	61
poussin, raw	Tesco	200	57
poussin, roasted	Tesco	228	65
quick roast, roasted	Bejam	229	65
roast, prepared	St Michael	124	35
roasted	Tesco	228	65
spring	St Michael	213	60
stuffed, raw	Tesco	198	56
stuffed, roasted	Tesco	247	70
tandoori flavour	St Michael	240	68
tandoori, raw	Tesco	240	68
whole	Waitrose	232	66

Product	Brand	Calories per 100g/ 100ml	Calories per oz/ pack/ portion
Chicken			
whole and portions, roast	St Michael	216	61
whole roasting, roasted	Bejam	233	66
whole spring, roasted	Bejam	233	66
with sage and onion, raw	Tesco	280	79
with stuffing, boneless (cooked)	Waitrose	130	37
with stuffing, cooked	Littlewoods	166	47
without skin, raw	Littlewoods	121	34
Chicken: breast	St Michael	186	53
	Waitrose	237	67
boneless	Waitrose	232	66
canned	Tesco	145	41
fillets	St Michael	116	33
	Waitrose	158	45
frozen	Waitrose	232	66
portions, boneless roasted, skin-on	Bejam	190	54
portions, boneless, casseroled	Bejam	145	41
portions, roasted	Bejam	190	54
pouch pack	Waitrose	232	66
skinless, in a crispy crumb	Waitrose	190	54
sliced	Tesco	145	41
slices, skinless, in crispy crumb	Waitrose	205	58
steaks	Bejam		per steak baked 254
stuffed boneless	St Michael	200	57

Product	Brand	Calories per 100g/ 100ml	Calories per oz/ pack/ portion
Chicken: drumsticks	Waitrose	237	67
cooked	Bejam		per drumstick as sold 87
frozen	Waitrose	237	67
goldenbake, baked	Bejam	229	65
pouch pack	Waitrose	237	67
roast	St Michael	216	61
roasted	Bejam	208	59
Chicken: legs	St Michael	237	67
	Waitrose	237	67
Chicken: portions	St Michael	92	26
	Waitrose	232	66
cooked (frozen)	Ross	260	74
goldenbake, baked	Bejam	208	59
goldenbake, southern-style, baked	Bejam	236	67
Chicken: quarters	Waitrose	232	66
wing (with bone)		74	21
cooked (frozen)	Ross	260	62
frozen	Waitrose	232	66
leg	Waitrose	232	66
pouch pack	Waitrose	237	67
roasted (frozen)	Bejam	208	59
Chicken: thighs	Waitrose	237	67
and drums, breaded	St Michael	289	82
frozen	Waitrose	237	67
pouch pack	Waitrose	237	67
roast	St Michael	216	61
roasted	Bejam	226	64
Chicken: wings	Waitrose	237	67
Chinese, baked	Bejam	265	75
pouch pack	Waitrose	232	66

Product	Brand	Calories per 100g/ 100ml	Calories per oz/ pack/ portion
Chicken a la king	Waitrose	108	31
Chicken a l'orange	Findus Lean Cuisine	119	34
Chicken and bacon pancakes	Findus	142	40
Chicken and chips snack	Bejam		per serving baked 510
Chicken and ham dinner	Heinz Baby Foods	66	per 128g can 84
Chicken and ham flaky bake pie	Birds Eye MenuMaster		per pie 525
Chicken and ham paste	Littlewoods	283	80
	Safeway	205	58
	Tesco	225	64
Chicken and ham pie	Bejam		per pie as sold 519
	Safeway	226	64
	Tesco	278	79
mini	St Michael	314	89
Chicken and ham soup with croutons	Knorr Quick Soup	419	119
Chicken and ham spread	Shippams	219	62
Chicken and leek plate pie	St Michael	248	70
Chicken and leek soup, dried as sold	Batchelors Cup-a-Soup	408	per 24g sachet 98
	Knorr Quick Soup	414	117
	Waitrose	376	per 44g pack 165
low calorie	Batchelors Slim-a-Soup	317	per 12g sachet 38
made up	Chef Box	27	8

Product	Brand	Calories per 100g/ 100ml	Calories per oz/ pack/ portion
Chicken and lemon soup, dried, low calorie	Knorr Quick Soup	292	83
Chicken and mushroom casserole	Birds Eye MenuMaster		per pack 160
Chicken and mushroom Chinese style meal	Bejam		per serving baked 143
Chicken and mushroom pancakes	Birds Eye Snacks		per pancake shallow-fried 150
Chicken and mushroom pie	Birds Eye		per pie for one 350
	Fray Bentos	196	56
	Littlewoods	293	per 283g pack of two 414
plate	St Michael	212	60
Chicken and mushroom pie filling	Fray Bentos	106	30
Chicken and mushroom soup, dried	Knorr Quick Soup	403	114
Chicken 'n' mushroom soup with croutons	Batchelors Snack-a-Soup	423	per 47.5g sachet as sold 201
Chicken and mushroom Toast Topper	Heinz	54	15
Chicken and oriental vegetables	Findus Lean Cuisine	81	23
Chicken and potato bake	St Michael	111	31
Chicken and stuffing sandwichmaker	Shippams	141	40

Product	Brand	Calories per 100g/ 100ml	Calories per oz/ pack/ portion
Chicken and sweetcorn savoury rice	Safeway	353	100
Chicken and sweetcorn soup	Waitrose	53	15
condensed	Campbell's	88	25
low calorie	Waistline	26	7
Chicken 'n' sweetcorn soup with croutons	Batchelors Snack-a-Soup	385	per 39g sachet as sold 150
Chicken and vegetable broth with rice	Granny's	37	as served 25
Chicken and vegetable pie	Tesco	285	81
individual	Littlewoods	271	77
Chicken and vegetable soup	Campbell's Main Course	51	14
	Heinz Big Soups	41	12
	St Michael	58	16
low calorie	Heinz Weight Watchers	21	per 286g can 60
	Waitrose	14	per 295g can 41
dried	Batchelors	404	per 74g pint pack as sold 299
dried, with croutons	Knorr Quick Soup	406	115
instant, dried	Tesco	382	108
instant, made up	Safeway	41	12
Chicken and vegetable stewpot pie, individual	Ross	224	64
Chicken and watercress quiche	St Michael	227	64

Product	Brand	Calories per 100g/ 100ml	Calories per oz/ pack/ portion
Chicken, bacon and mushroom flan	Bejam		per flan as sold 288
Chicken biryani	Waitrose	115	33
Chicken bites	Bejam		per bite baked 36
Chicken broth	Baxters	33	per 425g can 141
Chicken broth supper			
3-9 months	Heinz Baby Foods	58	per 128g jar 74
7-15 months	Heinz Baby Foods	69	per 170g jar 117
Chicken burgers, breaded	St Michael	289	82
Chicken cacciatore	Findus Lean Cuisine	81	23
Chicken casserole cooking mix, traditional	Colman's	335	95
Chicken casserole with vegetables			
3-9 months	Heinz Baby Foods	67	per 128g can 86
7-15 months	Heinz Baby Foods	65	per 170g jar 111
Chicken chasseur and rice	St Michael	111	31
	Bejam		per serving baked 362
Chicken chasseur Cook in Sauce	Homepride	42	12
Chicken chasseur Cook in the Pot	Crosse & Blackwell	389	110
Chicken chasseur cooking mix	Colman's	245	69
	Tesco	362	103

Product	Brand	Calories per 100g/ 100ml	Calories per oz/ pack/ portion
Chicken chow mein	Birds Eye MenuMaster		per pack 320
	Waitrose	88	per 255g pack 224
Chicken cordon bleu	Bejam		per serving baked 499
	St Michael	204	58
	Waitrose	206	58
Chicken cream soup	Knorr "No Simmer"	500	142
Chicken crisps	Christies	520	per 26g bag 130
Chicken croquettes	Safeway	260	74
Chicken curry, with bones		209	59
without bones		237	67
Chicken curry	Campbell's Quick Snack	85	24
	Findus	110	31
	St Michael	159	45
	Tesco Snack Meal	117	33
	Vesta	372	per 232g pack for two as served 864
and rice	Bejam		per serving baked 432
	Branston Snackatak	360	102
canned	Tyne Brand	101	29
	Tesco	107	30
canned, extra hot	Tesco	98	28
canned, mild	St Michael	112	32
canned, with separate rice	Crosse & Blackwell	111	31
with pilau rice	St Michael	401	114

Product	Brand	Calories per 100g/ 100ml	Calories per oz/ pack/ portion
Chicken curry with rice	Birds Eye MenuMaster		per meal 400
Chicken curry pancakes	Findus	160	45
Chicken dinner	Boots Baby Foods	395	112
	Cow and Gate	62	per 110g jar 68, 150g jar 93
Chicken drink	Knorr	274	78
Chicken escalope with bacon, raw	Tesco	297	84
cooked	Tesco	278	79
Chicken fingers, goldenbake, baked	Bejam		per finger baked 44
Chicken flavour Chinese noodles, instant	Sharwood	420	119
Chicken flavour soya wurst	Granose	300	85
Chicken Florentine en-croute	Bejam		per serving baked 416
Chicken fricassee	St Michael	97	27
Chicken, ham and mushroom pie in a white wine sauce	Waitrose	245	per 142g pie 345
	Waitrose	239	68
Chicken Hawaiian style	Waitrose	171	48
Chicken in sweet chilli sauce	St Michael	135	38
Chicken Italienne	St Michael	174	49

Product	Brand	Calories per 100g/ 100ml	Calories per oz/ pack/ portion
Chicken Kashmir	Birds Eye MenuMaster		per meal 305
Chicken Kiev	Bejam		per serving baked 648
	St Michael	260	74
	Waitrose	252	71
Chicken-like flavour protein food	Soyapro	242	69
Chicken liver pate	St Michael	224	64
Chicken livers	Waitrose	135	38
Chicken masala	Waitrose	154	per 320g pack 493
	Vesta	317	per 267g pack for two 846
Chicken moghlai	Waitrose	201	per 320g pack 643
Chicken nibbles	Waitrose	224	64
Goldenbake	Bejam		per nibble baked 120
Indian style	Waitrose	70	20
smokey barbeque	Waitrose	70	20
Chicken noodle soup, dried		329	93
made up		20	6
Chicken noodle soup canned, low calorie	Heinz Weight Watchers	19	per 316g can 60
condensed	Campbell's	36	10
dried	Batchelors	327	per 41g pint pack as sold 134
(made up)	Chef Box	26	7
	Knorr	347	98
	Tesco	368	104
	Waitrose	303	per 66g pack as sold 200

Product	Brand	Calories per 100g/ 100ml	Calories per oz/ pack/ portion
Chicken nuggets			
goldenbake	Bejam		per nugget baked 40
in breadcrumbs, cooked	Waitrose	165	47
Chicken olives	Waitrose	240	68
Chicken paste	Littlewoods	282	80
Chicken pasties	Ross	270	77
Chicken Peking	Birds Eye MenuMaster		per meal 330
Chicken pie	Tesco	323	92
family	Bejam		per 1/4 pie baked 402
	Birds Eye		per pie for 2/3 1075
	Ross	270	77
frozen	Tesco	286	81
individual	Bejam	272	per 142g pie 385
	Birds Eye		per pie 410
	Ross	280	79
shortcrust	St Michael	290	82
Chicken, pork and pate pie	Waitrose	237	67
Chicken provencale Cook in Sauce	Homepride	34	10
Chicken Provencale vegetable mix	Ross	70	20
Chicken rice soup, condensed	Campbell's	50	14
Chicken risotto	Birds Eye MenuMaster		per meal 455

Product	Brand	Calories per 100g/ 100ml	Calories per oz/ pack/ portion
Chicken risotto			
low calorie	Batchelors Slim-a-Meal	351	per 65.5g pack 230
Chicken risotto	Cow and Gate	71	per 110g jar 78; 150g jar 107
Chicken roll	Waitrose	136	39
cooked	Littlewoods	144	41
sliced	Tesco	130	37
Chicken Romane	Waitrose	186	53
Chicken salad meal	St Michael	175	50
Chicken samosa	Waitrose	226	64
Chicken sate sticks	Waitrose	156	44
Chicken Saucy Noodles	Batchelors	340	96
Chicken savoury rice	Batchelors	329	93
Chicken seasoning sauce mix	Colman's Cook In	360	102
	Colman's Pour Over	360	102
Chicken slices	Soyapro	210	60
Chicken soup	Campbell's Bumper Harvest	44	12
	Granny's	60	as served 40
	Littlewoods	58	16
low calorie	Heinz Weight Watchers	22	per 295g can 65
Chicken soup, dried	Batchelors Cup-a-Soup	428	per 25g sachet as sold 107
	Chef Chunky	44	12
	Knorr Quick Soup	420	119
	Littlewoods	380	per 37g pack as sold 141

Product	Brand	Calories per 100g/ 100ml	Calories per oz/ pack/ portion
Chicken soup, dried	Waitrose	287	per 69g pack as sold 198
instant	Safeway	395	112
low calorie	Batchelors Slim-a-Soup	317	per 12g sachet as sold 38
thick (made up)	Chef Box	30	9
Chicken spread	Littlewoods	205	per 35g pack 72
	Shippams	219	per 35g pack 77
Chicken spring roll	Waitrose	376	per average roll 267
Chicken stew, canned	Campbell's	66	19
Chicken stock cubes	Knorr	324	92
	Oxo	210	60
	Safeway	285	per cube 33
	Waitrose	322	91
Chicken stock powder	Knorr	198	56
Chicken style curry	Granose	57	16
Chicken Super Noodles	Batchelors	465	per pack as sold 460
Chicken supper	Boots Baby Foods	62	18
Chicken supreme	Campbell's Quick Snack	116	33
	St Michael	127	36
and rice (frozen)	Bejam		per serving baked 456
canned	Tesco	150	43
dried	Beanfeast	295	84
	Vesta	385	per 244g pack for two as served 940
with rice (frozen)	Birds Eye MenuMaster		per pack 460

Product	Brand	Calories per 100g/ 100ml	Calories per oz/ pack/ portion
Chicken supreme dinner	Heinz Baby Foods	77	per 128g can 99
Chicken tikka	Waitrose	226	64
Chicken, tomato and cucumber sandwich	Waitrose	285	81
Chicken with almonds	Waitrose	146	41
Chicken with courgettes and honey, canned	St Michael	90	26
Chicken with mushroom sauce crepes	Findus	135	38
Chicklets	Birds Eye Snacks		per chicklet grilled 160, fried 195
Chicory, raw		9	3
Chicory, fresh, raw	Tesco	20	6
cooked	Tesco	17	5
Children's assortment confectionery	St Michael	352	100
Children's pack			
boiled	Tesco	377	107
chews	Tesco	403	114
compressed	Tesco	365	103
Chilli: see Pepper, red			
Chilli and tomato Chinese sauce mix	Sharwood	275	78
Chilli beans, canned	Batchelors	65	18
Chilli Chinese pouring sauce, hot	Sharwood	138	39
sweet	Sharwood	186	53

Product	Brand	Calories per 100g/ 100ml	Calories per oz/ pack/ portion
Chilli con carne	Campbell's Quick Snack	124	35
	St Michael	119	34
	Tesco Ready Meal	138	39
	Waitrose	88	25
and rice	Branston Snackatak	377	107
and rice (frozen)	Tyne Brand	108	per 369g pack
canned	Crosse & Blackwell	125	35
	Old El Paso	134	per 418g can 560
	St Michael	110	31
	Tyne Brand	133	38
frozen	Bejam		per serving baked 346
with rice (frozen)	Birds Eye MenuMaster		per meal 375
Chilli con carne Cook in Sauce	Homepride	86	24
Chilli con carne pizza, pan bake	Waitrose	222	per 350g pizza 777
Chilli con carne sauce mix	Colman's	295	84
Cook in the Pot	Crosse & Blackwell	382	108
Chilli Dish of the Day, dried	Crosse & Blackwell	370	105
Chilli powder		314	89
Chilli sauce		21	6
Chilli sauce mix	Knorr	382	108
Chilli tortilla chips	Trappers	492	per 50g pack 246

Product	Brand	Calories per 100g/ 100ml	Calories per oz/ pack/ portion
Chilli vegeburger	Real Eats	200	per 70g burger 140
Chillies in brine, whole green	Old El Paso	25	per 113g can 28
Chilly Choc ice cream	Wall's		per portion 80
Chinese barbecue sauce			
ginger and honey	Sharwood	140	40
Hoi Sin	Sharwood	161	46
orange and ginger sherry	Sharwood	140	40
Chinese cakes and biscuits		415	118
Chinese chicken vegetable mix	Ross	80	23
Chinese chicken wings, baked	Bejam	23	7
Chinese crispy pancake roll	St Michael	178	50
Chinese fish balls, steamed		52	15
Chinese flaky pastries		392	111
Chinese fried special savoury rice	Batchelors		per 131g sachet as sold 632
		482	
Chinese glutinous rice flour cakes		290	82
Chinese herbs soup mixture: *see Ching bo leung*			
Chinese leaf and sweetcorn salad	Safeway	47	13
Chinese leaves (amaranth), raw		26	7
boiled	Tesco	6	2
Chinese meat buns (barbecued pork)		265	75
Chinese mushroom, dried		284	81
Chinese noodles (Sharwood): *see flavours*			

Product	Brand	Calories per 100g/ 100ml	Calories per oz/ pack/ portion
Chinese pork luncheon meat		288	82
Chinese pouring sauce			
hot chilli	Sharwood	138	39
light soy	Sharwood	24	7
oyster	Sharwood	66	19
rich soy	Sharwood	60	17
sesame oil	Sharwood	900	255
sweet chilli	Sharwood	186	53
Chinese prawns vegetable mix	Ross	50	14
Chinese salted fish, steamed, bone removed		155	44
Chinese sauce mixes (Sharwood): *see flavours*			
Chinese stir fry vegetable dish, sweet and sour	St Michael	25	7
Chinese stir-fry meal	Bejam		per portion stir-fried 280
Chinese style chicken	St Michael	229	65
Chinese style meals			
Indian stir-fry	Bejam		per portion stir-fried 331
prawn curry	Bejam		per serving baked 85
special fried rice	Bejam		per serving baked 217
spring rolls	Bejam		per roll baked 162
sweet 'n' sour chicken	Bejam		per serving baked 145
sweet 'n' sour pork	Bejam		per serving baked 338

Product	Brand	Calories per 100g/ 100ml	Calories per oz/ pack/ portion
Chinese style pork rib-steak	Bejam		per steak grilled 201
Chinese style rice	St Michael	151	43
Chinese tofu	Granose	60	17
Ching bo leung (Chinese herbs soup mixture)		23	7
Chip Shop battered fillet, cod	Ross	190	54
haddock	Ross	180	51
Chip Shop chips	Ross	70	20
Chip Shop mushy peas, canned	Batchelors	76	22
Chiplets, salt and vinegar	St Michael	487	138
Chipolata sausages	Waitrose	326	92
English recipe	Wall's Light and Lean	190	per two chipolatas 108
Chips	Findus	109	31
	Safeway	122	35
American fries	Bejam	236	per 170g portion deep-fried 402
Chip Shop	Ross	70	20
chunky	Ross	100	28
French fries	Ross	120	34
potato	Safeway	120	per 454g pack 544
steak fries	Bejam	150	per 170g portion 255
steakhouse	Tesco	207	59
Chips, crinkle cut	Bejam	176	per 170g portion deep-fried 300
	Littlewoods	137	per 454g pack 622
	Ross	130	37

Product	Brand	Calories per 100g/ 100ml	Calories per oz/ pack/ portion
Chips, crinkle cut	Tesco	112	32
deep-fried	Birds Eye	247	70
shallow-fried	Birds Eye	229	65
Chips, oven	Bejam	133	per 170g portion baked 227
	Ross	140	40
	Safeway	150	per 454g pack 688
	Tesco	150	43
	Waitrose	158	per 454g pack 720
baked or grilled	Birds Eye	194	55
cooked	Tesco	235	67
crinkle cut	Bejam	139	per 170g portion baked 237
Just Bake	St Michael	208	59
Oven Stars, baked or grilled	Birds Eye	229	65
Oven Stars, fried	Birds Eye	300	85
steak	Bejam	126	per 170g portion 214
Chips, straight cut	Bejam	162	per 170g portion deep-fried 277
	Ross	110	31
	Tesco	112	32
	Waitrose	118	per 454g pack 528
cooked	Tesco	290	82
deep-fried	Birds Eye	247	70
shallow-fried	Birds Eye	229	65
Chive mustard	Colman's	170	48
Chives and rosemary spreading cheese	Medley	319	per 75g pack 239
Cho cho (chayote, vegetable pear), raw		19	5
Choc-a-Mint	Wander	348	99

Product	Brand	Calories per 100g/ 100ml	Calories per oz/ pack/ portion
Choc 'n' cherry Arctic gateau	Birds Eye		per 1/5 gateau 100
Choc 'n' choc choc ice	Bejam		per ice 119
Choc 'n' mint mousse	Bejam		per tub as sold 76
Choc 'n' nut cornets	Bejam		per cornet 258
Choc and nut Cornetto	Wall's		per cone 220
Choc 'n' nut ice cream	Bejam	226	64
Cup	Wall's Italiano		per cup 170
slice	Wall's		per 1/5 of packet 105
Sweet Trolley	Wall's Italiano	125	per 1/10 litre pack 125
Choc 'n' nut split lolly	Bejam		per lolly 158
Choc 'n' nut sundae	Bejam		per sundae as sold 177
Choc 'n' nut Supermousse tub dessert	Birds Eye		per tub 150
Choc bars, double choc	Wall's		per bar 160
mint and crispy	Wall's		per bar 185
nutty choc	Wall's		per bar 190
Choc chip n' nut cookies	Huntley & Palmer	488	per biscuit 45
Choc chip choc ices	Waitrose	309	per ice 192
Choc ices			
choc 'n' choc	Bejam		per ice 119
dark	Bejam		per ice 115
dark and golden	Wall's		per ice 130
dark mint	Bejam		per ice 115
dark satin	Lyons Maid		per ice 128

Product	Brand	Calories per 100g/ 100ml	Calories per oz/ pack/ portion
Choc ices			
golden	Bejam		per ice 115
golden vanilla	Wall's		per ice 130
individual	Tesco	128	36
Neapolitan	Bejam		per ice 119
silky smooth	Lyons Maid		per ice 132
Choc mint Cup ice cream	Wall's Italiano		per cup 170
Choc orange with cointreau ice cream	Bejam	176	50
Chockle	Lyons Maid		each 72
Choco rico Cornetto	Wall's		per super cone 250
Chocolate and banana ice cream	Lyons Maid	181	51
Chocolate and blackcurrant gateau	Safeway	375	106
Chocolate and hazelnut spread	Tesco	533	151
Chocolate and mint mousse	Tesco	171	48
Chocolate and nut cookies	Littlewoods	502	142
	Waitrose	500	142
Chocolate and orange bombes	Bejam		per bombe 177
Chocolate and orange Caprice biscuits	Cadbury's	470	per biscuit 60
Chocolate and vanilla Swiss roll	Lyons	373	106
Chocolate biscuits, full-coated		524	149

Product	Brand	Calories per 100g/ 100ml	Calories per oz/ pack/ portion
Chocolate blancmange	Brown and Polson	335	95
Chocolate Brazil	Rowntree Mackintosh		per sweet 35
	Waitrose	574	163
Chocolate Break	Cadbury's	410	per 28g biscuit 115
Chocolate Buttons	Cadbury's	530	per 33g standard pack 175
Chocolate Cabaret biscuits	Cadbury's	470	per biscuit 45
Chocolate cake, iced layer	Tesco	428	121
	St Michael	340	96
Chocolate cake mix	Safeway	315	per 210g pack as sold 662
diabetic	Boots	463	131
Swiss style	Green's	401	made up per portion 300
Chocolate casket assortment	St Michael	537	152
Chocolate chip and orange cookies	Waitrose	495	140
Chocolate chip cookies	St Michael	494	140
	Tesco	479	136
	Waitrose	463	131
with fruit	Tesco	445	126
with nut	Tesco	465	132
Chocolate chip ice cream, American style	Waitrose	194	55
Chocolate chip muesli bar	Granose	484	per 25g bar 121

Product	Brand	Calories per 100g/ 100ml	Calories per oz/ pack/ portion
Chocolate chip shortbread	Waitrose	468	133
Chocolate chip shortbread biscuits	Tesco	512	145
Chocolate coated caramel bar biscuits	Tesco	463	131
Chocolate coated digestive bars	Tesco	504	143
Chocolate coated fruit and nut bars	Tesco	502	142
Chocolate coated muesli bars	Tesco	510	145
Chocolate coated orange filled bars	Tesco	503	143
Chocolate coated sandwich bar biscuits	Tesco	512	145
Chocolate coated shortcake bar biscuits	Tesco	498	141
Chocolate coated Swiss roll	Tesco	406	115
Chocolate coated tea cakes	Tesco	432	122
Chocolate coated toffee rolls	Tesco	458	130
Chocolate coated wafers, diabetic	Boots	560	159
Chocolate coconut flake ice cream	Lyons Maid Gold Seal	183	52
Chocolate Complan (powder)	Farley	440	per 57g sachet 251

Product	Brand	Calories per 100g/ 100ml	Calories per oz/ pack/ portion
Chocolate covered sponge roll	St Michael	412	117
Chocolate cream bar	Cadbury's	420	per 50g bar 210
Chocolate cream dessert	Young's	250	71
Chocolate cream gateau	Waitrose	259	73
Chocolate cream tartlets	St Michael	440	125
Chocolate creams, assorted	Safeway	485	137
Chocolate cup cakes	Lyons	338	96
Chocolate dairy cream sponge	Bejam		per 1/6 cake as sold 104
Chocolate dairy toffees	Trebor	468	per toffee 45
Chocolate delight dessert	St Michael	139	39
Chocolate dessert	St Michael	127	36
	Waitrose	432	per 72g pack 311
Lovely	Birds Eye		per tub 235
Supermousse	Birds Eye		per tub 120
Chocolate dessert	Heinz Baby Foods	90	per 128g jar 115
	Boots Baby Foods	92	26
Chocolate dessert cake	Tesco	444	126
Chocolate dessert sauce	Lyons Maid	283	80

Chocolate digestives: *see Digestive biscuits*

Product	Brand	Calories per 100g/ 100ml	Calories per oz/ pack/ portion
Chocolate drink			
diabetic	Boots	341	97
semi-skimmed	St Michael	66	19
Chocolate, drinking	Cadbury's	385	per portion 20
Chocolate drop teacake mix	Green's	419	per portion made up 61
Chocolate eclairs	Young's	440	125
	Trebor	470	per sweet 39
Chocolate fancies	Lyons	449	127
Chocolate filled Swiss roll	Tesco	406	115
Chocolate fingers	Lyons	414	117
Chocolate flake ice cream	Tesco	209	59
Chocolate flavour dessert mix	Dietade	292	83
Chocolate flavour fruit crisps	Littlewoods	360	102
Chocolate flavour limes	Littlewoods	406	115
Chocolate fruit roll	Trebor	382	per sweet 16
Chocolate fudge	Trebor	457	per sweet 43
Chocolate fudge brownie mix, American style	Green's	453	made up per portion 79
Chocolate fudge dessert	Ross	340	96
Chocolate gateau	Tesco	451	128
	St Michael	346	98
Chocolate ginger biscuits	Waitrose	384	109

Product	Brand	Calories per 100g/ 100ml	Calories per oz/ pack/ portion
Chocolate ginger crunch biscuits	Waitrose	472	134
Chocolate harlequin dessert	Wall's		per 1/5 pack 110
Chocolate ice cream	Waitrose	185	55
	Wall's Alpine		per 1/10 pack 125
dairy	Bertorelli	211	60
non-dairy	Lyons Maid	180	51
soft scoop	Safeway	167	49
Chocolate Jelly-Creams	Chivers	365	per portion 160
Chocolate King Cone	Lyons Maid		per cone 219
Chocolate lime roll	Trebor	382	per sweet 16
Chocolate log and buttercream cake	Safeway	428	121
Chocolate malted food drink, low fat instant	Horlicks	393	111
Chocolate menthe dairy ice cream	Bertorelli	233	66
Chocolate milkshake	St Michael	86	24
	Waitrose	73	22
Chocolate mint creams	Trebor	380	per sweet 38
Chocolate mint crunch mix	Royal	343	per 488g pack made up 1674
Chocolate mints	St Michael	406	115
	Trebor	381	per sweet 24
Chocolate mousse	Bejam		per tub as sold 76
	Safeway	166	49
	Tesco	188	53
	Waitrose	152	43
and mint swirl	Safeway	153	45

Product	Brand	Calories per 100g/ 100ml	Calories per oz/ pack/ portion
Chocolate mousse			
tub dessert	Birds Eye		per tub 110
wizard	St Ivel	186	53
Chocolate Munch Bunch	Eden Vale	108	per 125g pack 135
Chocolate nut cookies	Safeway	500	142
Chocolate Oliver biscuits	Fortts	359	per biscuit 88
Chocolate orange crunch mix, dry	Tesco	419	119
made up	Tesco	270	77
Chocolate orange dessert	Waitrose	432	per 69g pack 298
Chocolate orange ice cream, American style	Waitrose	195	58
Chocolate Pavlova cake	Waitrose	300	85
Chocolate peanuts and raisins	Tesco	489	139
Chocolate peppermint creams	Waitrose	414	117
Chocolate popcorn	Tesco	414	117
Chocolate pudding	St Michael	311	88
Chocolate pudding	Boots Baby Foods	92	26
	Heinz Baby Foods	83	per 128g can 106
	Cow and Gate	92	per 110g jar 101; 150g jar 138
with tapioca	Heinz Baby Foods	74	per 128g can 95

Product	Brand	Calories per 100g/ 100ml	Calories per oz/ pack/ portion
Chocolate ripple	St Michael	139	39
Chocolate ripple ice cream	Lyons Maid	181	51
Chocolate ripple mousse	Findus	177	50
Chocolate roll	Tesco	396	112
caramel	Lyons	437	124
jam and vanilla	Lyons	385	109
mini	Tesco	471	134
Chocolate sandwich cake	Waitrose	457	per 291g cake 1332
	Lyons	378	107
Chocolate sandwich cake mix	Granny Smiths	423	per 495g pack made up 2096
Chocolate sauce	Tesco	331	94
Chocolate souffle	St Ivel	191	54
	St Michael	167	47
Chocolate sponge and sauce pudding mix	Green's	402	made up per portion 323
Chocolate sponge cake mix	Granny Smiths	398	per 350g pack made up 1392
Luxury (dry)	Tesco	416	118
(made up)	Tesco	370	105
traditional recipe	Green's	344	per portion made up 91
Chocolate sponge pudding	Heinz	296	84
Chocolate sponge roll with buttercream	St Michael	403	114
Chocolate sponge slice cake	Littlewoods	363	103

Product	Brand	Calories per 100g/ 100ml	Calories per oz/ pack/ portion
Chocolate spread hazelnut	Cadbury's	315	per portion 45
	Cadbury's	570	per portion 85
	Sun-Pat	520	147
Chocolate sundae cups	Lyons Maid		each 156
Chocolate supershake	Eden Vale	75	per 194g pack 146
Chocolate supreme	Eden Vale	134	per 125g pack 168
Chocolate Supreme Delight	Safeway	423	120
Chocolate swirl ice cream	Lyons Maid Gold Seal	192	54
Chocolate Swiss roll with buttercream	St Michael	377	107
Chocolate teacakes	Littlewoods	427	121
Chocolate topped orange cakes	Waitrose	381	108
Chocolate tops cake mix	Granny Smiths	354	per 307g pack made up 1088
Chocolate Topsy Turvy	Ambrosia	103	29
Chocolate triple biscuits	Peek Frean	541	per biscuit 180
Chocolate truffles, fresh cream	St Michael	536	152
Chocolate yogurt low fat	Mr Men	100	28
	Tesco	107	30
	Waitrose	98	per 150g pack 147
Chocolate, fancy and filled		460	130
Chocomousse	Eden Vale	180	per 60g pack 108
Chop suey	Beanfeast	270	77
	Vesta	397	per pack for two as served 1020

Product	Brand	Calories per 100g/ 100ml	Calories per oz/ pack/ portion
Chopped cured pork			
in jelly	Littlewoods	367	104
slices	St Michael	194	55
Chopped ham and pork, canned		270	77
sliced	Tesco	237	67
Chopped ham with	Armour	306	per 198g can 606
pork	Littlewoods	294	per 170g pack 500
Chorizos	Waitrose	342	97
Chorley cakes	St Michael	408	116
	Waitrose	420	119
Choux buns	St Michael	330	94
dairy cream	Birds Eye		per bun 130
Choux pastry, raw		214	61
cooked		330	94
frozen, baked	Bejam	335	95
Choux ring dessert	St Michael	424	120
Chow mein	Vesta	361	per pack for two as served 679
low calorie	Batchelors Slim-a-Meal	301	per 80.5g pack 242
Chow mein style pot meal	Boots Shapers	332	94
Christmas cake			
all butter iced top and brandy, fully	Tesco	351	100
iced	Tesco	374	106
Christmas pudding		304	86
	Crosse & Blackwell	321	91
	Peek Frean	312	88
	Robertson's	296	84
	Tesco	338	96

Product	Brand	Calories per 100g/ 100ml	Calories per oz/ pack/ portion
Chuck steak: see Beef, chuck			
Chuckles roll	Trebor	363	per sweet 11
Chump chops: see lamb, pork, etc			
Chunks, vegetarian			
beef flavour	Direct Foods	273	77
natural flavour	Direct Foods	251	71
Chunky bar	Itona	540	153
Chunky chicken (canned)	St Michael	150	43
curry	Shippams	131	per 206g can 270
in barbecue sauce	Shippams	138	per 206g can 284
in mushroom sauce	Shippams	169	per 206g can 348
supreme	Shippams	152	per 206g can 313
Chunky chicken with bacon and ham pie	Waitrose	302	86
Chunky chips	Ross	100	28
Chunky curried beef (canned)	St Michael	99	28
Chunky haddock and mushroom crumble	St Michael	125	35
Chunky mixed fruits in natural syrup	Libby	52	15
Chunky steak in rich gravy (canned)	St Michael	100	28
Chunky steak with kidney pie	Waitrose	288	82
Chutney: see flavours			
Cider, dry		36	10
sweet		42	12
vintage		101	29

Product	Brand	Calories per 100g/ 100ml	Calories per oz/ pack/ portion
Cider	Autumn Gold	30	per pint 170 bottled or canned
	Autumn Gold	40	per pint 230, keg
	Blackthorn	34	per pint 200
	Diamond White	54	per pint 310
	Natch	34	per pint 200
	Special Vat	44	per pint 250
dry	Pommia	54	per pint 310
dry, traditional draught	Taunton	30	per pint 170
medium, traditional draught	Taunton	34	per pint 190
original	Bulmer	37	per half pint 104
sweet	Exhibition	59	per pint 330
	Pommia	65	per pint 370
Cider apple and herbs stuffing mix	Knorr	401	114
Cinnamon powder		261	74
Cinnamon	Safeway	337	96
	Tesco	267	76
Citric acid	Boots	247	70
Citro drink, lemon	St Michael	42	12
orange and apricot	St Michael	35	10
Citrus creams	Peek Frean	480	per biscuit 58
Citrus fruit drink, carbonated	Boots Shapers		per 330ml bottle 3
Clam chowder	Waitrose	43	12
Clams, seasoned, canned		112	32
Classic Chinese sauces (Homepride): see flavours			
Classic curry sauces (Homepride): see flavours			
Clear fruits	Waitrose	356	101
Clear mints	St Michael	362	103

Product	Brand	Calories per 100g/ 100ml	Calories per oz/ pack/* portion
Clear mints	Waitrose	356	101
Clear soup with croutons, low calorie, dried			
beef	Batchelors Slim-a-Soup	371	per 10.5g sachet 39
chicken	Batchelors Slim-a-Soup	390	per 10g sachet 39
Cloudy lemonade	Boots Shapers	1	per 330ml bottle 3
Clover dairy spread	Dairy Crest	682	per 250g pack 1705
Cloves, whole	Safeway	413	117
Club biscuits			
coffee	Jacobs	503	per biscuit 113
fruit	Jacobs	471	per biscuit 113
milk	Jacobs	510	per biscuit 117
mint	Jacobs	495	per biscuit 113
orange	Jacobs	497	per biscuit 113
plain	Jacobs	494	per biscuit 112
wafer	Jacobs	517	per biscuit 100
Cluster beans: see Guare			
Coat and cook sauces (Homepride): see flavours			
Coated caramel wafers	Littlewoods	490	139
Cob or hazelnuts		380	108
with shells		137	39
Coca-cola		39	11
Cock-a-Leekie soup	Baxters	24	per 425g can 102
	Heinz Classic Soups	20	6
	Waitrose	24	per 425g can 102
Cockles, boiled		48	14
cooked	Dan Maid	100	28
frozen, raw	Tesco	60	17

Product	Brand	Calories per 100g/ 100ml	Calories per oz/ pack/ portion
Cocktail biscuit assortment, savoury	St Michael	575	163
Cocktail cherries in syrup, bottled	Tesco	203	58
Cocktail gherkins	Tesco	11	3
	Waitrose	14	4
Cocktail onions	Tesco	13	4
	Waitrose	27	8
Cocktail sausage rolls	Birds Eye Snacks		per roll baked 65
	Littlewoods	425	per roll 106
	Waitrose	430	122
Cocktail sausages	Bejam		per sausage grilled 34
	St Michael	350	99
Coco Pops	Kellogg's	358	101
Coco Ready Brek	Lyons	388	110
Cocoa		312	88
	Rowntree's	308	87
	Safeway	312	88
	Waitrose	326	92
Bournville	Cadbury's	310	per portion 15
Cocoa puffs	Tesco	391	111
Coconut desiccated		604	171
fresh		351	100
kernel only		351	100
Coconut creamed desiccated	Sharwood	600	170
	Safeway	604	171
	Tesco	683	194
	Whitworths	604	171

Product	Brand	Calories per 100g/ 100ml	Calories per oz/ pack/ portion
Coconut			
flesh	Tesco	345	98
kernel	Littlewoods	351	100
sweetened	Tesco	398	113
Coconut milk		21	6
Coconut oil		883	250
Coconut and apricot slice	Lyons	454	129
Coconut and honey biscuits	Boots	541	153
Coconut and honey original crunchy bar	Jordans	416	per bar 138
Coconut and sultana muesli tubs	Jordans	366	104
Coconut biscuits	Huntley & Palmer	511	per biscuit 51
Coconut cake, all butter	Safeway	417	118
	Waitrose	375	106
with buttercream	St Michael	415	118
Coconut Coasters	Cadbury's	485	per biscuit 45
Coconut cookies	Littlewoods	490	139
	Waitrose	490	139
Coconut cream, prepared without water		330	94
Coconut crumble creams	Tesco	525	149
	Waitrose	521	148
Coconut crunch bar	Boots Second Nature	452	128
Coconut eclair	Rowntree Mackintosh		per sweet 45
Coconut flake	Lyons Maid		each 181

Product	Brand	Calories per 100g/ 100ml	Calories per oz/ pack/ portion
Coconut gateau with buttercream	Safeway	374	106
Coconut macaroons	Tesco	500	142
Coconut mallows	Peek Frean	384	per biscuit 46
Coconut mushrooms	Bassett's	407	115
Coconut Nice creams, assorted	Safeway	527	149
Coconut rings	Safeway	451	128
	Tesco	509	144
	Waitrose	489	139
Coconut sandwich cake	Waitrose	375	106
decorated	Littlewoods	435	per 275g cake 1196
Coconut snowballs	Littlewoods	449	127
Coconut sponge with buttercream	Safeway	430	122
Coconut yoghurt	Safeway	119	per 150g pack 179
	Tesco	96	27
Cod			
baked		96	27
baked (with bones and skin)		82	23
cooked		138	39
fried in batter		199	56
grilled		95	27
poached		94	27
smoked, poached		101	29
poached (with bones and skin)		82	23
smoked, raw		79	22
steamed		83	24
steamed (with bones and skin)		67	19

Product	Brand	Calories per 100g/ 100ml	Calories per oz/ pack/ portion
Cod	Littlewoods	76	22
battered (frozen)	Littlewoods	230	each 115
battered, oven (frozen)	Ross	200	57
battered, raw (frozen)	Tesco	170	48
battered, cooked (frozen)	Tesco	203	58
breaded (frozen)	Littlewoods	261	each, pack of two, 261
	Littlewoods	258	each, 240g pack of four, 155
breaded, cooked (frozen)	Tesco	110	31
breaded, raw (frozen)	Tesco	103	29
crispy battered	Ross	170	48
in batter (frozen)	Safeway	200	57
in breadcrumbs (frozen)	Safeway	125	35
in breadcrumbs	Young's	179	51
Cod chunks, battered	Ross	170	48
Cod, dried			
salted, boiled		138	39
salted, raw		130	37
Cod fillets			
fresh, raw		76	22
	Waitrose	83	24
battered, baked	Bejam	208	59
breaded, deep-fried	Bejam	208	59
breaded, in natural crumb	Ross	170	48
breaded, in wholemeal crumb	Ross	170	48

Product	Brand	Calories per 100g/ 100ml	Calories per oz/ pack/ portion
Cod fillets			
breaded	Waitrose	110	31
chilled	Young's	75	21
Chip Shop battered	Ross	190	54
frozen	Ross	80	23
	Safeway	80	23
	Waitrose	80	23
in breadcrumbs	St Michael	118	33
in breadcrumbs (frozen)	Safeway	140	40
ovencrisp	St Michael	250	71
prime, poached	Bejam	99	28
	Young's	78	22
	Waitrose	101	29
supercrumb, baked	Bejam	296	84
Cod fillet fish fingers	Birds Eye		per finger grilled 50, fried 60
Cod fingers			
battered, jumbo	Ross	190	54
crispy	Birds Eye		per finger fried 65
Cod fish cakes	Bejam		per fish cake fried 117
	Birds Eye		per cake grilled 90, fried 140
fresh	Young's	213	60
Cod fish fingers	Bejam		per finger grilled 44
	Littlewoods	209	per finger 52
	Littlewoods	209	per finger 52
	Safeway	184	52
	Waitrose	180	51
crumb crisp	Findus	172	49
minced	Waitrose	182	52

Product	Brand	Calories per 100g/ 100ml	Calories per oz/ pack/ portion
Cod fish fingers			
oven crispy	Birds Eye		each baked/grilled 70, shallow-fried 80
Cod: in butter sauce	Birds Eye		
	MenuMaster		per pack 155
	Safeway	90	per 150g 135
	Tesco	73	21
and parsley	St Michael	94	27
boil-in-bag	Bejam		per serving 138
Cod: in cheese sauce	Birds Eye		
	MenuMaster		per pack 175
boil-in-bag	Bejam		per serving 167
Cod: in cream sauce	Birds Eye		
	MenuMaster		per pack 125
Cod: in mushroom sauce	Birds Eye		
	MenuMaster		per pack 180
boil-in-bag	Bejam		per serving 179
Cod: in parsley sauce	Birds Eye		
	MenuMaster		per pack 140
	Safeway	80	per 150g pack 120
	Tesco	68	19
boil-in-bag	Bejam		per serving 136
Cod: in shrimp flavour sauce	Birds Eye		
	MenuMaster		per pack 165
Cod nuggets			
deep-fried	Birds Eye	247	70
grilled or baked	Birds Eye	212	60
shallow-fried	Birds Eye	229	65
Cod portions	Littlewoods	84	24
battercrisp	Findus	193	55
	St Michael	230	65
crumb crisp	Findus	206	58

Product	Brand	Calories per 100g/ 100ml	Calories per oz/ pack/ portion
Cod roe			
hard, raw		113	32
fried		202	57
Cod steak			
in butter sauce	Findus	81	23
	Ross	90	26
in cheese sauce	Findus	89	25
	Ross	110	31
in parsley sauce	Findus	65	18
	Ross	80	23
in seafood sauce	Findus	71	20
in sweetcorn sauce	Ross	80	23
Cod steaks			
frozen, raw		68	19
	Bejam		per steak grilled 51
	Birds Eye		per steak 80
	Ross	80	23
	Waitrose	70	per 142g steak 100
	Young's	75	21
battered	Findus	173	49
breaded	Bejam		per steak grilled 111
breaded, in natural crumb	Ross	170	48
breaded, in wholemeal crumb	Ross	170	48
crispy	Birds Eye		each shallow-fried 190, deep-fried 215
in breadcrumbs	Findus	105	30
in crisp crunch crumb	Birds Eye		each grilled/baked 185, shallow fried 210

Product	Brand	Calories per 100g/ 100ml	Calories per oz/ pack/ portion
Cod steaks			
in crispy batter	Bejam		per steak deep-fried 248
in wafer light batter	Birds Eye		each baked/grilled 195,shallow-fried 220
in wholemeal crumb	Birds Eye		each grilled/baked 195,shallow-fried 220
oven crispy	Birds Eye		per steak baked or grilled 215
Cod and broccoli mornay	Waitrose	83	per 454g pack 377
Cod and mushroom crumble	Littlewoods	117	per 400g pack 468
Cod and parsley croquettes	Young's	192	54
Cod and potato pie	Tesco	83	24
Cod and prawn crumble	Littlewoods	125	per 400g pack 500
Cod and prawn pasta	Bejam		per serving baked 274
Cod and prawn pie	Bejam		per serving baked 408
	Tesco	195	55
	Young's	195	55
individual	St Michael	150	43
Cod and ratatouille gratin	St Michael	125	35
Cod bake	Bejam		per serving baked 297
	Ross	120	34
Cod bites	Bejam		per bite baked 34

Product	Brand	Calories per 100g/ 100ml	Calories per oz/ pack/ portion
Cod bonne femme, raw			
(frozen)	Tesco	93	26
cooked	Tesco	83	24
Cod crumble	Bejam		per serving baked 485
	Ross	195	55
Cod liver oil		899	255
Cod mornay	Birds Eye MenuMaster		per pack 420
Cod provencal	Tesco	75	21
Coffee, ground, roasted		287	81
infusion, 5 minutes		2	1
instant		100	28
Coffee			
beans, all flavours	Waitrose	194	55
dandelion	Symingtons	320	91
Dandex	Lanes	385	109
freeze-dried	St Michael	90	26
freeze-dried, all flavours	Waitrose	100	28
Gold, dry	Safeway	330	94
granules, all flavours	Waitrose	100	28
granules, instant	Safeway	330	94
	St Michael	90	26
ground	Tesco	351	100
ground, all flavours	Waitrose	287	81
infused, all flavours	Safeway	2	1
instant, dry	Safeway	330	94
others	Tesco	324	92
powder	Safeway	330	94
Coffee, decaffeinated	Symingtons	155	44
beans	Waitrose	194	55

Product	Brand	Calories per 100g/ 100ml	Calories per oz/ pack/ portion
Coffee, decaffeinated			
filter fine	Waitrose	287	81
freeze-dried	Safeway	330	94
instant	Boots	100	30
	Waitrose	100	28
Coffee and chicory			
essence		218	62
	Waitrose	134	38
dry	Safeway	380	108
Coffee and hazelnut roll	Tesco	377	107
Coffee and mandarin gateau	Bejam		per 1/8 gateau 213
Coffee Break	Safeway	50	14
Coffee cake, fresh cream slice	Tesco	418	119
Coffee cake mix, Austrian style	Green's	388	made up per portion 292
Coffee Choice	Safeway	330	94
Coffee Club biscuits	Jacobs	503	per biscuit 113
Coffee Compliment	Cadbury's	540	per portion 10
Coffee cream	Rowntree Mackintosh		per sweet 30
Coffee creams	Peek Frean	480	per biscuit 56
	St Michael	534	151
	Tesco	464	132
	Waitrose	476	135
Coffee Crisp block	Needlers	494	per 45g pack 222
Coffee cup	Rowntree Mackintosh		per sweet 40
Coffee half cream portions	St Michael	136	39

Product	Brand	Calories per 100g/ 100ml	Calories per oz/ pack/ portion
Coffee ice cream	Bejam	166	47
	Waitrose	154	46
dairy	Bertorelli	196	56
Coffee-mate	Carnation	535	per rounded tsp in 10fl oz water 10
Coffee sugar crystals	Safeway	394	112
Coffee whitener	Tesco	539	153
Coffee yogurt, French style	Littlewoods	102	per 150g pack 153
Cola	Britvic	33	9
	Canada Dry	34	10
(1.5 litre pack)	Littlewoods	29	9
(330ml pack)	Littlewoods	31	9
	Safeway	40	12
	St Michael	46	14
bottled	Tesco	30	9
canned	Tesco	32	9
diabetic	Boots	1	
Diet	Canada Dry		per 175ml pack 0.3
	Safeway		
low calorie	Tesco	4	1
	Waitrose	4	1
Cola chews	Trebor	385	per sweet 15
Cola cubes	Littlewoods	367	104
Cola drink	Corona Coola	42	12
	Waitrose	35	10
Cola-flavoured concentrate	Safeway	218	65
low calorie	Safeway	1	
Cola quench	Lyons Maid		each 31
Cola sherbets	Trebor	359	per sweet 23

Product	Brand	Calories per 100g/ 100ml	Calories per oz/ pack/ portion
Cole, dried, boiled		12	3
Coleslaw	Littlewoods	106	30
	St Ivel	125	35
	St Michael	172	49
	Safeway	198	56
	Tesco	104	29
	Waitrose	128	36
apple	Tesco	157	45
apple and sultana	Safeway	202	57
canned	Heinz	126	36
classic	Eden Vale	127	36
coarse cut	Eden Vale	124	35
curried	Tesco	204	58
diet	Eden Vale	55	16
fruity	Eden Vale	207	59
reduced calorie dressing, other recipes	Tesco	52	15
in vinaigrette	Tesco	60	17
in vinaigrette, other recipes	Tesco	40	11
low calorie	St Ivel Shape	38	11
	Safeway	52	15
	Waitrose	62	18
mild	Eden Vale	200	57
other recipes	Tesco	124	35
premier	St Ivel	230	65
	Tesco	189	54
other recipes	Tesco	168	48
reduced calorie dressing	Littlewoods	54	15
	Tesco	44	12
spicy	Eden Vale	201	57

Product	Brand	Calories per 100g/ 100ml	Calories per oz/ pack/ portion
Coleslaw			
with cheese and chives	St Michael	286	81
Coleslaw dressing	Kraft	449	133
Coley			
fillets	Young's	74	21
	Waitrose	99	28
frozen	Littlewoods	97	per portion 89
frozen, cooked	Tesco	99	28
frozen, raw	Tesco	85	24
portions	Bejam	98	per 4oz portion poached 111
steaks	Waitrose	80	per 142g steak 115
steaks, frozen	Ross	80	23
Colocasia: *see Arvi*			
Comforters	Barratt	333	94
Complan powder			
butterscotch	Farley	436	124
chocolate	Farley	440	per 57g sachet 251
malted	Farley	444	per 57g sachet 253
natural	Farley	444	per 57g sachet 253
savoury	Farley	436	per 57g sachet 249
strawberry	Farley	444	per 57g sachet 253
Complete batter mix (as sold)	Green's	359	102
Compound cooking fat		894	253
Condensed milk			
sweetened, skimmed		267	76
sweetened, whole		322	91
full cream	Itona	310	88
sweetened	Nestle	325	92

Product	Brand	Calories per 100g/ 100ml	Calories per oz/ pack/ portion
Condensed milk			
sweetened, skimmed	Fussell's Blue Butterfly	267	76
Conference pears	Tesco	29	8
Consomme			
condensed	Campbell's	8	2
specialty soup	Crosse & Blackwell	22	6
Continental chocolate assortment, diabetic	Boots	519	147
Continental mix	Bejam	36	per 113g portion 41
Continental mixed vegetables	Safeway	57	per 397g pack 226
Continental salad	Eden Vale	186	53
Continental stir fry vegetables (as sold)	Birds Eye	42	12
fried	Birds Eye	53	15
Continental style pear flan	St Michael	233	66
Continental vegetable mix	Tesco	313	89
Cook In sauce (Colman's): *see flavours*			
Cook in Sauces (Homepride): *see flavours*			
Cook in the Pot (Crosse & Blackwell): *see flavours*			
Cookeen cooking fat	Van den Berghs	900	255
Cookie crunch biscuits	Tesco	452	128
Cookies	Tesco	304	86
Cooking chocolate			
milk	Tesco	532	151
plain	Tesco	540	153

Product	Brand	Calories per 100g/ 100ml	Calories per oz/ pack/ portion
Cooking chocolate			
white	Tesco	526	149
Cooking fat	Cookeen	900	255
compound		894	253
Cooking-in Sauces (Baxters): *see flavours*			
Cooking margarine	Safeway	726	206
Cooking mixes (Colman's): *see flavours*			
Cooking oil, blended	Tesco	875	248
Coolmints	Trebor	382	per sweet 6
Coq au vin cooking mix	Colman's	245	69
Coquilles mornay	St Michael	150	43
Coriander leaves, dried		279	79
seeds		298	84
Corn chips	Trappers	492	per 50g pack 246
Californian	St Michael	570	162
Corn cobs: *see also Corn on the cob*			
Corn cobs	Waitrose	127	per 397g pack of two 504
mini	Bejam		per two cobs boiled 174
	Safeway	127	per 907g pack 1152
	Waitrose	127	per 624g pack of four 792
Corn, cream style	Waitrose	82	23
Corn crisp cakes	St Michael	457	130
Corn curls	Tesco	528	150
Corn nuts	Letec	619	per 45g pack 260
Corn oil	Boots	899	255
	Mazola	900	255
	Safeway	900	255

Product	Brand	Calories per 100g/ 100ml	Calories per oz/ pack/ portion
Corn oil	Sunwheel	900	255
	Tesco	875	248
	Waitrose	900	266
Corn on the cob	Bejam	83	per 198g boiled 165
	Birds Eye	71	per 198g cob 140
	Findus	127	36
	Safeway	127	per 397g 504
Corn, popping	Holland and Barrett	375	106
Corn relish	Safeway	118	33
Corned beef		217	62
	Armour	225	64
	Fray Bentos	215	61
	Libby	200	57
	Tesco	178	50
	Waitrose	230	65
loaf	Armour	206	per 312g can
sliced	Tesco	178	50
slices	St Michael	217	62
with jelly	Littlewoods	165	47
Corned beef, cress and horseradish sandwich	Tesco	205	58
Cornets	St Michael	544	154
Cornetto			
Black Forest	Wall's		per super cone 230
choc & nut	Wall's		per cone 220
choco rico	Wall's		per super cone 250
mint choc chip	Wall's		per cone 235
strawberry	Wall's		per cone 205

Product	Brand	Calories per 100g/ 100ml	Calories per oz/ pack/ portion
Cornetto			
tutti frutti	Wall's		per super cone 240
Cornflakes		368	104
	Kellogg's	350	99
	Safeway	354	100
	Tesco	354	100
	Waitrose	345	98
Crunchy Nut	Kellogg's	378	107
Cornflakes and wheatflakes	St Michael	354	100
Cornflour		354	100
	Boots	354	100
	Safeway	331	94
	Tesco	350	99
	Waitrose	330	94
patent	Brown and Polson	330	94
Cornish butter	Safeway	731	207
Cornish crab bisque	Waitrose	78	22
Cornish creams	Safeway	502	142
Cornish dairy ice cream	Waitrose	173	51
Cornish dairy King Cone	Lyons Maid		per cone 229
Cornish ice cream	Safeway	169	50
dairy	Lyons Maid	202	57
vanilla	Safeway	169	50
	Tesco	181	51
Cornish pastie		332	94
	Littlewoods	315	89
	Ross	270	77

Product	Brand	Calories per 100g/ 100ml	Calories per oz/ pack/ portion
Cornish pastie			per pasty as sold
mini	Bejam		154
traditional	Bejam		per pasty baked 505
Cornish pasty pie	Littlewoods	321	per pie 353
	Tesco	247	70
Cornish puff pastry pasties	St Michael	239	68
Cornish seafood soup	Knorr	374	106
Cornish wafers	Jacobs	514	per biscuit 43
	Safeway	514	per biscuit 8
Cornmeal, sifted, raw		368	104
unsifted, raw		353	100
Coronation chicken	St Michael	232	66
Cotswold pasty	Littlewoods	276	78
Cottage cheese: *see also flavours*			
Cottage cheese	Holland and Barrett	110	31
	Littlewoods	96	per 227g pack 218
	Safeway	104	per 113g pack 116
	St Michael	97	27
	Waitrose	94	per 113g pack 108
creamy, natural	St Michael	133	38
creamy, with prawn	St Michael	175	50
crunchy	Eden Vale	114	32
diet, natural	Eden Vale	83	24
diet, onion and chive	Eden Vale	81	23
diet, pineapple	Eden Vale	90	26
natural	Eden Vale	97	27
	Raines	100	28
	St Ivel	94	27

Product	Brand	Calories per 100g/ 100ml	Calories per oz/ pack/ portion
Cottage cheese	St Ivel Shape	79	22
with apple, celery and nut	St Michael	157	45
with beef and horseradish	St Michael	147	42
with cheddar and onion	Raines	120	34
with chives	Raines	100	28
	Safeway	104	per 227g pack 232
with pineapple	Raines	95	27
	St Michael	107	30
with prawns	St Michael	167	47
with tuna, sweetcorn and pepper	St Michael	149	42
Cottage cheese flan	Tesco	243	69
Cottage cheese snack with prawn	St Michael	163	46
Cottage pie	Littlewoods	186	per pie 263
	Tesco	198	56
	Waitrose	136	per 425g pie 585
fresh potato, family	St Michael	168	48
large	St Michael	155	44
small	St Michael	144	41
Cough candy twists	Trebor	356	per sweet 26
Country cake	St Michael	405	115
Country casserole ready meal, vegetarian	Boots	78	22
Country cereal mix, vegetarian	Boots	367	104
Country chicken and ham dinner	Heinz Baby Foods	68	per 170g jar 116

Product	Brand	Calories per 100g/ 100ml	Calories per oz/ pack/ portion
Country chicken and leek soup	Crosse & Blackwell Pot Soup		per sachet made up 62
Country chicken casserole	Boots Baby Foods	62	18
Country chicken dinner	Heinz Baby Foods	57	per 128g jar 73
Country chicken/pork marinade	Knorr	290	82
Country crunch biscuits	Peek Frean	445	per biscuit 36
Country harvest brown bread mix	Granny Smiths	225	per 455g pack made up 1024
Country herb stuffing mix	Tesco	383	109
	Waitrose	320	91
Country lamb and liver dinner	Heinz Baby Foods	71	per 128g can 91
Country lamb with carrots	Heinz Baby Foods	75	per 128g can 96
Country Maid instant milk	Wander	355	101
Country mix vegetables	Findus	55	16
	Ross	30	9
Country muesli	Jordans	345	98
Country mushroom Potato Saucery	Batchelors	351	per 94g pack as sold 330
Country Potato Bake	Birds Eye		per pack 435
Country recipe sausages	Wall's Light and Lean	198	per sausage 99

Product	Brand	Calories per 100g/ 100ml	Calories per oz/ pack/ portion
Country stir fry vegetables (as sold)	Birds Eye	28	8
fried	Birds Eye	35	10
Country Store	Kellogg's	346	98
Country strawberry dairy ice cream	Safeway	223	66
Country style mixed fruit cake	St Michael	360	102
Country style savoury pudding	Granose	167	47
Country vegetable bake	Boots Baby Foods	380	108
Country vegetable soup	Knorr	337	96
Homestyle	Heinz Ready to Serve	43	12
thick, dried (made up)	Chef Box	32	9
with croutons	Knorr Quick Soup	399	113
Country vegetable with beef soup	Crosse & Blackwell	41	12
Courgette provencale	Waitrose	30	per 340g pack 102
Courgettes (zucchini, squash), raw		25	7
frozen	Safeway	25	per 454g pack 112
sliced (frozen)	Bejam	16	per 113g portion boiled 18
stir fry	Safeway	86	per 340g pack 288
Couscous		227	64
	Bewell	342	97
Cow peas: *see* Blackeye beans			

Product	Brand	Calories per 100g/ 100ml	Calories per oz/ pack/ portion
Cow's milk yoghurt, natural	Holland and Barrett	50	14
fruit	Holland and Barrett	95	27
Cox's apples	Tesco	46	13
Crab			
boiled (with shell)		25	7
canned		81	23
boiled		127	36
claws	Waitrose	80	23
	Young's	127	36
whole	St Michael	127	36
Crab bisque			
condensed	Campbell's	74	21
Cornish	Waitrose	78	22
Crabmeat in brine	Armour	80	per 170g can 136
Crab paste	Shippams	183	per 75g pack 137
	Safeway	205	per 75g pack 154
Crab pate	St Michael	226	64
Crab spread	Littlewoods	141	per 35g pack 49
Crab thermidor	Young's	130	37
Cracked wheat	Holland and Barrett	311	88
Cracker barrel Cheddar cheese	Kraft	406	115
Crackers			
Hovis	Tesco	484	137
wholemeal	St Michael	459	130
Cracknels	Rowntree Mackintosh		per sweet 40
Cranberries, raw		15	4

Product	Brand	Calories per 100g/ 100ml	Calories per oz/ pack/ portion
Cranberry sauce			
	Pan Yan	132	37
	Safeway	137	39
	Tesco	148	42
and wine	O.K.	215	61
jellied	Baxters	258	73
whole fruit	Baxters	143	41
Crawlies	Trebor	607	per sweet 17
Cream			
brandy	Safeway	443	126
non-dairy	Tesco	253	72
rum	Safeway	446	126
spooning	Eden Vale	363	103
	Waitrose	295	87
whipped	Young's	345	98
Cream, clotted	Eden Vale	510	145
	St Ivel	570	162
	Young's	520	147
Cornish	St Michael	570	162
Cornish	Tesco	551	156
Devon	Tesco	577	164
Cream, double	Eden Vale	450	128
	Raines	450	128
	Safeway	462	137
	St Ivel	445	126
	St Michael	449	127
	Tesco	444	126
	Waitrose	450	133
	Young's	450	128
double		447	127
extra thick	Safeway	447	132
	Tesco	285	81
	Waitrose	450	133

Product	Brand	Calories per 100g/ 100ml	Calories per oz/ pack/ portion
Cream			
thick brandy	St Michael	435	123
thick, with rum	Tesco	402	114
UHT	Eden Vale	450	128
	St Ivel	445	126
Cream, half	Safeway	137	41
	St Michael	135	38
	Tesco	134	38
	Waitrose	130	38
UHT	Eden Vale	136	39
	St Ivel	140	40
Cream, single	Eden Vale	190	54
	Raines	190	54
	Safeway	190	56
	St Ivel	200	57
	St Michael	212	60
	Tesco	186	53
	Waitrose	190	56
	Young's	180	51
single		212	60
UHT	Eden Vale	190	54
	Safeway	190	56
	St Ivel	200	57
	St Michael	190	54
Cream, soured	Eden Vale	190	54
	Raines	190	54
	Safeway	190	56
	St Ivel	185	52
	Tesco	186	53
	Waitrose	178	53
Cream, sterilised (canned)		230	65
	Fussell's Golden Butterfly	233	66
	Littlewoods	240	68

Product	Brand	Calories per 100g/ 100ml	Calories per oz/ pack/ portion
Cream, sterilised (canned)	Nestle	233	66
	Safeway	230	65
Cream, whipping	Eden Vale	363	103
	Raines	387	110
	Safeway	387	115
	St Ivel	375	106
	St Michael	379	107
	Tesco	373	106
	Waitrose	380	112
		332	94
dairy	Young's	330	94
UHT	Eden Vale	363	103
	Safeway	387	200ml pack
	St Ivel	335	95
Cream alternative			
single	Elmlea	195	55
whipping	Elmlea	330	94
Cream and mushroom cooking sauce	St Michael	81	23
Cream caramel dessert	Heinz Baby Foods	88	per 128g can 113
Cream cheese			
and chives	Waitrose	435	123
soft	St Ivel	460	130
Cream cheese and cucumber sandwich	Waitrose	211	60
Cream chicken with pasta	Findus	143	41
Cream crackers		440	125
	Jacobs	431	per biscuit 33
	Safeway	443	126
	Tesco	459	130

Product	Brand	Calories per 100g/ 100ml	Calories per oz/ pack/ portion
Cream crackers	Waitrose	431	122
for cheese	Safeway	431	per biscuit 8
	Tesco	430	122
Cream dessert, chocolate	Young's	250	71
raspberry	Young's	200	57
Cream doughnuts	St Michael	365	103
Cream fruit trifle, individual	St Michael	158	45
Cream of asparagus soup	Baxters	66	per 425g can 281
	Heinz Classic Soups	43	12
	St Michael	64	18
	Waitrose	55	per 425g can 234
dried	Nestle Bonne Cuisine	329	93
dried, with croutons	Batchelors Cup-a-Soup Special	430	per 32.5g pack as sold 140
	Knorr Quick Soup	467	132
Cream of celery soup	Heinz Ready to Serve	43	12
	Tesco	44	12
	Waitrose	54	15
condensed	Campbell's	82	23
Cream of chicken and sweetcorn soup with croutons	Batchelors Cup-a-Soup Special	455	per 27.5g pack as sold 125
Cream of chicken and vegetable soup with croutons	Batchelors Cup-a-Soup Special	456	per 27g pack as sold 123
	Knorr Quick Soup	472	134

Product	Brand	Calories per 100g/ 100ml	Calories per oz/ pack/ portion
Cream of chicken soup, canned		58	16
condensed		98	28
condensed, as served		49	14
Cream of chicken soup	Baxters	67	per 425g can 283
	Crosse & Blackwell	63	18
	Heinz Ready to Serve	46	13
	Safeway	52	per 425g can 221
	St Michael	55	16
	Tesco	73	21
	Waitrose	58	per 425g can 247
condensed	Campbell's	99	28
dried	Batchelors	467	per 71.5g pint pack as sold 334
	Nestle Bonne Cuisine	327	93
dried, with croutons	Knorr Quick Soup	466	132
Cream of chicken with white wine soup	Heinz Classic Soups	50	14
Cream of Cornish ice cream	Wall's	90	32
blue ribbon vanilla	Wall's	95	34
sliceable	Wall's	100	36
vanilla	Wall's		per 1/5 pack 95
Cream of leek soup	Baxters	52	per 425g can 221
Cream of mushroom soup, canned		53	15
Cream of mushroom soup	Baxters	53	per 425g can 225
	Crosse & Blackwell	54	15

Product	Brand	Calories per 100g/ 100ml	Calories per oz/ pack/ portion
Cream of mushroom soup	Heinz Ready to Serve	45	13
	Safeway	68	per 425g can 289
	St Michael	50	14
	Tesco	55	16
	Waitrose	53	per 425g can 225
condensed	Campbell's	86	24
dried	Batchelors Cup-a-Soup Special	414	per 29g pack as sold 120
	Nestlé Bonne Cuisine	320	91
dried, with croutons	Knorr Quick Soup	464	132
Cream of pheasant soup	Baxters	62	per 425g can 264
Cream of scampi soup	Baxters	64	per 425g can 272
Cream of smoked salmon soup, condensed	Campbell's	106	30
Cream of smoked trout soup	Baxters	64	per 425g can 272
	St Michael	63	18
Cream of tartar	Boots		
Cream of tomato and vegetable soup, dried	Batchelors	393	per 89g pint pack as sold 350
Cream of tomato soup, canned, ready to serve		55	16
condensed		123	35
condensed, as served		62	18
Cream of tomato soup	Baxters	70	per 425g can 298
	Heinz Ready to Serve	60	17
	Safeway	68	per 425g can 289

Product	Brand	Calories per 100g/ 100ml	Calories per oz/ pack/ portion
Cream of tomato soup	St Michael	55	16
	Tesco	36	10
	Waitrose	63	per 425g can 268
condensed	Campbell's	124	35
dried	Batchelors	388	per 93g pint pack as sold 361
dried, with croutons	Knorr Quick Soup	458	130
with pasta shapes	Heinz Invaders	71	20
Cream of vegetable soup, dried	Batchelors	404	per 76g pint pack as sold 307
	Nestle Bonne Cuisine	324	92
with croutons	Batchelors Cup-a-Soup Special	415	per 32.5g pack as sold 135
	Knorr Quick Soup	465	132
Cream puff pastry slices	St Michael	435	123
Cream scones	St Michael	340	96
Cream soda	Whites	20	6
	Corona	26	8
Cream soda-flavoured concentrate	Safeway	193	57
Cream sponge, dairy whipping	Ross	270	77
	Ross	380	108
Cream style corn	Waitrose	82	23
Cream wafers, assorted	Safeway	505	143
Creamed coconut	Sharwood	600	170
Creamed horseradish	O.K.	200	57
	Safeway	185	per 156g jar 286

Product	Brand	Calories per 100g/ 100ml	Calories per oz/ pack/ portion
Creamed horseradish	Waitrose	190	per 145g jar 276
Creamed leeks	Bejam		per five mini portions boiled 52
Creamed macaroni	Ambrosia	92	26
Creamed mushrooms, canned	Tesco	87	25
Creamed porridge	Cow and Gate	69	per 110g jar 76, 150g jar 104
Creamed rice	Ambrosia	91	26
	Libby	89	25
	Safeway	88	per 439g can 388
traditional	Safeway	102	per 439g can 450
Creamed rice pudding, 3-9 months	Heinz Baby Foods	96	per 128g can 123
7-15 months	Heinz Baby Foods	97	per 128g can 124
Creamed sago	Ambrosia	81	23
Creamed semolina	Ambrosia	83	24
Creamed smatana	Raines	129	37
Creamed spinach	Bejam		per five mini portions boiled 54
Creamed tapioca	Ambrosia	83	24
Creamed tomato, onion and pepper soup	Crosse & Blackwell	74	21
Creamed tomato soup	Crosse & Blackwell	71	20
with herbs	Crosse & Blackwell	73	21
with mint	Crosse & Blackwell	70	20

Product	Brand	Calories per 100g/ 100ml	Calories per oz/ pack/ portion
Creamed tomato soup with spices	Crosse & Blackwell	71	20
Creamola foam crystals	Creamola	323	92
Creamy cottage cheese, natural	St Michael	133	38
with prawn	St Michael	175	50
Creamy leek Potato Saucery	Batchelors	339	per 93g pack as sold 315
Creamy mushroom flan	St Michael	195	55
Crediou cheese	Waitrose	335	95
Creme biscuits, orange	Cadbury's	500	per biscuit
Creme caramel	Eden Vale	139	39
	Ross	130	37
	Safeway	110	31
	St Ivel	104	29
	St Michael	157	45
individual	Young's	115	33
Creme caramel	Cow and Gate	58	per 110g jar 64; 150g jar 87
Creme orange	Eden Vale	141	40
Creme raspberry	Eden Vale	141	40
Crepes			
asparagus with ham	Findus	141	40
beef burgundy	Findus	140	40
chicken with mushroom sauce	Findus	135	38
Swiss cheese with ham	Findus	182	52

Product	Brand	Calories per 100g/ 100ml	Calories per oz/ pack/ portion
Crespolini in a pottery bowl	Waitrose	130	37
Crinkle cut chips: see Chips, crinkle cut			
Crinkles	St Michael	530	150
Crisp 'n' Dry			
solid cooking oil	Spry	900	255
vegetable oil	Spry	900	255
Crisp bake pork pies	St Michael	349	99
individual	St Michael	339	96
Crisp blocks (Needlers): see flavours			
Crisp corn cake	Tesco	477	135
Crisp puffed rice	Tesco	366	104
Crisp rice cake	Tesco	483	137
Crisp rice chocolate bar	Tesco	522	148
Crispbread, rye		321	91
wheat, starch reduced		388	110
Crispbread	Littlewoods	392	111
ideal bran	Holland and Barrett		per biscuit 20
rye light	St Michael	375	106
scan bran	Holland and Barrett		per biscuit 10
wheat	Tesco	390	111
whole rye	Boots Shapers	391	111
	Tesco	375	106
wholewheat	Allinson		per biscuit 90
Crisps: see also flavours			
Crisps	Littlewoods	552	per 25g pack 138
	Sooner	533	per 27g pack 144
crinkle cut	Tesco	568	161
	Waitrose	520	147

Product	Brand	Calories per 100g/ 100ml	Calories per oz/ pack/ portion
Crisps			
crinkle cut, ready salted	Littlewoods	534	per 75g pack 401
	Safeway	543	per 75g pack 407
ready salted	Christies	520	per 26g bag 130
	Hunters	520	per 26g bag 130
	Littlewoods	561	per 25g pack 140
	Nature's Snack	530	per 50g pack 265
	Safeway	500	per 25g pack 125
	St Michael	545	155
	Tesco	547	155
	Waitrose	520	per 75g pack 390
ready salted lower-fat	St Michael	485	137
Shakers	St Michael	56	16
wholewheat	Nature's Snack	550	per 20g pack 110
wholewheat cheese	Nature's Snack	550	per 20g pack 130
Worcester sauce	Hunters	520	per 26g bag
Crispy bacon pizza			
4 inch	Ross	250	71
pack of 4 (frozen)	Safeway	230	65
Crispy base pizza			
cheese and tomato	Findus	208	59
ham	Findus	168	48
Crispy batter mix	Green's	341	97
Crispy cod, haddock, etc: *see Cod, Haddock, etc*			
Crispy Crosses, potato	Ross	180	51
Crispy mushrooms	St Michael	162	46
Crispy squares	Safeway	472	per 50g pack 236
Crispy thins	Waitrose	484	137
Crispy vegetables with bacon salad meal	St Michael	165	47
Criss Cross	Cadbury's	454	per portion 65

Product	Brand	Calories per 100g/ 100ml	Calories per oz/ pack/ portion
Crofters' thick vegetable soup	Knorr	310	88
Croissants	St Michael	383	109
Croquette potatoes	Findus	91	26
baked or grilled	Birds Eye	71	20
fried	Birds Eye	159	45
Croquettes			
cod and parsley	Young's	192	54
potato	St Michael	216	61
potato	Ross	100	28
Croutons	St Michael	558	158
Crumble mix	Granny Smiths	454	per 225g pack made up 1022
(as sold)	Tesco	673	191
(made up)	Tesco	459	130
	Whitworths	466	132
Crumpets	Sunblest	182	per crumpet 80
	Tesco	168	48
fruited treacle	St Michael	280	79
Scottish	Tesco	260	74
Crunch bar	St Michael	450	128
Crunch bar mix, apple	Green's	355	made up per portion 224
apple and blackcurrant	Green's	408	made up per portion 220
Crunch creams	Peek Frean	482	per biscuit 58
Crunch mixes: see flavours			
Crunch nut cake topping	Tesco	491	139
Crunchie bar	Cadbury's	465	per small 24g bar 110, standard bar 195

Product	Brand	Calories per 100g/ 100ml	Calories per oz/ pack/ portion
Crunchy Bemax	Beecham	310	88
Crunchy bran	Allinson	360	102
Crunchy bran flakes	St Michael	308	87
Crunchy cereal	Safeway	438	124
Crunchy coated peanuts	Sooner	490	per 40g pack 196
Crunchy cookies	Waitrose	443	126
Crunchy cottage cheese	Eden Vale	114	32
Crunchy creams	Waitrose	506	143
Crunchy crumble mix	Tesco	460	130
Crunchy nut	Tesco	375	106
Crunchy nut cereal	Granose	493	140
Crunchy Nut Corn Flakes	Kellogg's	378	107
Crunchy sandwich bars	St Michael	499	141
Crunchy sticks, ready salted	Littlewoods	483	per 50g pack 242
	Safeway	481	per 75g pack 361
salt and vinegar	Littlewoods	481	per 50g pack 241
	Safeway	487	per 75g pack 365
Crunchy toffee ice cream	Bejam	201	57
Crusty bun pizza	Findus	231	65
Crusty white rolls	Bejam		per roll baked 105
Cryovac salmon	Marine Harvest		35-55 per oz
Crystals	Trebor	357	per sweet 5
Cub Lion bar	Rowntree Mackintosh	495	per bar 80

Product	Brand	Calories per 100g/ 100ml	Calories per oz/ pack/ portion
Cube sugar, white	Tate and Lyle	394	112
Cucumber (khira, kakdi), raw		10	3
fresh	Littlewoods	10	3
pickled, sliced	Safeway	28	8
Cucumber dressing	Heinz All Seasons	276	78
Cucumber relish	Safeway	118	33
Cucumber sandwich spread	Heinz	183	52
Cumberland pie	Findus	153	43
family	St Michael	145	41
Cumin seeds		375	106
Cup-a-Soup (Batchelors): see flavours			
Cup-a-Soup Special (Batchelors): see flavours			
Cup cakes, chocolate	Lyons	338	96
orange and lemon	Lyons	361	102
Cup Italiano ice cream (Wall's): see flavours			
Curacao		311	88
Curd cheese	Waitrose	158	45
medium fat	Tesco	176	50
natural, with walnut	Tesco	308	87
Cured pork pies	St Michael	348	99
individual	St Michael	348	99
Curly wurly	Cadbury's	470	per 29g bar 135
Currant bun mix (as sold)	Tesco	410	116
made up	Tesco	347	98
Currant buns		302	86
Currant crisp biscuits	Peek Frean	440	per biscuit 30

Product	Brand	Calories per 100g/ 100ml	Calories per oz/ pack/ portion
Currant crunch biscuits	Safeway	450	128
Currant crunch creams	Tesco	498	141
Currants, dried		243	69
	Holland and Barrett	240	68
	Safeway	243	69
	Tesco	249	71
	Whitworths	243	69
Greek	Waitrose	243	69
Currants, white, raw		26	7
stewed with sugar		57	16
stewed without sugar		22	6
Curried beans	Safeway	101	per 227g can 229
with sultanas	Heinz	88	25
Curried chicken, canned	St Michael	120	34
Curried chicken Toast Topper	Heinz	73	21
Curried coleslaw	Tesco	204	58
Curried fruit chutney	Pan Yan	144	41
	Sharwood	141	40
	Tesco	141	40
Curried meat, cooked		160	45
Curried turkey sandwich	St Michael	227	64
Curry	Granose	76	22
chicken style	Granose	57	16
Curry accompaniment, Indian vegetable	Sharwood	27	8

Product	Brand	Calories per 100g/ 100ml	Calories per oz/ pack/ portion
Curry chutney	Waitrose	193	per 300g jar 579
Curry cooking sauce, medium	St Michael	41	12
Curry crisps	St Michael	547	155
Curry dressing	St Michael	327	93
Curry flavour Chinese noodles, instant	Sharwood	420	119
Curry leaves, raw		88	25
Curry powder		325	92
	Safeway	535	152
	Tesco	353	100
Curry Prawnaise	Lyons Seafoods	200	57
Curry rice, mild, cooked	Uncle Ben's	136	cooked
Curry sauce	Tesco	367	104
Bombay Dhansak	Sharwood	127	36
Cook in	Homepride	112	per 376g pack 421
Goan Vindaloo	Sharwood	79	22
Moghulai Korma	Sharwood	190	54
Pour Over	Crosse & Blackwell	95	27
Rogan Josh	Sharwood	117	33
Tamatar Madras	Sharwood	126	36
Curry sauce mix, Cook In	Colman's	350	99
Pour Over	Colman's	350	99
Curry savoury rice	Whitworths	287	81
	Safeway	342	97
Curry style pot meal	Boots Shapers	327	93
Custard powder		354	100

Product	Brand	Calories per 100g/ 100ml	Calories per oz/ pack/ portion
Custard pudding, egg		118	33
powder, made up		118	33
Custard			
canned	Itona	149	per 412g can 615
instant mix	Brown and		
	Polson	404	115
	Rowntree's	416	118
	Safeway	428	121
mix	Granny Smiths	79	per 516g pack made up 408
powder	Boots	358	101
	Creamola	354	100
	Nestle	330	94
	Safeway	333	94
	Tesco	324	92
	Waitrose	330	94
quick	Batchelors	424	per 90g pack 382
Custard apple, raw		92	26
Custard creams	Peek Frean	483	per biscuit 53
	Rakusen	469	133
	Safeway	507	144
	St Michael	505	143
	Tesco	464	132
	Waitrose	507	144
assorted	Safeway	502	142
diabetic	Boots	555	157
Custard tart		287	81
Cuttlefish, raw		81	23
Cwm Dale Water, natural	Tesco		
sparkling	Tesco		
Dairy Cassata Bombe	Bertorelli	215	61

Product	Brand	Calories per 100g/ 100ml	Calories per oz/ pack/ portion
Dairy cheese, soft	Tesco	271	77
with chives	Tesco	290	82
with pineapple	Tesco	358	101
Dairy cream and chocolate sponge	Birds Eye		per 1/6 sponge 110
Dairy cream choux buns	Birds Eye		per bun 130
Dairy cream doughnuts	Birds Eye		per doughnut 170
Dairy cream eclairs	Bejam		per eclair 103
	Birds Eye		per eclair 145
	Safeway	388	110
Dairy cream fingers	Tesco	486	138
Dairy cream sponge	Bejam		per 1/6 cake as sold 104
	Birds Eye		per 1/6 sponge 130
	Ross	270	77
	Tesco	313	89
Dairy elite carte d'or cup ice cream	Wall's		per portion 155
Dairy fudge	Trebor	457	per sweet 43
Dairy ice cream		167	47
chocolate scooping	Wall's Italiano	95	per 1/40 4-litre 95
strawberry scooping	Wall's Italiano	90	per 1/40 4-litre pack 90
vanilla	St Michael	176	50
vanilla scooping	Wall's Italiano	90	per 1/40 4-litre pack 90
Dairy Milk chocolate bar	Cadbury's	530	per 20g bar 105
Dairy milk ices	Lyons Maid	124	35

Product	Brand	Calories per 100g/ 100ml	Calories per oz/ pack/ portion
Dairy Milk miniatures	Cadbury's	530	per miniature 30
Dairy spread	Sun-Pat	268	76
Clover	Dairy Crest	682	193
Delight	Van den Berghs	398	113
low fat	Outline	370	105
	Tesco	393	111
original Clover	Dairy Crest	682	193
Summer County	Van den Berghs	650	184
Dairy spread processed cheese	St Michael	300	85
Dairy toffees	Rowntree Mackintosh		per sweet 30
	Trebor	456	per sweet
Dairy whipping cream sponge	Ross	380	108
Dairylea cheese spread	Kraft	273	per 85g pack 232
Dal masala	Waitrose	171	48
Damson jam	Waitrose	248	70
Damson preserve	Tesco	255	72
Damsons			
raw		38	11
raw (with stones)		34	10
stewed without sugar		32	9
stewed without sugar (with stones)		29	8
stewed with sugar		69	20
stewed with sugar (with stones)		63	18
	Hartley's	85	per 112g can 95
Danbo cheese	Waitrose	272	77
Dandelion and burdock	Corona	20	6
	Whites	25	7

Product	Brand	Calories per 100g/ 100ml	Calories per oz/ pack/ portion
Dandelion coffee	Symingtons	320	91
Dandex coffee	Lanes	385	109
Danish blue cheese	St Ivel	350	99
	St Michael	355	101
	Waitrose	350	99
extra mature	Waitrose	350	99
gold	Tesco	401	114
mild	Waitrose	350	99
Danish cookies	Tesco	505	143
Danish salami	Waitrose	520	per 113g pack 588
Dansak Classic curry sauce	Homepride	103	per 383g pack 394
Darjeeling tea, infused	Safeway	1	
Dark and aromatic Chinese sauce mix	Sharwood	270	77
Dark and golden choc ice	Wall's		per ice 130
Dark Bournville chocolate bar	Cadbury's	510	per 50g bar 255
Dark choc ice	Bejam		per choc ice 115
	Waitrose	290	per 62ml ice 180
Dark chocolate carte d'or cup ice cream	Wall's		per portion 160
Dark mint choc ice	Bejam		per choc ice 115
Dark satin choc ice	Lyons Maid		per ice 128
Date and apple dessert bar	Prewetts Fruit Bars	238	per 42g bar 100
Date and apple slice	Lyons	371	105
Date and apricot bar	Granose	340	per 25g bar 85
Date and coconut bar	Granose	412	per 25g bar 103

Product	Brand	Calories per 100g/ 100ml	Calories per oz/ pack/ portion
Date and fig bar	Granose	320	per 25g bar 80
Date and fig dessert bar	Prewetts	262	per 42g bar 110
Date and muesli bar	Boots	324	92
Date and nut bar	Granose	380	per 25g bar 95
Date and sesame bar	Granose	372	per 25g bar 93
Date and walnut cake	Waitrose	406	115
Date and walnut cottage cheese	Safeway	119	34
Date bar	Granose	352	per 25g bar 88
Dates			
raw		144	41
	Tesco	137	39
Dates, dried			
raw		248	70
(with stones)		213	60
chopped	Whitworths	273	77
dessert	Whitworths	213	60
stoned	Holland and Barrett	240	68
	Whitworths	248	70
sugar rolled	Tesco	279	79
Decaffeinated coffee			
beans	Waitrose	194	55
filter fine	Waitrose	287	81
freeze-dried	Safeway	330	94
instant (freeze-dried)	Waitrose	100	28
Decorated Genoa cake	Littlewoods	323	92
Delight dairy spread	Van den Berghs	398	113
Delights, all flavours			
dry	Tesco	405	115

Product	Brand	Calories per 100g/ 100ml	Calories per oz/ pack/ portion
Delights, all flavours made up	Tesco	142	40
Deltas	St Michael	515	146
De luxe bean mix (dried)	Holland and Barrett	265	75
Deluxe muesli	Prewetts	360	102
	Sunwheel	390	111
	Sunwheel	392	111
Demerara sugar		394	112
	Holland and Barrett	380	108
	Safeway	394	112
	Tate and Lyle	394	112
dark	Waitrose	389	110
light	Waitrose	389	110
Derby cheese	Dairy Crest	400	113
	Tesco	367	104
Desiccated coconut		604	171
	Safeway	604	171
	Tesco	683	194
	Whitworths	604	171
Dessert bars (Prewetts): see flavours			
Dessert logs, Sonata	Wall's		per 1/6 log 130
Viennetta	Wall's		per 1/6 log 135
Dessert mixes (Dietade): see flavours			
Dessert pies, apple	Lyons	349	99
Dessert sauces (Lyons Maid): see flavours			
Dessert topping, dry	Tesco	512	145
made up	Tesco	181	51
Dessert white sauce	Ambrosia	97	27
Devon butter	Safeway	731	207
Devon creams	Peek Frean	487	per biscuit 58

Product	Brand	Calories per 100g/ 100ml	Calories per oz/ pack/ portion
Devon custard	Ambrosia	100	28
Devon sponge cake mix (dry)	Green's	396	made up per portion 223
Devon toffees	Littlewoods	416	118
	Waitrose	430	122
Devonshire cheesecake			
blackcurrant	St Ivel	250	71
strawberry	St Ivel	250	71
Devonshire cream cheesecake	Young's	260	74
Devonshire cream torte and raspberries	Young's	270	77
Devonshire trifles, individual	Ross	160	45
Dextrosol tablets, all varieties	Dextrosol	347	98
Diabetic bourbon creams	Boots	467	132
Diabetic cake mix (dry)			
chocolate	Boots	463	131
plain	Boots	459	130
Diabetic cherry truffles	Boots	420	119
Diabetic chocolate coated wafers	Boots	560	159
orange	Boots	555	157
Diabetic chocolate drink	Boots	341	97
Diabetic Cola	Boots	1	
Diabetic continental chocolate assortment	Boots	519	147

Product	Brand	Calories per 100g/ 100ml	Calories per oz/ pack/ portion
Diabetic custard creams	Boots	555	157
Diabetic dressing	Boots	155	44
Diabetic drinks (Boots): see flavours			
Diabetic fruit cocktail	Boots	24	7
Diabetic fruit flavour drops	Boots	367	104
Diabetic ginger creams	Boots	468	133
Diabetic hazelnut biscuits	Boots	428	121
Diabetic honey spread	Boots	256	73
Diabetic jams (Boots, Dietade): see flavours			
Diabetic jelly crystals (Boots): see flavours			
Diabetic Lincoln biscuits	Boots	402	114
Diabetic marmalade	Dietade	230	65
fine cut	Boots	239	68
thick cut	Boots	239	68
Diabetic marzipan bars	Boots	465	132
Diabetic milk chocolate	Boots	512	145
coffee cream	Boots	574	163
hazelnut	Boots	518	147
strawberry cream	Boots	552	156
yogurt cream	Boots	556	158
Diabetic milk chocolate drops	Boots	512	145
Diabetic milk chocolate wafers			
caramel	Boots	523	148

Product	Brand	Calories per 100g/ 100ml	Calories per oz/ pack/ portion
Diabetic mint imperials	Boots	371	105
Diabetic muesli biscuits	Boots	437	124
Diabetic pastilles			
fruit flavours	Boots	100	28
peppermint	Boots	99	28
Diabetic peach slices	Boots	20	6
Diabetic pear quarters	Boots	21	6
Diabetic plain chocolate	Boots	500	142
Diabetic praline truffles	Boots	582	165
Diabetic preserves	Thursday Cottage	140	40
Diabetic sweetener (powder)	Boots	360	102
Diamond White cider	Taunton	54	per pint 310
Diet cola	Safeway	-1	litre bottle
Diet cottage cheese			
natural	Eden Vale	83	24
onion and chive	Eden Vale	81	23
pineapple	Eden Vale	90	26
Diet drinks: see flavours			
Diet lemonade	Safeway	-1	litre bottle
Diet muesli chocolate bar	Boots Shapers Meal	478	136
Diet Ski yogurt (Eden Vale): see flavours			
Dietade (Appleford): see products			
Digestive bars, chocolate coated	Tesco	504	143

Product	Brand	Calories per 100g/ 100ml	Calories per oz/ pack/ portion
Digestive biscuits			
chocolate		493	140
plain		471	134
	Boots	457	130
	Huntley & Palmer	463	per biscuit 63
	Mitchellhill		per biscuit 60
	Rakusen	484	137
	Safeway	493	140
	St Michael	499	141
	Tesco	496	141
	Waitrose	490	139
Bourneville	Cadbury's	480	per biscuit 45
for cheese, small	Safeway	490	per biscuit 10
fruit	Huntley & Palmer	451	per biscuit 50
Hovis	Nabisco	486	per biscuit 57
	Tesco	481	136
milk chocolate	Cadbury's	490	per biscuit 50
	Safeway	505	143
	St Michael	500	142
	Tesco	504	143
	Waitrose	499	141
	Waitrose	499	141
milk half coated	Huntley & Palmer	502	per biscuit 65
plain chocolate	Safeway	500	142
	St Michael	505	143
	Tesco	508	144
	Waitrose	505	143
plain half coated	Huntley & Palmer	496	per biscuit 65
small	Peek Frean	490	per biscuit 48
sweetmeal	Tesco	470	133

Product	Brand	Calories per 100g/ 100ml	Calories per oz/ pack/ portion
Digestive creams	Boots	497	141
Digestive finger creams	Waitrose	489	139
Dijon mustard	Colman's	170	48
Dill cucumber, pickled	Tesco	14	4
Dill seeds		305	86
Dill, sliced	Tesco	17	5
Dinner balls	Granose	145	41
Dish of the Day (Crosse & Blackwell): *see flavours*			
Disneys Cartoons cake mix	Green's	408	made up per portion 64
Dixie crackers	Safeway	431	per biscuit 4
Dogfish			
fried in batter		265	75
fried (with waste)		244	69
Dolcelatte cheese	Tesco	325	92
	Waitrose	330	94
Dolly mixtures	Bassett's	366	104
	Littlewoods	377	107
cubes	Tesco	389	110
jellies	Tesco	378	107
squares	Tesco	389	110
Dolmio (as sold)			
original	Dolmio	41	11
with mushrooms	Dolmio	39	11
with peppers	Dolmio	40	11
Double choc Arctic circles	Birds Eye		per piece 165
Double choc choc bar	Wall's		per bar 160
Double Decker	Cadbury's	465	per 51g bar 235

Product	Brand	Calories per 100g/ 100ml	Calories per oz/ pack/ portion
Double decker			
black cherry	St Michael	124	35
tropical	St Michael	124	35
Double Gloucester	Dairy Crest	405	115
cheese	Safeway	405	115
	St Ivel	405	115
	Tesco	371	105
	Waitrose	380	108
and chives, mini	Safeway	406	115
farmhouse	Waitrose	390	111
mini	Waitrose	380	108
with chives and onion	St Ivel	400	113
	Waitrose	398	113
with onion and chives	Tesco	371	105
Double Top dessert topping (canned)	Nestle	178	50
Doublemint chewing gum	Wrigley		per stick 9
Doughnut mix	Granny Smiths	425	per 392g pack made up 1664
Doughnuts		349	99
cream	St Michael	365	103
dairy cream	Birds Eye		per doughnut 170
iced ring	Tesco	420	119
Doux de Montagne cheese	St Michael	325	92
Dover sole	St Michael	95	27
	Tesco	85	24
cooked	Tesco	129	37
whole	Waitrose	81	23

Product	Brand	Calories per 100g/ 100ml	Calories per oz/ pack/ portion
Dover sole			
whole	Young's	80	23
Dressing			
diabetic	Boots	155	44
reduced calorie	Heinz Weight Watchers	148	42
Drifter	Rowntree Mackintosh	460	per biscuit 130
junior	Rowntree Mackintosh	460	per biscuit 75
Drinking chocolate		366	104
	Cadbury's	385	per portion 20
	Ovaltine	387	110
	Safeway	358	101
	Tesco	390	111
	Waitrose	395	112
fat reduced	Boots	345	98
granules	St Michael	366	104
instant	Ovaltine	400	113
Dripping			
beef		891	253
beef	Waitrose	900	255
refined	Tesco	875	248
Driver's			
gin and tonic	Britvic	31	per 180ml pack 55
whisky and			
American ginger ale	Britvic	31	per 180ml pack 57
white rum and cola	Britvic	37	per 180ml pack 66
Drumstick: *see Horseradish*			
Dry ginger	Tesco	19	6
low calorie	Tesco	6	2
Dry ginger ale	Hunts	16	5
	Safeway	24	7

Product	Brand	Calories per 100g/ 100ml	Calories per oz/ pack/ portion
Dry ginger ale	Schweppes	15	4
	Waitrose	22	7
low calorie	Safeway	5	1
Dry roasted peanuts	Safeway	570	per 100g pack 570
	Sooner	602	per 50g pack 301
	Waitrose	625	per 225g pack 1406
Duchess mince pies	Tesco	415	118
Duchesse dessert	St Michael	224	64
Duchesse potatoes	Ross	110	31
Duck			
meat only, raw		122	35
meat only, roast		189	54
meat, fat and skin, raw		430	122
meat, fat and skin, roast		339	96
Duck liver pate	Tesco	256	73
Duckling			
breast quarters, frozen, roasted	Bejam	332	94
fresh	Waitrose	400	113
frozen	Waitrose	400	113
frozen, roasted	Bejam	332	94
Duckling a l'orange	St Michael	187	53
Dumplings		211	60
apple	Ross	250	71
apple and blackberry	Ross	250	71
Dundee cake	Safeway	312	88
	Tesco	336	95
butter	Safeway	382	108
large	Safeway	312	88

Product	Brand	Calories per 100g/ 100ml	Calories per oz/ pack/ portion
Dutch cheese			
Edam	Safeway	305	86
Gouda	Safeway	346	98
Dutch finger creams	St Michael	507	144
Dutch shortcake biscuits	Huntley & Palmer	539	per biscuit 40
Earl Grey tea, infused	Safeway	1	per 125g pack 1
Eastern Choice	Waitrose	376	107
Easy cook rice	Safeway	364	103
	Waitrose	360	102
American	Waitrose	360	102
cooked	Tesco	120	34
raw	Tesco	353	100
Eccles cakes, all butter	Waitrose	390	111
Echo margarine	Van den Berghs	740	210
Eclairs		376	107
	Waitrose	410	116
chocolate	Young's	440	125
dairy cream	Birds Eye		per eclair 145
milk chocolate	Cadbury's	450	each pocket pack 20, standard pack 40
Economy burgers	Birds Eye		per burger grilled
	Steakhouse		100, fried 110
	Safeway	264	75
Edam cheese	St Ivel	335	95
	St Michael	310	88
	Tesco	301	85
Dutch	Safeway	305	86
	Waitrose	310	88
wedges	Safeway	305	86

Product	Brand	Calories per 100g/ 100ml	Calories per oz/ pack/ portion
Eddoes, fresh, cooked	Tesco	181	51
Eel			
raw		168	48
raw, flesh only		168	48
stewed		201	57
Egg and bacon breakfast			
3-9 months	Heinz Baby Foods	75	per 128g can 96
7-15 months	Heinz Baby Foods	70	per 128g can 90
Egg and bacon sandwich	St Michael	325	92
Egg and cheese savoury	Boots Baby Foods	405	115
Egg and cress sandwich	St Michael	204	58
Egg, bacon and mayonnaise sandwich	Waitrose	209	59
Egg, cheese and bacon flan	Findus	239	68
Egg custard	Boots Baby Foods	405	115
with rice, 3-9 months	Heinz Baby Foods	81	per 128g 104
with rice, 7-15 months	Heinz Baby Foods	97	per 128g jar 124
with tapioca	Heinz Baby Foods	94	per 128g can 120
Egg custard dessert mix, no bake (as sold)	Green's	380	per portion made up 148
Egg custard tarts	St Michael	267	76

Product	Brand	Calories per 100g/ 100ml	Calories per oz/ pack/ portion
Egg, ham, cheese and tomato quiche	Tesco	247	70
Egg lasagne: see Lasagne			
Egg mayonnaise sandwich	Waitrose	285	81
Eggnog and raisin dairy ice cream	Safeway	224	66
Eggplant: see Aubergine			
Eggs			
boiled		147	42
dried		564	160
fried		232	66
omelette		190	54
poached		155	44
raw, white only		36	10
raw, whole		147	42
raw, yolk only		339	96
scrambled		246	70
all sizes	Waitrose	147	42
brown fresh	St Michael	147	42
brown size 3	St Michael	147	42
free range	St Michael	147	42
size 2	Safeway	96	27
size 3	Safeway	88	25
size 4	Safeway	81	23
Eggs, ducks'			
raw, whole		188	53
salted whole, boiled, without shell		198	56
"Eight" fruit muesli	Granose	408	116
8 varieties; biscuits for cheese	Waitrose	452	128

Product	Brand	Calories per 100g/ 100ml	Calories per oz/ pack/ portion
Elderberry and cherry yoghurt	Safeway	86	per 150g pack 129
11 + fruit drink, long life	Safeway	46	13
Elmlea cream alternative			
single	Van den Berghs	195	55
whipping	Van den Berghs	330	94
Emmental cheese	Tesco	383	109
Swiss	Waitrose	272	77
Emmentaler cheese	Waitrose	330	94
Endive, raw		11	3
English apple juice: *see Apple juice*			
English breakfast	Boots Baby Foods	400	113
English butter	Safeway	731	207
English Cheddar: *see Cheddar cheese, English*			
English fruit squash	Boots	202	60
English mustard	Safeway	95	per 95g pack 90
as sold	Colman's	480	136
made up	Colman's	180	51
English recipe sausages	Wall's Light and Lean	190	per sausage 95
chipolata	Wall's Light and Lean	190	per two chipolatas 108
Esrom cheese	Waitrose	272	77
Evaporated milk unsweetened, whole		158	45
	Carnation	160	45
	Libby	158	45
	Safeway	159	45
	Tesco	183	52

Product	Brand	Calories per 100g/ 100ml	Calories per oz/ pack/ portion
Evaporated milk			
full cream	Waitrose	159	per 170g can 270
	Nestle Ideal	160	45
Everton mints	Trebor	365	per sweet 23
Exhibition sweet cider	Taunton	59	per pint 330
Exotic fruit and nut mix			
dried	Tesco	269	76
tub	Tesco	467	132
Exotic fruit and nuts	Waitrose	445	126
Exotic juice	St Ivel Real	47	14
Extra hot chicken curry	Tesco	98	28
Extra Jam, all flavours	Chivers	255	per portion 40
Extra strong mints	Needlers	364	per 113g pack 411
roll	Trebor	378	per mint 10
Fab	Lyons Maid	133	each 69
Faggots		268	76
	Littlewoods	265	75
	Tesco	159	45
	Safeway	166	369g/13oz pack
in rich sauce	Birds Eye MenuMaster	187	per 369g tray 611
in rich sauce	Ross	180	51
Faggots 'n' peas (canned)	Crosse & Blackwell	112	32
Family Favourites processed cheese (average)	Saint Ivel	280	79
Family shortcake biscuits	Littlewoods	502	142
Fancies, chocolate	Lyons	449	127
Fancy iced cakes		407	115

Product	Brand	Calories per 100g/ 100ml	Calories per oz/ pack/ portion
Farex weaning food	Farley	388	110
Farmhouse biscuits	Jacobs	488	per biscuit 39
Farmhouse Bran apple and apricot	Weetabix	326	92
honey and nut	Weetabix	335	95
toasted	Weetabix	300	85
Farmhouse cake	Waitrose	359	102
Farmhouse casserole Ready Meal	Tesco	77	22
Farmhouse chicken and leek soup	Knorr	338	96
Farmhouse crackers	Safeway	488	per biscuit 8
Farmhouse fruitcake mix	Granny Smiths	388	per 439g pack made up 1704
Farmhouse Hot Pot	Branston Snackatak	363	103
Farmhouse lamb cooking mix	Colman's	325	92
Farmhouse lentil mix, vegetarian	Boots	349	99
Farmhouse mixed vegetables	Ross	30	9
Farmhouse pate	St Michael	238	67
Farmhouse pork dinner	Heinz Baby Foods	79	per 128g can 101
Farmhouse potato and vegetable soup	Crosse & Blackwell Pot Soup		per sachet made up 64
Farmhouse steak dinner	Heinz Baby Foods	51	per 170g jar 87

Product	Brand	Calories per 100g/ 100ml	Calories per oz/ pack/ portion
Farmhouse-style mix vegetables			per 113g portion
	Bejam	22	25
Farmhouse vegetable soup			
dried	Batchelors	283	per 52g pint pack as sold 147
	Hera	376	107
thick	Crosse & Blackwell	53	15
	Heinz Ready to Serve	48	14
Farmhouse vegetable soup mix			1/6 serving boiled
	Bejam		65
Fast Pints	Safeway	490	139
Fat Frog	Wall's		each 50
Feast	Wall's		each 260
Fennel seeds		345	98
Fennel, fresh, cooked	Tesco	22	6
Fenugreek			
leaves, raw		35	10
seeds		323	92
Ferguzade	Beecham	94	28
Feta cheese		245	69
Fibre bran	Safeway	248	per 40g pack 99
Fiesta fruit jellies	Needlers	304	per 125g pack 380
'55' Juice			
'55' Apple	Britvic	43	12
'55' Grapefruit	Britvic	50	14
'55' Orange	Britvic	51	14
'55' Pineapple	Britvic	51	14
Fig and orange biscuits, hand-baked	Boots	484	137

Product	Brand	Calories per 100g/ 100ml	Calories per oz/ pack/ portion
Fig and prune bar	Granose	312	per 25g bar 78
Fig and raisin bar	Granose	340	per 25g bar 85
Fig bar biscuits	Tesco	362	103
Fig biscuits	Prewetts		per biscuit 79
Fig rolls	Jacobs	355	per biscuit 54
	Littlewoods	348	per biscuit 58
	Safeway	350	99
Figs			
fresh, raw		41	12
dried, raw		213	60
dried, stewed without sugar		118	33
dried, stewed with sugar		136	39
green, raw		41	12
dried	Holland and Barrett	200	57
	Whitworths	180	51
Filled green pepper	St Michael	95	27
Filled plaice			
with butter sauce	Young's	158	45
with mornay sauce	Young's	158	45
Fillet of cod Florentine	Findus Lean Cuisine	85	24
Fillet of cod with broccoli	Findus Lean Cuisine	78	22
Fillet steak, frozen, grilled	Bejam	159	45
Fine beans, fresh, cooked	Tesco	34	10
Fine cut marmalade: see Marmalade			
Finger biscuits	Cadbury's	495	per biscuit 25
Finger creams	Safeway	478	136

Product	Brand	Calories per 100g/ 100ml	Calories per oz/ pack/ portion
Finger sandwich	Waitrose	155	44
Finnan haddock			
frozen, raw	Tesco	89	25
frozen, steamed	Tesco	101	29
Fish 'n' chips, oven crispy	Birds Eye		per pack baked 470
Fish 'n' Chips candy	Trebor	540	per sweet 54
Fish batter mix (as sold)	Green's	341	97
Fish bonne femme Cook in the Pot	Crosse & Blackwell	379	107
Fish cakes: see also Cod, Haddock, etc			
Fish cakes			
frozen		112	32
fried		188	53
	Findus	118	33
	Safeway	121	34
	Waitrose	112	per fish cake 56
cod	Bejam		per cake fried 117
	Birds Eye		each grilled 90, fried 140
cod, chilled	Young's	213	60
raw	Tesco	112	32
salmon	Birds Eye		each grilled 100, fried 160
traditional	Ross	120	34
Fish fingers: see also Cod, Haddock, etc.			
Fish fingers			
frozen		178	50
fried		233	66
	Ross	190	54

Product	Brand	Calories per 100g/ 100ml	Calories per oz/ pack/ portion
Fish fingers and chips snack, jumbo	Bejam		per serving baked 478
Fish fingers	Safeway	184	52
	St Michael	169	48
	Tesco	174	49
cod	Bejam		per finger grilled 44
	Safeway	184	52
	Waitrose	180	51
cod fillet	Birds Eye		each grilled 50, fried 60
cod, crisp crumb	Findus	172	49
cod, minced	Waitrose	182	52
cod, oven crispy	Birds Eye		each baked/grilled 70, shallow-fried 80
economy	Findus	180	51
haddock fillet	Birds Eye		each grilled 50, shallow-fried 55
haddock, crisp crumb	Findus	191	54
value	Birds Eye		each grilled 45, fried 55
value	Littlewoods	199	per finger 50
Fish in cheese sauce	Cow and Gate	46	per 110g jar 51, 150g jar 69
Fish kebabs			
fresh	Young's	56	16
smoked	Young's	134	38
Fish paste		169	48
Fish pie		128	36
traditional	St Michael	112	32

Product	Brand	Calories per 100g/ 100ml	Calories per oz/ pack/ portion
Fish steaks			
battered	Findus	217	62
in butter sauce	Ross	90	26
Fishburgers, Captain's	Birds Eye		each fried 100, grilled/baked 135
Fisherman's Choice	Birds Eye MenuMaster		per pack 290
Fisherman's pie	St Michael	136	39
Five Centre bar	Cadbury's	425	per bar 215
Five fruit juice	Waitrose	52	15
Fivepints milk powder (as sold)	St Ivel	470	per pint made up 270
	St Ivel	46	per pint made up
Fizza chews	Trebor	359	per sweet 14
Fizzy Bears	Trebor	283	per sweet 17
Fizzy Cola roll	Trebor	341	per sweet 14
Flageolet beans, dried	Holland and Barrett	252	71
Flake			
Flake	Cadbury's	530	per 34g bar 180
Flake 99	Cadbury's	530	per 13g bar 65
Flaky bake pie			
chicken and ham	Birds Eye MenuMaster		per pie 525
seafood	Birds Eye MenuMaster		per pie 445
steak and mushroom	Birds Eye MenuMaster		per pie 505
Flaky pastries, Chinese		392	111

Product	Brand	Calories per 100g/ 100ml	Calories per oz/ pack/ portion
Flaky pastry mix (as sold)	Tesco	558	158
Flan case	Lyons	320	91
all sizes	Tesco	323	92
Flan fillings (Armour): see flavours			
Flans: see flavours			
Flapjack biscuits	Tesco	442	125
Flash fry steak	St Michael	128	36
Flora			
cooking fat, white sunflower	Van den Berghs	900	255
margarine	Van den Berghs	740	210
sunflower oil	Van den Berghs	900	255
Florentines chocolate biscuits	St Michael	545	155
Florida cocktail yogurt, low calorie	Diet Ski	54	per 150g pack 81
Florida orange mini juice	Wall's		per portion 30
Florida salad	Littlewoods	125	per 227g pack 284
	St Michael	205	58
	Tesco	102	29
	Waitrose	163	per 227g pack 370
Florida spring vegetable soup, dried	Knorr	280	79
Flour			
brown (85%)		327	93
chapati, brown, coarse		331	94
chapati, white, plain		332	94
millet		354	100
patent (40%)		347	98
rice		366	104

Product	Brand	Calories per 100g/ 100ml	Calories per oz/ pack/ portion
Flour			
white (72%) household, plain		350	99
white (72%) self-raising		339	96
white breadmaking (72%)		337	96
wholemeal (100%)		318	90
brown	Tesco	333	94
buckwheat	Holland and Barrett	330	94
carob	Holland and Barrett	180	51
maize	Holland and Barrett	370	105
plain	Safeway	327	93
	Tesco	321	91
	Whitworths	350	99
plain, traditional	Waitrose	341	97
plain, superfine	Waitrose	340	96
rice, brown	Holland and Barrett	360	102
rye	Holland and Barrett	335	95
self-raising	Safeway	327	93
	Tesco	310	88
	Whitworths	339	96
self-raising, traditional	Waitrose	341	97
self-raising superfine	Waitrose	340	96
soya, low fat	Holland and Barrett	350	99
wheatmeal, strong brown	Safeway	327	93
white, strong plain	Waitrose	342	97
white, strong plain	Safeway	337	96
white	Tesco	333	94

Product	Brand	Calories per 100g/ 100ml	Calories per oz/ pack/ portion
Flour			
wholemeal	Boots Second Nature	306	87
wholemeal 100%	Holland and Barrett	320	91
wholemeal 85%	Holland and Barrett	330	94
wholewheat, strong 100%	Safeway	318	90
wholewheat	Tesco	338	96
	Waitrose	318	90
wholewheat 100%	Jordans	300	85
Foam crystals, all flavours	Creamola	323	92
Fondant fancies	Littlewoods	373	106
	St Michael	339	96
Food, wholemeal	Boots Second Nature	306	87
Foo-juk: see Soya thread			
Forest fruit crush	St Michael	47	14
50% juice	St Michael	53	16
Forest fruit juice drink	Ribena	52	15
Forest fruit Sweet Trolley Italiano ice cream	Wall's		per 1/10 litre pack
Forest fruits yogurt	Gold Ski	115	per 150g pack 172
	Ski (Eden Vale)	85	150g pack 128
Four fruit cocktail drink, long-life	Waitrose	54	per 200ml pack 108
Four fruits in water	Dietade	21	6
Fox's Glacier Fruits	Rowntree Mackintosh	380	per sweet, stickpack, 12

Product	Brand	Calories per 100g/ 100ml	Calories per oz/ pack/ portion
Fox's Glacier Fruits	Rowntree		
	Mackintosh	380	per sweet, bag, 20
Fox's Glacier Mints	Rowntree		per sweet,
	Mackintosh	380	stickpack, 12
	Rowntree		
	Mackintosh	380	per sweet, bag, 20
Frankfurters		274	78
	St Michael	295	84
sliced	Tesco	302	86
Freedent chewing gum			
peppermint	Wrigley		per stick 9
spearmint	Wrigley		per stick 9
French beans, boiled		7	2
French bread pizza: *see also flavours*			
French bread pizza	Birds Eye		
	MenuMaster		per pizza 330
	Ross	270	77
French Brie cheese	Tesco	306	87
French dressing		658	187
	Heinz	511	145
classic	Kraft	496	147
oil-free	Waistline	13	4
French fries	Ross	120	34
French half baguettes	Bejam		per half baguette 263
French mayonnaise	St Michael	753	213
French mushroom flan	Findus	224	64
French mustard	Colman's	115	33
	Safeway	75	21

Product	Brand	Calories per 100g/ 100ml	Calories per oz/ pack/ portion
French mustard and honey roast ham	Waitrose	173	49
French oil dressing	Safeway	480	142
French onion flan	Findus	231	65
French onion quiche	St Michael	260	74
French onion soup	Baxters	24	per 425g can 102
	Waitrose	15	per 295g can 44
condensed	Campbell's	29	8
dried	Tesco	334	95
	Waitrose	315	per 27g pack 85
dried instant special	Safeway	38	11
dried, with croutons	Batchelors Cup-a-Soup Special	338	per 16g pack as sold 54
instant	Tesco	328	93
French rolls	Bejam		per roll baked 130
French sandwich cake	Lyons	369	105
jam	Littlewoods	375	106
	Waitrose	399	113
French style yogurt: see also flavours			
French style yogurt, all varieties	Eden Vale	87	per 125g pack 109
French vegetable mix	Ross	25	7
Fresh cream apple slice cake	Tesco	312	88
Fresh cream apple strudel cake	Tesco	156	44
Fresh cream apricot and apple cake	Tesco	148	42
Fresh cream cheesecake	Tesco	275	78

Product	Brand	Calories per 100g/ 100ml	Calories per oz/ pack/ portion
Fresh cream chocolate truffles	St Michael	536	152
Fresh cream coffee slice cake	Tesco	418	119
Fresh cream fruit cocktail	Safeway	141	40
Fresh cream fruit trifle	St Michael	165	47
Fresh cream lemon slice cake	Tesco	406	115
Fresh cream liqueur truffles	St Michael	522	148
Fresh cream meringues	St Michael	338	96
Fresh cream rum baba cake	Tesco	256	73
Fresh cream slice cake	Tesco	430	122
Fresh cream sponge bar cake	Tesco	332	94
Fresh cream trifle	Tesco	176	50
Fresh fruit marmalade	St Michael	240	68
Fresh garlic dressing	St Michael	330	94
Fresh mints	Boots Cadbury's	363	per 125g pack 454 per mint 25
Fresh orange marmalade, thick cut	Waitrose	248	70
Fresh vegetable dip	St Michael	718	204
Fresh vegetable flan	St Michael	228	65
Freshly squeezed orange juice	Tesco	42	12

Product	Brand	Calories per 100g/ 100ml	Calories per oz/ pack/ portion
Fricassee	Granose	130	37
Frikaletts	Granose	120	34
Fritters, Scotch			
with beans	Ross	240	68
with cheese	Ross	240	68
Frittini rissole mix, vegetarian	Costa	348	99
Frosties	Kellogg's	355	101
Frosties	Trebor	365	per sweet 23
Fructose	Holland and Barrett	400	113
Fruit and bran bar	Prewetts	202	per 42g bar 85
Fruit and bran biscuits	Boots Second Nature	418	119
Fruit and cereal breakfast	Cow and Gate	58	per 110g jar 64, 150g jar 87
	Heinz Baby Foods	79	per 128g jar 101
Fruit 'n Fibre	Kellogg's	338	96
Fruit and fibre muesli	Waitrose	293	83
Fruit and nut bar	Cadbury's	470	per 57g bar 270
Fruit and nut bar, chocolate coated	Tesco	502	142
Fruit and nut bar with honey	Boots	447	127
Fruit and nut biscuits	Holland and Barrett		per biscuit 60
carob coated	Holland and Barrett		per biscuit 70

Product	Brand	Calories per 100g/ 100ml	Calories per oz/ pack/ portion
Fruit and nut carob bar			
no added sugar	Sunwheel Kalibu	483	per 60g bar 290
with raw sugar	Sunwheel Kalibu	503	per 60g bar 302
Fruit and nut cereal bar	St Michael	444	126
Fruit and nut chocolate bar	Boots Shapers Meal	504	143
	Tesco	529	150
Fruit and nut chocolates	Nestle	475	135
Fruit and nut cookies	Barbaras		per biscuit 210
	Cadbury's	450	per biscuit 45
Fruit and nut creams	St Michael	460	130
Fruit and nut dessert bar	Prewetts	310	per 42g bar 130
Fruit and nut loaf mix, wholemeal (as sold)	Green's	370	made up per portion 150
Fruit and nut muesli	Sunwheel	364	103
	Waitrose	354	100
35%	Safeway	326	92
sugar-free	Sunwheel	360	102
Fruit and syrup cake	Lyons	401	114
Fruit batch cake	Tesco	306	87
Fruit BonBons	Cadbury's	380	each pocket pack 20, standard pack 25
Fruit bran	Granose	302	86
Fruit bread	Granose	310	88
Fruit buns	Tesco	300	85

Product	Brand	Calories per 100g/ 100ml	Calories per oz/ pack/ portion
Fruit cake			
plain		354	100
rich		332	94
rich, iced		352	100
all butter wholemeal	Safeway	348	99
iced	Waitrose	375	106
Fruit cheesecake	Birds Eye		per 1/6 cake 260
Fruit chews	St Michael	370	105
Fruit chutney, curried	Tesco	141	40
Fruit Club biscuits	Jacobs	471	per biscuit 113
Fruit cocktail	Libby	79	22
	Safeway	95	per 114g can 170
diabetic	Boots	24	7
fresh cream	Safeway	141	per 397g pack 560
in apple juice	Waitrose	50	14
in fruit juice	Del Monte	47	13
in natural juice	Tesco	48	14
in syrup	Del Monte	67	19
	Tesco	74	21
	Waitrose	95	per 411g can 390
low calorie	Boots Shapers	22	6
Fruit cocktail trifle	Littlewoods	135	per 397g pack 536
	Waitrose	134	per 400g pack 536
Fruit creams	Trebor	333	per sweet 31
Fruit delight dessert	Cow and Gate	62	per 110g jar 68, 150g jar 93
Fruit dessert with tapioca	Heinz Baby Foods	69	per 128g can 88
Fruit digestive biscuits	Huntley & Palmer	451	per biscuit 50
Fruit fillings (Morton): *see flavours*			

Product	Brand	Calories per 100g/ 100ml	Calories per oz/ pack/ portion
Fruit flavour drops	Boots	363	103
	Littlewoods	357	101
diabetic	Boots	367	104
Fruit flavour pastilles			
diabetic	Boots	100	28
Fruit flavoured jellies	Littlewoods	296	84
Fruit flavoured toffees	Trebor	456	per sweet 31
Fruit For-All (Chivers): see flavours			
Fruit gums		172	49
	Rowntree Mackintosh	265	per gum, tube 5, carton 6
Mr Men	Bassett's	308	87
real	Bassett's	293	83
	St Michael	340	96
soft	Wilkinson	319	90
Fruit harvest ice cream (Lyons Maid): see flavours			
Fruit jellies	Tesco	367	104
	Waitrose	296	84
Fruit loaf, sliced	Tesco	310	88
Fruit loaf cake mix (as sold)	Green's	396	made up per portion 110
Fruit malt loaf	Littlewoods	262	74
Fruit mixture, dried	Whitworths	245	69
Fruit muesli bar	Boots	377	107
Fruit mushrooms	Bassett's	406	115
Fruit, nuts and seeds	Waitrose	470	133
Fruit of the forest low fat yogurt	Tesco	106	30
Fruit pastilles	Needlers	322	91
	Rowntree Mackintosh	350	each, tube 11, carton 14

Product	Brand	Calories per 100g/ 100ml	Calories per oz/ pack/ portion
Fruit pastilles	Rowntree Mackintosh	350	per sweet, carton
	Tesco	322	91
	Waitrose	322	91
assorted	St Michael	253	72
real	Bassett's	303	86
Fruit pie			
individual, pastry top and bottom		369	105
pastry top		180	51
Fruit pie filling, canned		95	27
Fruit pie fillings (Tesco): *see flavours*			
Fruit pies (Lyons): *see flavours*			
Fruit salad			
canned		95	27
	Heinz Baby Foods	52	per 128g can 67
dried	Holland and Barrett	192	54
	Whitworths	159	45
in syrup	Waitrose	91	per 425g can 387
Fruit salad chews	Trebor	385	per sweet 15
Fruit salad fruity juice dessert	Heinz Baby Foods	87	per 128g jar 111
Fruit salad hard gums	Bassett's	277	79
Fruit sauce	Tesco	67	19
	Waitrose	120	34
Fruit scones	Tesco	286	81
Fruit sensations	Needlers	334	95
Fruit shortcake	Tesco	460	130
	Waitrose	476	135
Fruit shortcake biscuits	Peek Frean	443	per biscuit 36
	Safeway	477	135

Product	Brand	Calories per 100g/ 100ml	Calories per oz/ pack/ portion
Fruit shortcake biscuits			
	St Michael	476	135
Fruit shorties biscuits	Boots	452	128
Fruit snack bar, carob coated	Sunwheel Kalibu	340	per 30g bar 102
Fruit softy			
apricot	Eden Vale	129	37
strawberry	Eden Vale	129	37
Fruit sponge pudding mix (as sold)	Green's	386	made up per portion 292
Fruit spread			
pear 'n' apple	Sunwheel	239	68
pear 'n' apricot	Sunwheel	264	75
pear 'n' black cherry	Sunwheel	258	73
pear 'n' strawberry	Sunwheel	242	69
Fruit squash, English	Boots	202	60
Fruit sugar	Dietade	394	112
Fruitcake mix, farmhouse (as sold)	Granny Smiths	388	per 439g pack made up 1704
Fruited lardy cake	St Michael	419	119
Fruited malt loaf	Waitrose	243	69
Fruited treacle crumpets	St Michael	280	79
Fruits of the forest cheesecake mix, made up	Lyons	232	made up
Fruits of the forest ice cream, scooping	Wall's Italiano	90	per 1/40 4-litre 90

Product	Brand	Calories per 100g/ 100ml	Calories per oz/ pack/ portion
Fruits of the forest ministick chocolate bar	St Michael	473	134
Fruits of the forest pies	Tesco	398	113
Fruits of the forest yoghurt creamy	Waitrose	143	per 125g pack 179
Fruits of the forest yogurt	St Ivel	81	23
low calorie	St Ivel	41	12
Fruity apple spreading cheese	Medley	305	per 75g pack 229
Fruity juice dessert apple	Heinz Baby Foods	74	per 128g jar 95
apple and banana	Heinz Baby Foods	53	per 128g jar 68
apple and blackcurrant	Heinz Baby Foods	62	per 128g jar 79
apple and orange	Heinz Baby Foods	60	per 128g jar 77
fruit salad	Heinz Baby Foods	87	per 128g jar 111
pear and cherry	Heinz Baby Foods	61	per 128g jar 78
Fruity sauce	Branston	90	26
	O.K.	90	26
	Safeway	98	28
Fruity sherbets	Needlers	345	98
Fruties (Birds Eye): see flavours			
Fudge	Cadbury's	435	per 30g bar 130
	Littlewoods	398	113

Product	Brand	Calories per 100g/ 100ml	Calories per oz/ pack/ portion
Fudge	Rowntree Mackintosh		per sweet 45
	Tesco	413	117
bars	St Michael	447	127
Fudge yogurt	Mister Men	100	28
	Munch Bunch	92	per 125g pack 115
Funtime	Safeway	95	per 150g pack 143
Funny Feet	Wall's		per portion 80
Funtime yoghurts (Safeway): see flavours			
Fusille bianche	Waitrose	222	63
Fussell's Blue Butterfly condensed milk, skimmed, sweetened	Nestle	267	76
Fussell's Golden Butterfly sterilized cream	Nestle	233	66
Gala egg pie	Littlewoods	350	99
Gala slice	Tesco	241	68
Galaxy	Mars	547	155
Gambit	Cadbury's	520	per 40g bar 210
Game consomme	Baxters	9	per 425g can 36
Game pie	Waitrose	221	63
Game soup, dried	Nestle Bonne Cuisine	208	59
Gammon			
joint, sweetcure	St Michael	199	56
joint, unsmoked Danish	St Michael	160	45
joint with bacon fat, Danish	St Michael	160	45
roll, baked	Waitrose	288	82
smoked, sliced	St Michael	112	32

Product	Brand	Calories per 100g/ 100ml	Calories per oz/ pack/ portion
Gammon			
steaks	Tesco	179	51
steaks, grilled	Bejam	138	39
steaks, smoked	St Michael	195	55
steaks smoked, British	St Michael	195	55
steak, sweetcure	St Michael	199	56
steaks, unsmoked Danish	St Michael	160	45
Gammon and pork steaks	Safeway	240	68
Garden mint sauce	Safeway	10	3
Garden peas: see Peas, garden			
Garden vegetable casserole	Boots Baby Foods	415	118
Garden vegetable soup, thick (dried, made up)	Chef Box	25	made up
Gari, raw		351	100
Garibaldi biscuits	Peek Frean	358	per biscuit 32
	Tesco	373	106
	Waitrose	370	105
Garlic, raw		117	33
Garlic and herb Dish of the Day, dried	Crosse & Blackwell	457	130
Garlic and herbs stuffing mix	Knorr	411	117
Garlic bread	Bejam		per baguette baked 690
Garlic butter	Safeway	695	197
Garlic dressing	Duchesse	33	10
fresh	St Michael	330	94
Italian	Kraft	426	126

Product	Brand	Calories per 100g/ 100ml	Calories per oz/ pack/ portion
Garlic dressing			
Italian style	St Michael	138	39
Italian	Tesco	450	128
Garlic mayonnaise	Hellmanns	720	204
	Safeway	745	211
	Waitrose	734	208
Garlic oil dressing	Safeway	440	130
Garlic pate	Tesco	397	113
Garlic Prawnaise	Lyons Seafoods	185	52
Garlic prawns	Young's	75	21
Garlic sauce mix	Knorr	435	123
Garlic sausage	Waitrose	262	74
French	Waitrose	262	74
German	Waitrose	330	94
sliced	Tesco	238	67
Gateau roule, various fillings	Waitrose	354	100
Gelatin		338	96
Genoa cake	Tesco	362	103
decorated	Littlewoods	323	92
Georgia pecan pie ice cream	Safeway	246	73
German mustard	Colman's	135	38
German salami	Waitrose	427	121
German sausage, Extrawurst	Waitrose	350	99
Ghee			
butter		898	255
palm		897	254
vegetable		898	255
Gherkins			
raw		11	3

Product	Brand	Calories per 100g/100ml	Calories per oz/pack/portion
	Haywards	5	1
	Waitrose	14	4
cocktail	Tesco	11	3
	Waitrose	14	4
pickled	Safeway	6	2
Ginger			
ground		258	73
	Tesco	342	97
ground	Safeway	364	103
roots, raw		46	13
Ginger ale	Canada Dry	38	11
low calorie	Canada Dry Slim	1	per 113ml pack 1
American	Hunts	36	11
	Schweppes	21	6
	Tesco	28	8
American, low calorie	Diet Hunts	1	
	Tesco	6	2
dry	Hunts	16	5
dry	Schweppes	15	4
Ginger and bran biscuits, carob coated	Holland and Barrett		per biscuit 70
Ginger and hazelnut Caprice biscuits	Cadbury's	485	per biscuit 65
Ginger and honey Chinese barbecue sauce	Sharwood	140	40
Ginger and lemon biscuits, hand-baked	Boots	514	146
Ginger and pear bar	Boots	344	98

Product	Brand	Calories per 100g/ 100ml	Calories per oz/ pack/ portion
Ginger bar	Shepherd Boy Bars		per bar 162
Ginger beer	Corona	29	9
	Idris Old English	35	10
	Safeway	49	15
	Schweppes	34	10
	St Michael	47	14
	Tesco	48	14
	Whites	29	8
with lemonade	Idris Old English	37	11
Ginger biscuits, plain chocolate	St Michael	490	139
Ginger creams	Safeway	488	138
	Waitrose	488	138
diabetic	Boots	468	133
Ginger crunch creams	Tesco	477	135
Ginger extra jam	Waitrose	248	70
Ginger fingers	Boots	439	124
Ginger fudge snack bar, carob coated	Sunwheel Kalibu	403	per 30g bar 121
Ginger nuts		456	129
	Peek Frean	431	per biscuit 36
	Safeway	426	121
	Tesco	433	123
Ginger pear bar	Granose	366	per 30g bar 110
Ginger preserve	Safeway	256	73
Ginger preserve marmalade	Tesco	275	78
Ginger snaps	St Michael	423	120
	Waitrose	428	121

Product	Brand	Calories per 100g/ 100ml	Calories per oz/ pack/ portion
Ginger thins	Waitrose	456	129
Gingerbread		373	106
Glace cherries		212	60
	Safeway	218	62
	Tesco	341	97
	Waitrose	212	60
	Whitworths	212	60
Glace fruit drops	Needlers	375	106
Glacier Fruits, Fox's	Rowntree Mackintosh	380	each, stickpack 12, bag 20
Glacier Mints, Fox's	Rowntree Mackintosh	380	each, stickpack 12, bag 20
Glazed chicken	Findus Lean Cuisine	110	31
Glitter fruits	Trebor	349	per sweet 22
mints	Trebor	349	per sweet 22
Globe artichoke: see *Artichoke, globe*			
Glucodin	Farley	340	96
Glucose drink, sparkling	Boots	77	23
Glucose energy tablets	Lucozade	339	96
Glucose health drink	Safeway	80	24
Glucose liquid, BP		318	90
Glucose powder	Boots	340	96
with vitamin C	Boots	340	96
Gluten-free biscuits	Farley	535	per biscuit 54
Glycerin soft pastilles			
honey and lemon	Boots	318	90
honey and orange	Boots	318	90
Goan Vindaloo curry sauce	Sharwood	79	22

Product	Brand	Calories per 100g/ 100ml	Calories per oz/ pack/ portion
Gold margarine	St Ivel	390	111
Gold Seal ice cream (Lyons Maid): *see flavours*			
Gold Ski yogurts (Eden Vale): *see flavours*			
Gold Spinner processed cheese	St Ivel	280	79
Gold coffee, dry	Safeway	330	94
Golden breadcrumbs	Tesco	371	105
Golden chicken and mushroom soup	Heinz Ready to Serve	42	12
Golden chicken and vegetable soup	Heinz Ready to Serve	34	10
Golden chicken dinner	Heinz Baby Foods	62	per 128g can 79
Golden choc ice	Bejam		per choc ice 115
Golden churn	Kraft	680	193
Golden cooking crumbs	Waitrose	340	96
Golden crunch creams	Safeway	506	143
	Tesco	502	142
Golden cup	Rowntree Mackintosh	450	per small cup 100
Golden cutlets	St Michael	83	24
Golden Delicious apples	Tesco	46	13
Golden marzipan	Waitrose	408	116
Golden mints	Boots	363	103
Golden plums	Waitrose	58	per 568g pack 329
Golden Ready Brek	Lyons	391	111
Golden savoury rice	Batchelors	328	per 134g sachet as sold 439

Product	Brand	Calories per 100g/ 100ml	Calories per oz/ pack/ portion
Golden savoury rice	Whitworths	340	96
Golden Shred marmalade	Robertson's	251	71
Golden spread	St Michael	710	201
Golden sweetcorn, no salt added	Del Monte	101	29
Golden syrup		298	84
	Tate and Lyle	298	84
Golden syrup preserve	Tesco	303	86
Golden toffee	Rowntree Mackintosh	460	per sweet 30
Golden vanilla choc ice	Wall's		per ice 130
Golden vegetable hotpot	Boots Baby Foods	405	115
Golden vegetable rice (frozen), cooked	Uncle Ben's	105	30
Golden vegetable savoury rice	Safeway	336	per 125g pack 420
Golden vegetable soup	Heinz Big Soups	37	10
	Heinz Ready to Serve	41	12
	Knorr	340	96
	Knorr Quick Soup	427	121
condensed	Campbell's	47	13
dried	Batchelors	360	per 65g pint pack as sold 234
	Batchelors Cup-a-Soup	357	per 21g sachet as sold 75
	Safeway	338	96

Product	Brand	Calories per 100g/ 100ml	Calories per oz/ pack/ portion
Golden vegetable soup			
dried, instant (as sold)	Safeway	363	103
dried, low calorie	Batchelors Slim-a-Soup	300	per 13g sachet 39
dried, made up	Chef Box	29	8
dried, with croutons	Batchelors Snack-a-Soup	365	per 43g sachet as sold 157
Golden vegetables	Heinz Baby Foods	71	per 128g can 91
Goldenbake (Bejam): see products, flavours			
Googles	Wall's		per portion 100
Goose, roast		319	90
Gooseberries			
green, raw		17	5
green, stewed without sugar		14	4
green, stewed with sugar		50	14
ripe, raw		37	10
	Hartley's	70	per 114g can 80
Gooseberry cream	Rowntree Mackintosh		per sweet 40
Gooseberry crumble	Waitrose	160	45
Gooseberry flan filling	Armour	89	25
Gooseberry fruit fool	St Michael	160	45
Gooseberry fruit pie filling	Tesco	95	27
Gooseberry slice	St Michael	318	90
Gooseberry yoghurt	Safeway	91	per 150g pack 137
	Waitrose	90	per 150g pack 135
Gorgonzola cheese, mountain	Waitrose	390	111

Product	Brand	Calories per 100g/ 100ml	Calories per oz/ pack/ portion
Gouda cheese	St Ivel	370	105
	Tesco	341	97
Dutch	Safeway	346	98
	Waitrose	390	111
Goulash	Granose	54	15
Goulash mix (dry)	Tesco	310	88
Goulash sauce mix	Knorr	380	108
Goulash soup	Waitrose	67	per 425g can 285
condensed	Campbell's	86	24
Gourd			
bitter (karela), fresh, raw		9	3
bitter (karela), canned, drained		7	2
bottle (chapni kaddu), raw		16	5
ridge (turia), raw		16	5
round (tinda)		21	6
Grain pilaff	Bewell Amazing Grains	340	96
Granny Smith apples	Tesco	46	13
Granulated sugar	Tate and Lyle	394	112
Granules	Bovril	186	53
Granymels			
caramel	Itona	390	111
liquorice	Itona	395	112
mint	Itona	370	105
treacle	Itona	400	113
Grape and blackcurrant juice	Waitrose	71	21
Grape juice			
red	Prewetts	66	20
red long life	Safeway	55	16
red sparkling long life	Safeway	47	14

Product	Brand	Calories per 100g/ 100ml	Calories per oz/ pack/ portion
Grape juice			
red	Schloer	49	15
red sparkling	Schloer	49	15
red	Volonte	60	18
red, 700ml pack	Waitrose	70	21
red, litre pack	Waitrose	55	16
white long life	Safeway	55	16
white sparkling long life	Safeway	47	14
white	Schloer	48	14
white sparkling	Schloer	49	15
white, 700ml pack	Waitrose	70	21
white, litre pack	Waitrose	59	17
Grapefruit			
raw		22	6
canned		60	17
whole fruit, raw		11	3
without skin	Littlewoods	22	6
Grapefruit and pineapple drink	Britvic	40	11
Grapefruit 'C'			
reduced calories	Libby	32	9
sweetened	Libby	58	16
Grapefruit drink	Waitrose	92	27
dilutable	Boots Shapers	8	2
sparkling	Tango	42	12
with pineapple juice	Corona	99	29
Grapefruit fruit juice	Del Monte	38	11
sweetened (canned)	Heinz	64	19
Grapefruit juice			
sweetened canned		38	11
unsweetened canned		31	9
	Boots	31	9
	Britvic	54	15

Product	Brand	Calories per 100g/ 100ml	Calories per oz/ pack/ portion
Grapefruit juice	Prewetts	31	9
	Schweppes	46	14
	St Ivel Mr Juicy	31	9
	St Ivel Real	31	9
chilled concentrated (frozen)	Tesco	42	12
	Tesco	136	39
	Waitrose	40	12
long life	Tesco	42	12
	Waitrose	36	11
pure, chilled	Waitrose	30	9
pure, long life	Safeway	35	10
sweetened	Hunts	62	18
	Libby	38	11
unsweetened	Libby	31	9
Grapefruit juice bar	Lyons Maid		each 39
Grapefruit marmalade	Baxters	249	per 340g jar 846
medium cut	Waitrose	248	70
Grapefruit segments in juice	Libby	30	9
	St Michael	41	12
	Waitrose	36	10
in natural juice	Tesco	34	10
in syrup	Tesco	63	18
	Waitrose	62	18
Grapefruit squash diluted	Quosh	43	13
real, undiluted	Quosh	123	36
Grapefruit whole fruit drink	Robinsons	95	28
Grapenuts		355	101

Product	Brand	Calories per 100g/ 100ml	Calories per oz/ pack/ portion
Grapes			
black, raw		61	17
black, whole, raw		51	14
white, raw		63	18
white, whole, raw		60	17
black, without skin	Littlewoods	61	17
white, without skin	Littlewoods	63	18
Gravy			
cubes	Knorr	348	99
granules (as sold)	Safeway	438	124
granules (made up)	Safeway	35	10
granules	Tesco	490	139
	Waitrose	507	144
mix	Tesco	265	75
powder	Waitrose	263	75
Gravy Madeira	Nestle Bonne Cuisine	359	102
Gravy paysan	Nestle Bonne Cuisine	348	99
Greek kebab marinade	Knorr	275	78
Green and white pasta shells (as sold)	Signor Rossi	309	88
Green banana: *see Plantain*			
Green beans			
canned	Tesco	14	4
cut (frozen)	Bejam	25	per 57g portion boiled 14
cut (canned)	Del Monte	19	5
cut	Waitrose	19	per 397g pack 75
cut (canned), no salt added	Del Monte	19	5

Product	Brand	Calories per 100g/ 100ml	Calories per oz/ pack/ portion
Green beans			
dried	Batchelors Surprise	130	per 33g sachet as sold 43
frozen	Ross	25	7
sliced (frozen)	Bejam	34	per 57g portion boiled 19
sliced (frozen)	Birds Eye	28	8
sliced (frozen)	Findus	30	9
sliced (canned)	Morton	20	6
sliced (canned)	Safeway	19	per 284g can 54
sliced (frozen)	Safeway	35	per 227g pack 80
sliced (frozen)	Tesco	14	4
sliced	Waitrose	35	per 454g pack 160
whole (frozen)	Birds Eye	35	10
whole (canned)	Safeway	40	per 397g can 159
whole (frozen)	Safeway	45	per 454g pack 208
whole (canned)	Tesco	33	9
whole (frozen)	Tesco	28	8
whole (frozen)	Waitrose	26	per 397g pack 103
whole (canned)	Waitrose	35	per 454g pack 160
Green Label mango chutney	Sharwood	217	62
Green pepper, filled	St Michael	95	27
Green peppers, fresh	Littlewoods	15	4
	Tesco	24	7
Green rye with mushroom soup	Boots Second Nature	319	90
Greengages			
raw		47	13
raw (with stones)		45	13
stewed without sugar		40	11
stewed without sugar (with stones)		38	11
stewed with sugar		75	21
stewed with sugar (with stones)		72	20

Product	Brand	Calories per 100g/ 100ml	Calories per oz/ pack/ portion
Grillsteaks	Ross	320	91
beef	Birds Eye Steakhouse		each grilled or fried 185
beef	Findus	233	66
	St Michael	279	79
beef joint (frozen), cooked	Tesco	284	81
beef, low fat	Birds Eye Steakhouse		each grilled or baked 155
jumbo	Ross	220	62
lamb	Bejam		each grilled 229
	Birds Eye Steakhouse		each grilled or fried 190
quick	Ross	320	91
steak	Bejam		each grilled 203
value	Birds Eye Steakhouse		each grilled 175, fried 190
Grissini (breadsticks)	Buitoni	360	per 125g pack 450
Grizzly bars, all varieties	Grizzly Bars		per bar 100
Ground beef steaklet	St Michael	128	36
Ground ginger: see *Ginger, ground*			
Groundnut oil	Boots	899	255
	Waitrose	900	266
Grouse, roast (with bone)		173 114	49 32
Gruyere cheese	Tesco	437	124
Swiss	St Michael	400	113
	Waitrose	272	77
Guare (cluster beans)		23	7
Guava and apple juice	Copella	36	11

Product	Brand	Calories per 100g/ 100ml	Calories per oz/ pack/ portion
Guavas			
fresh, raw		62	18
in syrup, canned		60	17
Gulab jamen (jambu)		357	101
home made		348	99
Gum-emu, soft	Barratt	292	83
Gum novelties	Barratt	324	92
Haddock			
fresh, raw		73	21
fresh, fried		174	49
fresh, fried (with bones)		160	45
fresh, steamed		98	28
fresh, steamed (with bones and skin)		75	21
	Waitrose	98	28
	Waitrose	75	per 142g steak 105
battered, Chip Shop	Ross	180	51
breaded	Waitrose	141	40
crispy battered	Ross	170	48
dippers	Young's	193	55
Finnan	Waitrose	101	29
fresh	Littlewoods	73	21
frozen	Safeway	85	24
frozen, raw	Tesco	75	21
frozen, steamed	Tesco	88	25
golden cutlets	St Michael	83	24
goujons	Waitrose	140	40
in batter (frozen)	Safeway	200	57
in breadcrumbs (chilled)	Young's	193	55
in breadcrumbs (frozen)	Safeway	140	40
ovencrisp Scottish	St Michael	225	64

Product	Brand	Calories per 100g/ 100ml	Calories per oz/ pack/ portion
Haddock			
portions (frozen)	Littlewoods	100	per portion 92
portions, batter crisp	Findus	224	64
portions, battercrisp	St Michael	170	48
portions, crumb crisp	Findus	221	63
Haddock fillets	Ross	80	23
	Young's	75	21
breaded	Bejam	222	deep-fried
	St Michael	119	34
breaded, in natural crumb	Ross	170	48
crispy breaded	St Michael	179	51
prime (frozen), poached	Bejam	99	28
skinless	St Michael	80	23
Haddock steaks	Bejam		per steak grilled 58
	Ross	80	23
battered	Findus	158	45
breaded	Bejam		per steak grilled 111
breaded, in natural crumb	Ross	170	48
crispy	Birds Eye		each shallow-fried 180, deep-fried 200
in breadcrumbs	Findus	107	30
in butter sauce	Findus	89	25
	Ross	80	23
in crisp crunch crumb	Birds Eye		each grilled/baked 185, fried 210/216

Product	Brand	Calories per 100g/ 100ml	Calories per oz/ pack/ portion
Haddock steaks			
in crispy batter	Bejam		per steak deep-fried 216
in parsley sauce	Findus	66	19
oven crispy	Birds Eye		per steak baked or grilled 215
Haddock, smoked			
steamed		101	29
steamed (with bones and skin)		66	19
buttered (frozen)	Birds Eye	106	30
croquettes	Young's	188	53
cutlets (chilled)	Young's	87	25
fillets (frozen) boil-in-bag	Bejam		per serving 238
fillets	Ross	80	23
	Waitrose	99	28
fillets (chilled)	Young's	78	22
	Young's	87	25
fillets, with butter	Ross	100	28
fillets/cutlets (frozen), poached	Bejam	85	24
Finnan, frozen, raw	Tesco	89	25
Finnan, frozen, steamed	Tesco	101	29
golden cutlets	Waitrose	99	28
raw (frozen)	Tesco	90	26
with butter	Findus	101	29
steamed (frozen)	Tesco	101	29
Haddock and mushroom crumble, Chunky	St Michael	125	35
Haddock and prawn crumble	Ross	180	51

Product	Brand	Calories per 100g/ 100ml	Calories per oz/ pack/ portion
Haddock and prawn pasta	Ross	100	28
Haddock curry		254	72
Haddock en-croute	Bejam		per serving baked 343
Haddock fillet fish fingers	Birds Eye		each grilled 50, shallow-fried 55
Haddock fish fingers crumb crisp	Findus	191	54
Haddock mornay	St Michael	125	35
	Tesco	101	29
Haddock, mushroom and tomato flan	St Michael	213	60
Haddock pastry lattice	Birds Eye MenuMaster		per pack 525
Haddock provencal	Tesco	208	cooked
	Tesco	86	24
Haggis, boiled		310	88
Hake fillets, skinless, poached	Bejam	92	26
Halibut			
raw		92	26
steamed		131	37
steamed (*with bones and skin*)		99	28
Halva, Greek		615	174
Halwa, Asian		381	108
Ham			
canned		120	34
	Armour	122	per 454g can 554
	Tesco	94	27
	Waitrose	108	31

Product	Brand	Calories per 100g/ 100ml	Calories per oz/ pack/ portion
Ham			
Bavarian slices	St Michael	160	45
Blackforest	Waitrose	371	105
Brunswick	Waitrose	176	50
Buckingham	Waitrose	121	34
Danish, slices	St Michael	130	37
French mustard and			
honey roast	Waitrose	173	49
honey roast	Waitrose	121	34
honey roast double			
loin, cooked	Littlewoods	151	43
honey roast thin			
sliced	St Michael	124	35
honey roast,			
continental	Waitrose	199	56
honey roast, sliced	Tesco	134	38
Italian dry cured			
sliced	St Michael	300	85
joints, Bavarian	St Michael	161	46
Maryland	Waitrose	156	44
mild cure, cooked	Littlewoods	130	37
mild cure, sliced	Tesco	103	29
oak smoked, English	Waitrose	163	46
Old English			
Virginia	Waitrose	163	46
peppered	Waitrose	173	49
premier smoked,			
sliced	Tesco	162	46
premier, sliced	Tesco	168	48
roast, cooked	Littlewoods	132	37
shoulder	Waitrose	121	34
shoulder, cured			
(cooked)	Waitrose	256	73
smoked	Waitrose	121	34

Product	Brand	Calories per 100g/ 100ml	Calories per oz/ pack/ portion
Ham			
smoked spiced			
sliced	St Michael	220	62
traditional matured			
York	Waitrose	176	50
Ham and bacon			
sandwichmaker	Shippams	134	per 95g can 127
Ham and beef paste	Shippams	198	per 35g pack 69
Ham and beef roll,	Crosse &		
canned	Blackwell	226	64
Ham and cheese			
quiche	Waitrose	211	60
Ham and cheese			
savoury toasts	Findus	220	62
Ham and cheese Toast			
Topper	Heinz	141	40
Ham and chicken roll,	Crosse &		
canned	Blackwell	220	62
Ham and mushroom			
French bread pizza	Waitrose	201	per 150g pack 302
Ham and mushroom	Birds Eye		
pizza	MenuMaster	242	per 265g pizza 640
(frozen)	Safeway	227	per 300g pizza 681
(frozen) pack of 4	Safeway	230	65
	Tesco	224	64
five inch	Bejam		per pizza grilled 225
Ham and Swiss cheese			per 397g quiche
quiche	Waitrose	213	840
Ham and tongue roll	Crosse &		
	Blackwell	270	77
Ham, asparagus and			
carrot quiche	St Michael	224	64

Product	Brand	Calories per 100g/ 100ml	Calories per oz/ pack/ portion
Ham, cheese and watercress sandwich	Tesco	206	58
Ham, chicken and lettuce sandwich with mayonnaise	Waitrose	285	81
Ham crispy base pizza	Findus	168	48
Ham cubes	Knorr	251	71
Ham, mushroom and cheese pizza, 4-inch	Ross	220	62
Ham salad wholemeal bap	Waitrose	203	58
Ham sandwich	Waitrose	211	60
Ham sausage	Waitrose	195	55
sliced	Tesco	164	46
Ham spread	Shippams	173	per 35g pack 61
	St Michael	193	55
Hand raised pork pie	Littlewoods	380	108
Hanging candy assortment	St Michael	392	111
Hanging fruit assortment	St Michael	339	96
Hard gums			
American	Bassett's	327	93
	Littlewoods	325	92
	Tesco	377	107
fruit salad	Bassett's	277	79
Hare			
stewed		192	54
stewed (with bones)		139	39
Haricot beans			
raw		271	77

Product	Brand	Calories per 100g/ 100ml	Calories per oz/ pack/ portion
Haricot beans			
boiled		93	26
(canned)	Boots	95	27
	Tesco	329	93
cooked	Tesco	135	38
dried	Holland and		
	Barrett	270	77
	Safeway	271	77
	Waitrose	271	77
Haricot verts	Findus	67	19
	Waitrose	25	7
Harlequin dessert			
chocolate	Wall's		per 1/5 pack 110
strawberry	Wall's		per 1/5 pack 110
Harvest bran brown rolls	Bejam		per roll baked 97
Harvest bran French roll	Bejam		per roll baked 120
Harvest fruit pie	Lyons	384	109
Harvest nut mix, vegetarian	Boots	410	116
Harvest rings	Sooner	453	per 30g pack 136
Harvest salad	Eden Vale	148	42
Harvest vegetable and beef soup	Crosse & Blackwell Pot Soup		per sachet made up 74
Hash browns	Ross	70	20
Haslet	Waitrose	153	43
Haunted House spaghetti shapes in tomato sauce	Heinz	72	20
Havarti cheese	Waitrose	344	98

Product	Brand	Calories per 100g/ 100ml	Calories per oz/ pack/ portion
Hawaiian drink	Safeway	43	13
Hawaiian fried special savoury rice	Batchelors	470	per 140.5g sachet as sold 660
Hawaiian Punch ice cream	Wall's	85	per 1/20 2-litre pack 85
Hazelnut and almond muesli bar	Granose	460	per 25g bar 115
Hazelnut and herbs stuffing mix	Knorr	428	121
Hazelnut and raisin cluster	Lyons	418	119
Hazelnut bar	Granose	476	per 50g bar 238
Hazelnut biscuits	Boots Second Nature	448	127
diabetic	Boots	428	121
Hazelnut carob bar	Kalibu	507	per 75g bar 380
Hazelnut chocolate bar	Boots Shapers	542	154
Hazelnut chocolate spread	Cadbury's	570	per portion 85
	Sun-Pat	520	147
	Waitrose	530	150
Hazelnut cluster	Rowntree Mackintosh		per sweet 45
Hazelnut confectionery bar, no added sugar	Sunwheel Kalibu	533	per 42g bar 224
Hazelnut cookies	Waitrose	493	140
Hazelnut muesli bar	Granose	476	per 25g bar 119
Hazelnut roll	Tesco	384	109
Hazelnut torte	Young's	320	91
Hazelnut yoghurt	Safeway	98	per 150g pack 147

Product	Brand	Calories per 100g/ 100ml	Calories per oz/ pack/ portion
Hazelnut yoghurt	Waitrose	98	per 150g pack 147
Hazelnut yogurt	Littlewoods	94	per 150g pack 141
	Raines	91	26
	Ski	88	per 150g pack 132
Hazelnuts	Holland and Barrett	380	108
	Tesco	625	177
	Whitworths	639	181
kernels	Littlewoods	380	108
Healthy life biscuits	Mitchellhill		per biscuit 60
Heart			
lamb, raw		119	34
ox, raw		108	31
ox, stewed		179	51
pig, raw		93	26
sheep, roast		237	67
lamb, braised	Bejam	194	55
Hedgehog crisps, natural	Hedgehog	407	per 27g pack 110
Hens and cocks (meat and skin), raw		251	71
Herb and garlic dressing	Heinz All Seasons	302	86
	Safeway	229	65
Herb and vegetable vegeburger	Real Eats	200	per 70g burger 140
Herb butter, Welsh	Safeway	704	200
Herb cream dressing	Waitrose	224	64
Herb crisps, natural	Hedgehog	407	per 27g pack 110
Herb salad dressing	St Michael	105	30
Herb thins	St Michael	522	148

Product	Brand	Calories per 100g/ 100ml	Calories per oz/ pack/ portion
Herb toss 'n' serve dressing	Crosse & Blackwell	11	3
Herb vegebanger	Real Eats	828	235
Herbs and garlic spreading cheese	Medley	319	90
Herbs sandwich spread	Granose	263	75
Herring			
raw		234	66
fried		234	66
fried (with bones)		206	58
grilled		199	56
grilled (with bones)		135	38
roe, fried		244	69
roe, soft, raw		80	23
fillets, chilled	Young's	234	66
frozen, raw	Tesco	234	66
whole	Waitrose	190	54
whole, chilled	Young's	234	66
Herring curry		349	99
Hibran bread			
medium sliced	Vitbe	201	per slice 66
thick sliced	Vitbe	201	per slice 80
Hi-fi biscuits	Itona		per biscuit 90
High bake water biscuits	Jacobs	394	per biscuit 31
	Tesco	402	114
	Waitrose	393	111
High fibre Crunch and Slim			
with honey and almonds	Boots	460	130
with orange and raisins	Boots	420	119

Product	Brand	Calories per 100g/ 100ml	Calories per oz/ pack/ portion
High fibre Crunch and Slim with sultana and hazelnuts	Boots	460	130
High fibre muesli	Holland and Barrett	340	96
High fibre porridge	Boots Second Nature	335	95
High Juice orange squash, concentrated	Rose's	160	47
Highland lentil soup	Knorr	314	89
Highland shorties	Safeway	494	140
	Waitrose	495	140
Highland Spring water natural	Tesco		
sparkling	Tesco		
Highlander's broth	Baxters	50	per 425g can 213
Hi-Juice 66	Schweppes	51	15
Hilo biscuits	Rakusen	307	per biscuit 15
Hilsa		273	77
Hing: see Asafoetida			
Hoi Sin Chinese barbecue sauce	Sharwood	161	46
Hoi Sin spare ribs	Waitrose	165	47
Home made biscuits		469	133
Homestyle soup beef and vegetable	Heinz Ready to Serve	39	11
country vegetable	Heinz Ready to Serve	43	12
potato and leek	Heinz Ready to Serve	36	10
Hominy (maize grits), raw		362	103

Product	Brand	Calories per 100g/ 100ml	Calories per oz/ pack/ portion
Honey			
comb		281	80
in jars		288	82
	Holland and Barrett	280	79
Acacia	Waitrose	304	86
Australian	Waitrose	304	86
Australian, clear	Waitrose	304	86
Canadian	Waitrose	304	86
Canadian clover	St Michael	290	82
Canadian, set	Safeway	300	85
clear	Gales	310	88
clear	Safeway	300	85
comb	Holland and Barrett	280	79
cut comb	Waitrose	304	86
English	Waitrose	304	86
Greek	Waitrose	304	86
Mexican	Waitrose	304	86
Mexican, set	Safeway	300	85
pure, clear	Waitrose	304	86
pure, set	Waitrose	304	86
set	Gales	310	88
set	Safeway	300	85
several varieties	Boots	288	82
Tasmanian	Waitrose	304	86
whole range	Tesco	289	82
wild flower	St Michael	290	82
Honey, almond and raisins original crunch	Jordans	396	112
Honey and almond Caprice biscuits	Cadbury's	470	per biscuit 60

Product	Brand	Calories per 100g/ 100ml	Calories per oz/ pack/ portion
Honey and almond original crunchy bar	Jordans	412	per bar 135
Honey and blackcurrant Glycerin pastilles	Boots	322	91
Honey and lemon Glycerin soft pastilles	Boots	318	90
Honey and lemon sweets	Trebor	349	per sweet 22
Honey and malt soya milk	Provamel	50	15
Honey 'n' nut cornflakes	Tesco	379	107
Honey and nut farmhouse bran	Weetabix	335	95
Honey and oatmeal cookies	Tesco	479	136
	Waitrose	479	136
Honey and orange Glycerin soft pastilles	Boots	318	90
Honey biscuits	Boots Second Nature	441	125
	Holland and Barrett		per biscuit 60
Honey crunch bar	Boots	432	122
Honey menthol	Boots	363	per 33g stick pack 120
Honey muesli	Boots Second Nature	417	118
Honey rice crisps	St Michael	352	100
Honey Smacks	Kellogg's	346	98

Product	Brand	Calories per 100g/ 100ml	Calories per oz/ pack/ portion
Honey spread, diabetic	Boots	256	73
Honeycomb crunch bar	St Michael	450	128
Horlicks		396	112
	Beecham	386	114
Horlicks food drink			
malted	Beecham	386	114
malted chocolate, low fat, instant	Beecham	393	111
malted, low fat, instant	Beecham	382	113
Horlicks hot chocolate drink, low fat, instant	Beecham	402	119
Horlicks maltlets	Beecham	386	109
Horseradish (*drumstick*)			
raw		59	17
leaves		72	20
pods		42	12
Horseradish mustard	Colman's	140	40
Horseradish relish	O.K.	100	28
Horseradish sauce	Safeway	90	26
	Tesco	125	35
	Waitrose	80	23
cream	Tesco	187	53
creamed	O.K.	200	57
	Safeway	185	52
	Waitrose	190	54
Hostess ice cream	Lyons Maid	223	63
Hot brunch	Allinson	357	per 70g pack 250
Hot chocolate drink	Carnation	379	107
instant	Waitrose	385	109

Product	Brand	Calories per 100g/ 100ml	Calories per oz/ pack/ portion
Hot chocolate drink			
low fat, instant	Horlicks	402	119
sugar-free	Carnation	360	per 17.5g sachet 65
Hot oat cereal	Safeway	384	109
Hot pot			
cooked		114	32
	Tesco Ready Meal	84	24
frozen	Safeway	120	34
Hotpot pie	Littlewoods	127	per pie 225
Hovis bread		228	65
Hovis crackers	Nabisco	468	per biscuit 29
	Tesco	484	137
Hovis digestive	Nabisco	486	per biscuit 57
biscuits	Tesco	481	136
Hubba Bubba Bubble Gum, all flavours	Wrigley		15/24 per chunk
Humbug Italiano ice cream, scooping	Wall's	90	per 1/40 4-litre pack 90
Humbugs	Tesco	407	115
Hummus (chickpea spread)		185	52
100s and 1000s	Tesco	375	106
Hungry Hound	Lyons Maid		each 85
Hycal juice, ready to drink			
blackcurrant	Beecham	243	72
lemon	Beecham	243	72
orange	Beecham	243	72
raspberry	Beecham	243	72
Ice cream			
dairy		167	47
non-dairy		165	47

Product	Brand	Calories per 100g/ 100ml	Calories per oz/ pack/ portion
Ice cream: see also flavours			
blue ribbon vanilla	Wall's	90	per 1/10 litre pack 90
Ice cream bar			
blue ribbon vanilla	Wall's		per bar 85
Ice cream roll	Bejam		per 1/6 roll 82
	Birds Eye		per 1/6 of roll 55
	Safeway	178	50
Iced bun cluster	Tesco	316	90
Iced chocolate cake	Tesco	428	121
Iced fruit cake	Waitrose	375	106
Iced gem biscuits	Peek Frean	380	per biscuit 5
Iced Madeira sandwich cake	Waitrose	423	120
Iced marzipan sponge	Tesco	413	117
Iced ring doughnuts	Tesco	420	119
Iced rings	Safeway	443	126
	Waitrose	443	126
Iced sports biscuits	Tesco	443	126
Iced tarts	Lyons	417	118
Icing sugar	Tate and Lyle	392	111
Ideal sauce	Heinz Ploughman's	106	30
Imperial mints	Trebor	376	each, giant roll 18, small roll 10
	Waitrose	370	105
Indian tea		108	31
Indian chicken vegetable mix	Ross	90	26

Product	Brand	Calories per 100g/ 100ml	Calories per oz/ pack/ portion
Indian fried special savoury rice	Batchelors	465	per 147g sachet as sold 684
Indian prawns	Dan Maid	45	13
Indian stir-fry Chinese-style meal	Bejam		per portion stir fried 331
Indian tea infused		-1	
Indian tonic water	Britvic	32	per 150ml can 47
	Canada Dry	24	per 113ml pack 27
	Hunts	24	7
	Tesco	25	7
low calorie	Canada Dry Slim	1	per 113ml pack 1
	Diet Hunts	1	per 100ml pack 0.5
	Tesco	6	2
Indian vegetable curry accompaniment	Sharwood	27	8
Instant coffee: *see Coffee, instant*			
Instant custard: *see Custard*			
Instant mashed potatoes (as sold)	Cadbury's Smash	265	per portion 55
	Safeway	265	per 71g pack 188
(made up)	Safeway	60	17
dried, made up with full cream milk	Yeoman	52	15
dried, made up with water	Yeoman	49	14
dried, made up, complete mix with chopped onion, made up	Yeoman	52	15
	Yeoman	53	15

Product	Brand	Calories per 100g/ 100ml	Calories per oz/ pack/ portion
Instant mashed potatoes			
without added salt, made up	Yeoman	49	14
Instant milk: see Milk, brands			
Instant potatoes			
made up		70	20
powder		318	90
Instant soups: see flavours			
Invaders cream of tomato soup with pasta shapes	Heinz Ready to Serve	71	20
Invaders and meteors spaghetti shapes and meatballs in tomato sauce	Heinz	89	25
Invaders spaghetti shapes in tomato sauce	Heinz	65	18
Irish stew			
cooked		124	35
cooked (with bones)		114	32
canned	St Michael	78	22
	Tesco	124	35
	Tyne Brand	96	27
Irn bru	Barr	39	per 250ml can 100
low calorie	Barr	4	per 330ml can 14
Irn bru soft drink	Littlewoods	39	12
Iron brew-flavoured concentrate	Safeway	167	49
Island Blend fruit drink			
pineapple, grapefuit and lemon	Del Monte	46	14
pineapple, lemon and lime	Del Monte	41	12

Product	Brand	Calories per 100g/ 100ml	Calories per oz/ pack/ portion
Island Blend fruit drink pineapple, orange and mandarin	Del Monte	46	14
Island Fruits	Schweppes	38	11
Italian beef bolognaise vegetable mix	Ross	85	24
Italian dressing, low calorie	Boots Shapers	92	26
Italian garlic dressing	Kraft	426	126
	Tesco	450	128
Italian oil dressing	Safeway	440	130
Italian salami thin sliced	Waitrose	411	117
	St Michael	491	139
Italian style garlic dressing	St Michael	138	39
Italian style pizza bits	St Michael	473	134
Italian style sausage French bread pizza	Findus	183	52
Italiano ice cream (Wall's): *see flavours*			
Italiano sauce	Whole Earth	60	17
Ivory Coast tuna skipjack steak in oil	Armour	289	per 200g can 578
Jacket scallops	Ross	100	28
Jacket wedges	Ross	120	34
Jackfruit, canned, drained		101	29
Jaffa cakes	Littlewoods	395	per biscuit 40
	St Michael	369	105
	Tesco	378	107
Jaffa crunch biscuits	Peek Frean	444	per biscuit 30
Jaffa dessert cake	Tesco	422	120
Jaffa orange drink	St Michael	110	33

Product	Brand	Calories per 100g/ 100ml	Calories per oz/ pack/ portion
Jaffa orange drink	St Michael	104	31
colour free	St Michael	110	33
long life	Waitrose	37	11
Jaffa orange ice cream	Safeway	221	65
Jaffa orange juice	St Michael	38	11
	St Michael	35	10
	Waitrose	37	11
pressed, long life	Waitrose	39	12
pure	St Michael	38	11
Jaffa orange yoghurt	Safeway	96	per 150g pack 144
	Mr Men	98	28
	Raines	89	25
Jaggery		367	104
Jalapeno bean dip	Old El Paso	106	per 297g can 315
Jalapenos, pickled	Old El Paso	32	per 283g can 91
Jam			
fruit with edible seeds		261	74
stone fruit		261	74
all flavours	Moorhouse	255	per portion 40
all varieties	Robertson's	251	71
no sugar	Whole Earth	120	34
Jam and cream sandwich biscuits	Tesco	419	119
Jam and vanilla chocolate roll	Lyons	385	109
Jam creams	Waitrose	479	136
Jam roly poly	Ross	370	105
Jam sandwich creams	Safeway	470	133
	St Michael	475	135
Jam sponge pudding	Safeway	359	102
	Tesco	333	94

Product	Brand	Calories per 100g/ 100ml	Calories per oz/ pack/ portion
Jam Swiss roll	St Michael	312	88
Jam tarts		384	109
	Lyons	414	117
Jambon de Bayonne, sliced	St Michael	230	65
Jamboree mallows	Peek Frean	382	per biscuit 77
Japanese medlar: see Loquats			
Jarlsberg cheese	Tesco	339	96
	Waitrose	272	77
Jellabi, Asian		309	88
Jelly			
cubes		259	73
made with milk		86	24
made with water		59	17
	Rowntree's	268	76
Jelly animals	Waitrose	311	88
Jelly babies	Bassett's	321	91
	Littlewoods	341	97
	St Michael	323	92
	Tesco	372	105
	Waitrose	311	88
Jelly beans	Bassett's	335	95
	Littlewoods	362	103
	Tesco	340	96
Jelly buttons	Bassett's	315	89
Jelly-Creams			
chocolate	Chivers	365	per portion 160
other flavours	Chivers	370	per portion 160
Jelly crystals			
lemon flavour	Dietade	290	82
orange flavour	Dietade	290	82
raspberry flavour	Dietade	290	82

Product	Brand	Calories per 100g/ 100ml	Calories per oz/ pack/ portion
Jelly crystals strawberry flavour	Dietade	290	82
Jelly diamond cake decorations	Tesco	305	86
Jelly drops	Littlewoods	344	98
Jelly eggs	Bassett's	346	98
Jelly jam, Pure Fruit, all flavours	Hartley's	260	per portion 40
Jelly Jumbo	Wall's		per portion 105
Jelly, table, all flavours	Chivers	290	per portion 100
Jellytots	Rowntree Mackintosh	345	per 46g bag 160
Jersey butter toffees	Needlers	423	120
Jersey creams	Peek Frean	482	per biscuit 58
Jersey liquorice eclairs	Needlers	406	115
Jersey milk chocolate eclairs	Needlers	507	144
Jersey mint eclairs	Needlers	413	117
Jersey potatoes	Waitrose	80	300g/10*oz pack
	Waitrose	80	23
Jersey Royal potatoes, canned	Safeway	53	per 283g can 150
Jew's ear (wood ear), dried tender variety		279	79
tough variety		325	92
Juicy Fruit chewing gum	Wrigley		per stick 9
Jumbo cod fingers, battered	Ross	190	54

Product	Brand	Calories per 100g/100ml	Calories per oz/pack/portion
Jumbo fish fingers and chips snack	Bejam		per serving baked 478
Jumbo grills	Ross	220	62
vegetarian	Protoveg Menu	251	71
Jumbo pork and beef sausages	Bejam		per sausage grilled 281
Jumbo quarterpounders	Ross	265	75
Jumbo sausage rolls	Ross	350	99
Jumbo traditional pasties	Ross	275	78
Junior Drifter	Rowntree Mackintosh	460	per biscuit 75
Junior rolls with jam filling	Waitrose	290	82
Jusoda orange drink	Barr	28	per 250ml can 70
Just apple	Heinz Baby Foods	45	per 128g can or jar 58
Just mints	Tesco	406	115
Kaisar: see Saffron			
Kakdi: see Cucumber			
Kale, fresh, boiled	Tesco	33	9
Kantola			
fresh, raw		19	5
canned, drained		18	5
Karela: see Gourd, bitter			
Kebab (Indian cooked dish)		357	101
Kedgeree		151	43
	St Michael	161	46

Product	Brand	Calories per 100g/ 100ml	Calories per oz/ pack/ portion
Kennett syrup biscuits	Huntley & Palmer	500	per biscuit 63
Kenya coffee			
fine filter, infused	Safeway	2	1
ground, infused	Safeway	2	1
Khira: see Cucumber			
Kia-Ora drinks: see also flavours			
Kia-Ora low sugar drink, concentrated	Schweppes	26	8
Kidney			
lamb, raw		90	26
lamb, fried		155	44
ox, raw		86	24
ox, stewed		172	49
pig, raw		90	26
pig, stewed		153	43
lamb's	Bejam	141	grilled
pig's	Bejam	120	grilled
Kidney beans			
raw		272	77
cooked		76	22
black, dried	Holland and Barrett	272	77
Kidney Beans			
canned, American	Waitrose	82	per 300g pack 246
Kidney beans, red			
raw		272	77
canned	Batchelors	106	30
	Boots	109	31
	Hartley's	105	per 114g can 120
	Safeway	84	per 440g can 370
	St Michael	98	28

Product	Brand	Calories per 100g/ 100ml	Calories per oz/ pack/ portion
Kidney beans, red			
canned	Tesco	125	35
canned, in chilli sauce	Waitrose	95	439g/15*oz can
dried	Boots	272	77
	Holland and Barrett	270	77
	Tesco	311	88
dried, cooked	Tesco	130	cooked
King biscuits	St Michael	508	144
King Cone (Lyons Maid): see flavours			
King size sausage rolls	Bejam		per roll baked 179
	Birds Eye Snacks		per roll baked 190
Kippers			
whole, grilled	Bejam		per kipper 259
Kipper cutlets	Bejam		per cutlet grilled 212
	Waitrose	190	54
chilled	Young's	213	60
Kipper fillets	Ross	210	60
	Waitrose	190	54
boil-in-bag	Bejam		per serving 378
buttered	Birds Eye	194	55
with butter	Findus	191	54
with butter	Ross	200	57
with butter	St Michael	307	87
Kippered mackerel			
chilled	Young's	323	92
fillets	Ross	210	60
Kippers			
baked		205	58
baked (with bones)		111	31

Product	Brand	Calories per 100g/ 100ml	Calories per oz/ pack/ portion
Kippers	Young's	213	60
boned	Waitrose	190	54
frozen, raw	Tesco	237	67
Loch Fyne	St Michael	368	104
whole	Waitrose	152	43
Kiri sparkling apple juice	Bulmer	38	per half pint 109
Kit Kat	Rowntree Mackintosh	505	4-finger bar 250, 2-finger bar 110
Kiwi fruit, fresh	Tesco	63	18
Kiwi fruit yoghurt	Safeway	92	per 150g pack 138
Knickerbocker glory	Bejam		per dessert 272
Knock Knock chews	Trebor	364	per sweet 16
Kola Kubes	Trebor	354	per sweet 17
Kop Kop roll	Trebor	338	per sweet 16
Korma Classic curry sauce	Homepride	83	per 383g pack 318
Korma curry sauce mix	Knorr	382	108
Korma mild curry cooking mix	Colman's	335	95
Krakowska	Waitrose	184	52
Krona margarine	Van den Berghs	740	210
Silver	Van den Berghs	740	210
Krunchy carob bar, no added sugar	Sunwheel Kalibu	432	per 60g bar 259
Kumquats			
fresh	Tesco	80	23
canned		138	39
Lactic cheese, soft	St Ivel	300	85

Product	Brand	Calories per 100g/ 100ml	Calories per oz/ pack/ portion
Lady's fingers: see Okra			
Lager, bottled		29	8
Lager shandy	Corona	24	7
Lamb			
breast, lean and fat, raw		378	107
breast, lean and fat, roast		410	116
breast, lean only, roast		252	71
dressed carcase, raw		333	94
fat, cooked		616	175
fat, raw (average)		671	190
lean, raw (average)		162	46
leg, lean and fat, raw		240	68
leg, lean and fat, roast		266	75
leg, lean only, roast		191	54
scrag and neck, lean and fat, raw		316	90
scrag and neck, lean and fat, stewed		292	83
scrag and neck, lean only, stewed		253	72
scrag and neck, lean only, stewed (with fat)		128	36
shoulder, lean and fat, raw		314	89
shoulder, lean and fat, roast		316	90
shoulder, lean only, roast		196	56
chump chops, grilled	Bejam	272	77
frozen, cooked	Tesco	251	71
heart, braised	Bejam	194	55
home produced	St Michael	280	79
leg steaks, boneless, grilled	Bejam	183	52
leg, roasted	Bejam	236	67
minced, boiled	Bejam	183	52

Product	Brand	Calories per 100g/ 100ml	Calories per oz/ pack/ portion
Lamb			
neck, best end, grilled	Bejam	402	114
roast with mint	Waitrose	271	77
shoulder, roasted	Bejam	289	82
stewing, casseroled	Bejam	293	83
Lamb and liver casserole	Heinz Baby Foods	74	per 170g jar 126
Lamb and noodle casserole	Cow and Gate	70	per 150g jar 105
Lamb boulangere	Waitrose	83	24
Lamb casserole	Boots Baby Foods	65	18
with vegetables	Heinz Baby Foods	80	per 128g can 102
Lamb chops			
loin, lean and fat, raw		377	107
loin, lean and fat, grilled		355	101
loin, lean and fat, grilled (with bone)		277	79
loin, lean only, grilled		222	63
loin, lean only, grilled (with bone)		122	35
loin, grilled	Bejam	303	86
Lamb cubes	Knorr	318	90
Lamb curry	Waitrose	376	107
Lamb cutlets			
lean and fat, raw		386	109
lean and fat, grilled		370	105
lean and fat, grilled (with bone)		244	69
lean only, grilled		222	63
lean only (grilled with fat and bone)		97	27
shoulder, grilled	Bejam	240	68

Product	Brand	Calories per 100g/ 100ml	Calories per oz/ pack/ portion
Lamb dinner	Boots Baby Foods	400	113
	Cow and Gate	65	per 110g jar 72, 150g jar 98
Lamb en croute	Waitrose	341	97
Lamb fingers snack, Goldenbake	Bejam		per finger baked 38
Lamb grills	Bejam		each grilled 229
	Birds Eye Steakhouse		each, grilled or fried 190
Lamb hotpot	Boots Baby Foods	65	18
Lamb kheema		310	88
Lamb mixed grills	Waitrose	211	60
Lamb ragout Cook in the Pot	Crosse & Blackwell	389	110
Lamb rogan josh	Waitrose	136	per 320g pack 435
Lamb samosa	Waitrose	376	per 57g pack 214
Lamb stockpot with vegetables	Heinz Baby Foods	82	per 170g jar 139
Lamb's kidney, grilled	Bejam	141	40
Lamb's liver			
home produced sliced, fried	St Michael	179	51
	Bejam	180	51
Lancashire cheese	Dairy Crest	370	105
	St Ivel	370	105
	Tesco	353	100
	Waitrose	390	111
Lancashire hotpot	Heinz Baby Foods	68	per 128g jar 87
Land salami	Waitrose	436	124

Product	Brand	Calories per 100g/ 100ml	Calories per oz/ pack/ portion
Lard		891	253
	Safeway	899	255
	Tesco	875	248
Dutch	Waitrose	900	255
refined English	Waitrose	900	255
Lasagne	Boots Second Nature	354	100
	St Michael	150	43
	Waitrose	145	41
as sold	Signor Rossi	272	77
dry	Buitoni	350	99
	Buitoni Country Harvest	318	90
egg	Safeway	346	98
egg, Quick-Cook, cooked	Tesco	135	38
egg, Quick-Cook, raw	Tesco	343	97
egg, verdi	Safeway	346	98
frozen	Bejam		per serving baked 527
	Birds Eye MenuMaster	123	per 255g pack 315
	Buitoni	531	151
	Findus	121	34
	St Michael	136	39
Lasagne, vegetarian	Boots Ready Meal	103	29
	Prewetts Ready Meals	91	26
Lasagne verde			
as sold	Signor Rossi	309	88
dry	Buitoni	340	96

Product	Brand	Calories per 100g/ 100ml	Calories per oz/ pack/ portion
Lasagne verde			
egg, Quick-Cook, raw	Tesco	343	97
Lattice pie	Tesco	375	106
cherry and apple	Lyons	314	89
blackcurrant and apple	Lyons	324	92
Lattice sausage rolls	St Michael	396	112
Laverbread		52	15
Layered fish lasagne	St Michael	91	26
Lean roast beef and gravy	Birds Eye MenuMaster	84	per 113g pack 310
Leek and carrot jacket potato	St Michael	141	40
Leek, bacon and tomato savoury	Waitrose	78	397g/14oz pack
Leeks			
raw		31	9
boiled		24	7
	Littlewoods	31	9
creamed	Bejam		per 5 mini portions 52
cut	Bejam	25	per 113g portion boiled 28
Legumes mornay	Waitrose	75	per 397g pack 298
Leicester cheese	Dairy Crest	400	113
	St Ivel	400	113
red	Safeway	400	113
	Tesco	367	104
	Waitrose	390	111
red, farmhouse	Waitrose	390	111
Lemon and barley drink, undiluted	Tesco	107	32

Product	Brand	Calories per 100g/ 100ml	Calories per oz/ pack/ portion
Lemon and honey drink	Lanes	95	28
Lemon and honey health drink	Lanes	75	21
Lemon and lime drink	Littlewoods	34	10
	Quosh	28	8
diabetic low calorie,	Boots	5	2
diluted	Quosh	2	1
undiluted	Quosh	90	27
	Safeway	99	29
	Tesco	89	26
	Waitrose	85	25
Lemon/lime drink, concentrated	Kia-Ora	99	29
Lemon and lime drops	Boots	363	per 33g stick pack 120
Lemon and lime marmalade, fine-cut	Waitrose	248	70
Lemon and lime ripple	St Michael	127	36
Lemon and lime whole fruit drink	Robinsons	95	28
Lemon and lime-flavoured concentrate	Safeway	220	65
Lemon bar	Granose	368	per 50g bar 184
Lemon barley crush, ready to drink	Lucozade	72	21
Lemon barley drink	Boots	120	36
	Robinsons	30	9
diabetic	Boots	10	3
dilutable	Boots Shapers	10	3

Product	Brand	Calories per 100g/ 100ml	Calories per oz/ pack/ portion
Lemon barley drink			
undiluted	Quosh	94	28
Lemon barley water	Corona	91	27
	Robinsons	105	31
	Safeway	95	28
real, undiluted	Quosh	160	47
Lemon Bon Bons	Trebor	403	per sweet 27
Lemon bubble gum	Wrigley Hubba Bubba		15/24 per chunk
Lemon cheese	Moorhouse	295	per portion 45
	Waitrose	329	93
Pure Fruit	Hartley's	295	per portion 45
Lemon cheesecake, baked	St Michael	248	70
Lemon Chinese sauce mix, sweet and sour	Sharwood	296	84
Lemon cream flan	St Michael	365	103
Lemon cream pie	Findus	358	101
Lemon creams	Safeway	478	136
Lemon crisp biscuits	Littlewoods	465	per biscuit 40
	St Michael	465	132
	Tesco	463	131
Lemon curd			
home made		290	82
starch base		283	80
	Chivers	285	per portion 45
	Gales	280	79
	Moorhouse	285	per portion 45
	Robertson's	291	82
	Safeway	294	83
	Tesco	331	94
	Waitrose	276	78
Lemon drink	Lanes	6	2

Product	Brand	Calories per 100g/ 100ml	Calories per oz/ pack/ portion
Lemon drink	Lanes	13	4
	Robinsons	40	12
	Safeway	99	29
concentrated	Schweppes	108	32
	St Michael	117	35
low calorie	Safeway	14	4
	Waitrose	12	4
low calorie, undiluted	Tesco	21	6
undiluted	Tesco	101	30
whole	Boots	101	30
	Waitrose	87	26
whole, diabetic	Boots	7	2
whole, undiluted	Corona	93	28
	Quosh	95	28
with lime juice, sparkling	Tango	35	10
Lemon flavour dessert mix	Dietade	264	75
Lemon flavour jelly crystals	Waitrose	272	77
	Dietade	290	82
Lemon, honey and ginger drink	Boots	140	40
Lemon iced Madeira cake	St Michael	415	118
Lemon jelly	Littlewoods	260	74
	Safeway	268	76
	Tesco	57	16
diabetic crystals	Boots	365	103
Lemon jelly marmalade, fine-cut	Waitrose	248	454g/16oz jar
Lemon juice	Hycal	243	72
	Jif	15	4

Product	Brand	Calories per 100g/ 100ml	Calories per oz/ pack/ portion
Lemon juice	Safeway	7	2
	Tesco	8	2
	Waitrose	13	4
less sharp, dilutable	Boots Shapers	8	2
less sharp, undiluted	PLJ	25	7
longlife	Tesco	48	14
original sharp, undiluted	PLJ	25	7
sharp, dilutable	Boots Shapers	8	2
Lemon Madeira cake mix	Granny Smiths	326	per 365g pack made up 1190
Lemon marmalade, fine shred	Baxters	253	per 340g jar
Lemon mayonnaise	Hellmanns	720	204
	Safeway	745	211
	Waitrose	734	208
Lemon meringue crunch mix (as sold)	Granny Smiths	252	per 780g pack made up 1968
	Tesco	410	116
Lemon meringue pie		323	92
Lemon meringue pie mix	Green's	416	made up per portion 192
Lemon meringues	Lyons	382	108
Lemon mousse	St Michael	237	67
Lemon Pavlova	Young's	295	84
Lemon pie filling mix	Green's	353	made up per portion 55
	Royal	147	per 375g pack made up 552
Lemon puff biscuits	Tesco	492	139

Product	Brand	Calories per 100g/ 100ml	Calories per oz/ pack/ portion
Lemon puffs	Huntley & Palmer	521	per biscuit 80
Lemon shred marmalade	Safeway	251	71
	Tesco	286	81
Lemon slice cake, fresh cream	Tesco	406	115
Lemon sole			
raw		81	23
fried		216	61
fried (with bones)		171	48
steamed		91	26
steamed (with bones and skin)		64	18
fillets	Waitrose	80	23
fillets, chilled	Young's	82	23
fillets, poached	Bejam	102	29
goujons	Young's	223	63
goujons, breaded	Waitrose	150	43
whole	Waitrose	80	23
whole breaded	St Michael	132	37
whole, chilled	Young's	82	23
Lemon sole bonne femme	Young's	85	24
Lemon sorbet	Waitrose	114	34
Lemon sorbet ice cream	Tesco	61	17
	Wall's Alpine		per 1/10 pack 85
scooping	Wall's Italiano	80	per 1/40 4-litre pack 80
Lemon souffle	St Ivel	164	46
	Waitrose	250	71
Lemon squash	St Michael	172	51
diluted	Britvic	19	5

Product	Brand	Calories per 100g/ 100ml	Calories per oz/ pack/ portion
Lemon squash			
diluted	Britvic High Juice	26	7
low calorie	Dietade	2	1
undiluted	Britvic	97	27
	Britvic High Juice	129	37
Lemon Surprise	Bertorelli	225	per 70g pack 158
Lemon tops cake mix	Granny Smiths	355	per 311g pack made up 1104
Lemon torte	Ross	270	77
Lemon water ice	Bertorelli	109	31
Lemon whole fruit drink	Robinsons	95	28
original	Robinsons	140	41
Lemon with sultanas cheesecake	Young's	280	79
Lemon yoghurt	Safeway	92	per 150g pack 138
French style	Littlewoods	102	per 150g pack 153
	St Michael	103	29
Lemonade, bottled		21	6
Lemonade	Barr	30	per 250ml can 75
	Britvic	23	per 150ml can 35
	Corona	24	7
	Hunts	24	7
	Littlewoods	26	8
	Safeway	26	8
	Safeway	23	per 330ml can 76
	Schweppes	23	7
	St Michael	44	13
	Tesco	22	6
	Waitrose	28	8
	Whites	20	per 150ml pack 30

Product	Brand	Calories per 100g/ 100ml	Calories per oz/ pack/ portion
Lemonade			
diabetic	Boots		per 100ml 0.6
Diet	Safeway	-1	
	Whites	2	per 250ml bottle 5
low calorie	Diet Corona	1	per 100ml 0,5
	Schweppes Slimline		per 100ml 0.38
	Tesco	4	1
	Waitrose	5	1
old fashioned	Waitrose	43	13
traditional	Corona	39	12
traditional flavour	Whites	28	per 250ml bottle 70
Lemonade and beer shandy			
low calorie	Schweppes Slimline	6	2
Lemonade and cider	Top Deck	38	11
Lemonade dipper	Barratt	341	97
Lemonade plus	St Michael	39	12
Lemonade shandy	Safeway	13	per 330ml can 43
	Schweppes	25	7
	Top Deck	25	7
Lemonade Sparkles	Wall's		per portion 30
Lemonade with beer, low calorie	Diet Top Deck	11	3
Lemonade-flavoured concentrate	Safeway	193	57
low calorie	Safeway	41	12
Lemons			
juice, fresh		7	2
whole		15	4
Lentil and lamb soup with croutons	Knorr Quick Soup	321	91

Product	Brand	Calories per 100g/ 100ml	Calories per oz/ pack/ portion
Lentil and vegetable casserole	Granose	100	28
Lentil roast	Granose	336	95
Lentil soup		99	28
	Baxters	50	per 425g can 210
	Campbell's Bumper Harvest	45	13
	Granny's	56	as served 37
	Heinz Ready to Serve	35	10
	Tesco	59	17
	Waitrose	49	per 425g can 208
condensed	Campbell's	88	25
dried, as sold	Prewetts Soup in Seconds	296	84
Lentils			
raw		304	86
masur dahl (red), cooked		90	26
masur dahl (red), raw		304	86
split, boiled		99	28
dried	Holland and Barrett	300	85
green, cooked	Tesco	140	40
green, dried	Boots	340	96
green, raw	Tesco	339	96
orange, cooked	Tesco	111	31
orange, raw	Tesco	338	96
red, dried	Boots	340	96
split	Safeway	304	86
split, boiled	Whitworths	99	28
split, dried	Waitrose	304	86
split, raw	Whitworths	304	86

Product	Brand	Calories per 100g/ 100ml	Calories per oz/ pack/ portion
Lettuce			
raw		12	3
	Littlewoods	12	3
iceberg	Tesco	13	4
round Cos crisp	Tesco	12	3
Lico-jet	Barratt	302	86
Licorice chewing gum	PK		per pellet 6
Liga rusks, all flavours	Cow and Gate	381	per rusk 27
Light rice pudding	Ambrosia	76	22
Lilva, canned, drained		65	18
Lime, fresh, raw		36	10
Lime and lemonade	Whites	22	per 250ml bottle 55
Lime cordial drink, undiluted	Tesco	89	25
Lime drink	Safeway	99	29
Lime flavour cordial			
concentrated	Schweppes	101	30
diluted	Britvic	17	5
undiluted	Britvic	86	24
	Corona	89	26
	Quosh	89	26
Lime flavour jelly	Waitrose	272	77
Lime jelly	Safeway	268	76
	Tesco	57	16
table	Littlewoods	260	74
Lime juice cordial			
undiluted		112	32
	Robinsons	90	27
	Waitrose	87	26
concentrated	Rose's	101	30

Product	Brand	Calories per 100g/ 100ml	Calories per oz/ pack/ portion
Lime juice cordial			
diluted	Britvic High Juice	27	8
undiluted	Britvic High Juice	134	38
Lime marmalade	Baxters	248	per 340g jar
	Safeway	251	71
fine-cut	Waitrose	248	70
Lime shred marmalade	Tesco	278	79
Limeade	Corona	23	7
	Safeway	24	7
	Tesco	20	6
Limeade and lager	Top Deck	32	9
Limmits apricot lunchpack	Limmits		per pack 210
Limon, sparkling	Schweppes	44	13
low calorie	Schweppes Slimline	1	
Lincoln biscuits	Peek Frean	486	per biscuit 35
	Tesco	485	137
diabetic	Boots	402	114
Lincoln pea soup, dried	Batchelors	312	per 84g pint pack as sold 262
Lincolnshire sausage	St Michael	350	99
Lion bar	Rowntree Mackintosh	495	per bar 210
Cub	Rowntree Mackintosh	495	per bar 80
Liqueur truffles	St Michael	519	147
fresh cream	St Michael	522	148
Liquid cherry	Rowntree Mackintosh		per sweet 30

Product	Brand	Calories per 100g/ 100ml	Calories per oz/ pack/ portion
Liquorice allsorts		313	89
	Bassett's	342	97
	Littlewoods	368	104
	St Michael	361	102
	Waitrose	368	104
coconut	Tesco	401	114
jellies	Tesco	372	105
liquorice	Tesco	344	98
squares	Tesco	395	112
Liquorice comfits	Bassett's	354	100
Liquorice drops	Boots	402	per 33g stick pack 133
Liquorice Granymels	Itona	395	112
Liquorice novelties	Tesco	321	91
Liquorice pipes	Barratt	295	84
Liquorice powder		212	60
Liquorice toffees	Littlewoods	414	117
	Trebor	456	per sweet 31
Liquorice torpedoes	Bassett's	354	100
Liquorice twists	Tesco	349	99
Lite fat-reduced spread	St Michael	540	153
Little Big Feet jellies	Trebor	289	per sweet 13
Liver			
calf, raw		153	43
calf, fried		254	72
chicken, raw		135	38
chicken, fried		194	55
lamb, raw		179	51
lamb, fried		232	66
ox, raw		163	46
ox, stewed		198	56

Product	Brand	Calories per 100g/ 100ml	Calories per oz/ pack/ portion
Liver			
pig, raw		154	44
pig, stewed		189	54
chicken (frozen)	Waitrose	135	38
lamb's, sliced, fried	Bejam	180	51
lamb, home produced	St Michael	179	51
pig	St Michael	154	44
pig's, fried	Bejam	152	43
turkey (frozen)	Waitrose	145	41
Liver and bacon casserole	Boots Baby Foods	60	17
Liver and bacon dinner	Boots Baby Foods	60	17
	Heinz Baby Foods	65	per 128g can 83
Liver and bacon paste	Shippams	194	per 35g pack 68
Liver casserole cooking mix	Colman's	350	99
Liver sausage		310	88
Liver with onion and gravy	Birds Eye MenuMaster		per pack 190
Lobster			
boiled		119	34
boiled (with shell)		42	12
whole	Waitrose	119	34
Lobster bisque	Baxters	59	per 425g can 251
	St Michael	50	14
	Waitrose	51	per 425g can 217
dried	Nestle Bonne Cuisine	268	76
Lobster flavour crisps	St Michael	533	151
Loch Fyne kippers	St Michael	368	104

Product	Brand	Calories per 100g/100ml	Calories per oz/pack/portion
Lockets	Mars	351	100
Log dessert, Cassata Denise	Wall's		per 1/6 log 105
Loganberries			
raw		17	5
stewed without sugar		16	5
stewed with sugar		54	15
canned		101	29
Lollies			
choc 'n' nut split	Bejam		per lolly 158
orange	Bejam		per lolly 20
raspberry split	Bejam		per lolly 61
Lollipops	Barratt	362	103
Lolly bag	Trebor	411	each, large bag 37, small bag 32
Lollyades	Trebor	363	per sweet 109
London grill (canned)	Crosse & Blackwell	157	45
Long grain and wild rice, made with butter	Uncle Ben's	112	32
Long grain rice	Tesco	356	101
(cooked)	Tesco	99	28
	Whitworths	361	102
American	St Michael	349	99
cooked	Uncle Ben's	115	32
frozen, cooked	Uncle Ben's	131	37
frozen, ready cooked	Bejam	91	per 142g portion 129
three minute, cooked (canned)	Uncle Ben's	113	32
Longan			
canned		63	18

Product	Brand	Calories per 100g/ 100ml	Calories per oz/ pack/ portion
Longan			
dried		256	73
Loquats (Japanese medlar), canned		84	24
Lorne sausage			
sliced	Littlewoods	396	112
sliced Scottish	St Michael	355	101
slicing	Littlewoods	304	86
Lotus tubers, canned		15	4
Low fat spread		366	104
	Safeway	365	103
	Tesco	340	96
with cheese	Sun-Pat	176	50
with cheese and garden herbs	Sun-Pat	176	50
with cheese and onion	Sun-Pat	176	50
Low sugar drink, concentrated	Kia-Ora	26	8
Lucozade		68	19
	Beecham	72	21
Lumachine verde bianche	Waitrose	222	63
Luncheon meat			
canned		313	89
sliced	Tesco	310	88
Luxury all butter rich fruit cake	Tesco	345	98
Luxury cheesecake mix (Tesco): see flavours			
Luxury mincemeat	Safeway	267	76
with brandy, glace cherries and almonds	Waitrose	275	78
Luxury pizza	Tesco	226	64

Product	Brand	Calories per 100g/ 100ml	Calories per oz/ pack/ portion
Luxury sponge mix	Granny Smiths	342	per 355g pack made up 1216
	Whitworths	425	120
dry	Tesco	431	122
made up	Tesco	370	105
Lychee yoghurt	Safeway	94	per 150g pack 141
Lychees			
fresh, raw		64	18
canned in syrup		68	19
Lymeswold cheese	Dairy Crest	425	120
white	Dairy Crest	425	120
Lys bleu cheese	Waitrose	303	86
M & Ms			
peanut	Mars	500	142
plain	Mars	483	137
Macadamia nuts	Holland and Barrett	760	215
	St Michael	691	196
Macaroni			
raw		348	99
boiled		117	33
	Boots Second Nature	354	100
	Buitoni Country Harvest	318	90
	Waitrose	378	107
cooked	Tesco	167	47
frozen	St Michael	140	40
quick, dry	Buitoni	340	96
Quick-Cook	Tesco	348	99
Quick-Cook, cooked	Tesco	152	43
raw	Tesco	348	99
short-cut	Safeway	344	98

Product	Brand	Calories per 100g/ 100ml	Calories per oz/ pack/ portion
Macaroni			
wholewheat	Waitrose	325	92
Macaroni cheese		174	49
	Birds Eye MenuMaster		per pack 470
canned	Crosse & Blackwell	102	29
	Heinz	106	30
Macaroni cheese	Heinz Baby Foods	89	per 128g can 114
Macaroni, creamed	Ambrosia	92	26
Macaroni Verdi, Quick-Cook	Tesco	343	97
Mackerel			
raw		223	63
fried		188	53
fried (with bones)		138	39
canned in brine	Shippams	201	per 425g can 854
canned in tomato sauce	Shippams	198	per 425g can 842
frozen, cooked	Tesco	310	88
frozen, raw	Tesco	302	86
hot peppered (frozen), cooked	Tesco	363	103
kippered	Young's	323	92
kippered fillets	Ross	210	60
	St Michael	310	88
peppered	Young's	333	94
smoked fillets	Ross	300	85
	St Michael	300	85
	Waitrose	256	73
smoked fillets, hot	Bejam	296	84

Product	Brand	Calories per 100g/ 100ml	Calories per oz/ pack/ portion
Mackerel			
smoked, with crushed peppercorns	Waitrose	256	73
steaks canned in brine	Armour	229	per 200g can 458
whole	Young's	275	78
Madeira cake		393	111
	Tesco	365	103
	Waitrose	437	124
all butter	Safeway	376	107
	Waitrose	370	105
butter	Lyons	378	107
cherry	Tesco	350	99
lemon iced	St Michael	415	118
with buttercream filling	Waitrose	309	88
Madeira cake mix			
classic	Green's	431	per portion made up 135
lemon	Granny Smiths	326	per 365g pack made up 1190
Madeira sandwich cake, iced	Waitrose	423	120
Madeira wine Cooking-in Sauce	Baxters	63	per 425g can 268
Madeleines			
apricot	Lyons	335	95
raspberry	Lyons	333	94
Madras Classic curry sauce	Homepride	82	per 383g pack 314
Madras curry, dry	Beanfeast	269	76

Product	Brand	Calories per 100g/ 100ml	Calories per oz/ pack/ portion
Madras curry Cook in the Pot	Crosse & Blackwell	442	125
Madras curry mix	Tesco	337	96
Madras hot curry Cooking-in Sauce	Baxters	83	per 425g can 353
Madras medium curry cooking mix	Colman's	335	95
Main Course soups (Campbell's): *see flavours*			
Maize flour	Holland and Barrett	370	105
Major Grey chutney	Sharwood	217	62
Makes Five Pints	Tesco	485	137
Mallard, fresh	Waitrose	400	113
Mallow tea cakes	Littlewoods	446	per biscuit 46
Mallows			
coconut	Peek Frean	384	per biscuit 46
jamboree	Peek Frean	382	per biscuit 77
milk coated	Peek Frean	433	per biscuit 52
orange coated	Peek Frean	433	per biscuit 52
Malt crunch biscuits	Peek Frean	420	per biscuit 35
Malt loaf	St Michael Sunblest Sun Malt	267	76
		262	74
fruited	Waitrose	243	69
wholemeal	Allinson	247	70
Malt loaf bread	Tesco	262	74
Malt vinegar	Tesco	4	1
	Waitrose	4	1
traditional	Tesco	4	1
Malted chocolate drink	Tesco	390	111

Product	Brand	Calories per 100g/100ml	Calories per oz/pack/portion
Malted Complan powder	Farley	444	per 57g sachet 253
Malted drink	Boots	358	101
	Tesco	398	113
	Waitrose	385	109
instant	Boots	394	112
instant, with honey flavour	Boots	392	111
Malted food drink	Horlicks	386	114
low fat, instant	Horlicks	382	113
Malted milk (as sold)	Safeway	385	109
Malted milk biscuits	St Michael	466	132
	Tesco	501	142
	Waitrose	466	200g/7oz pack
Malted milk chocolate sandwich bar	St Michael	496	141
Malted milk creams	Tesco	474	134
Malted white drink	Wander	385	109
Maltesers	Mars	500	142
Maltlets	Horlicks	386	109
Mandarin crush	St Michael	44	13
Mandarin juice			
long life	Waitrose	40	12
pure	St Michael	37	11
Mandarin orange fruit harvest ice cream	Lyons Maid	149	42
Mandarin oranges			
canned in syrup		56	16
in light syrup	Waitrose	67	19
in natural juice	Waitrose	45	13
Mandarin yoghurt	Safeway	93	per 150g pack 140

Product	Brand	Calories per 100g/ 100ml	Calories per oz/ pack/ portion
Mandarin yoghurt	St Ivel Shape	42	12
	Waitrose	93	per 150g pack 140
low fat	Diet Ski	56	per 150g pack 84
	Littlewoods	82	per 150g pack 123
Mandarins, Spanish	Safeway	56	per 312g can 176
Mange tout			
fresh, cooked	Tesco	34	10
frozen	Bejam	47	per 85g portion 40
Mango and ginger chutney	Sharwood	223	63
Mango chutney			
oily, whole contents		285	81
	Pan Yan	196	56
	Waitrose	221	63
Green Label	Sharwood	217	62
Mango fruit cocktail ice cream	Tesco	165	47
Mango juice		44	12
Mangoes			
fresh, raw		59	17
canned in syrup		77	22
Maple and walnut ice cream	Safeway	234	litre pack
	Tesco	186	53
American style	Waitrose	171	51
Marathon	Mars	508	144
Marble cake	Tesco	429	122
Marcona almonds	St Michael	565	160
Margarine, all kinds		730	207
	Granose	750	213
	Holland and Barrett	730	207

Product	Brand	Calories per 100g/ 100ml	Calories per oz/ pack/ portion
Margarine	Littlewoods	2960	839
	Rakusen	740	210
	Tesco	734	208
blended	Waitrose	730	207
blended soft	Waitrose	735	208
Blue Band	Van den Berghs	740	210
cooking	Safeway	726	206
de Luxe	Safeway	733	208
Echo	Van den Berghs	740	210
Flora Sunflower	Van den Berghs	740	210
Gold	St Ivel	390	111
Krona	Van den Berghs	740	210
Krona Silver	Van den Berghs	740	210
low fat spread	Littlewoods	1480	420
low salt	Granose	750	213
Luxury	Kraft	730	207
premier	Tesco	734	208
salt free	Tesco	734	208
soft	Tesco	734	208
soft, Dutch	Littlewoods	733	208
soya	Safeway	730	207
soya soft	Waitrose	735	208
special soft tub	Kraft	730	207
Stork	Van den Berghs	740	210
Stork Special Blend	Van den Berghs	740	per 250g pack
sunflower	Granose	720	204
	Littlewoods	740	210
	Safeway	735	208
	Tesco	734	208
	Waitrose	735	208
sunflower salt-free	Safeway	735	208
sunflower soft	St Michael	730	207
Superfine	Kraft	730	207
supersoft	Tesco	734	208

Product	Brand	Calories per 100g/ 100ml	Calories per oz/ pack/ portion
Margarine			
superspread soft	St Michael	730	207
table	Safeway	733	208
Tomor	Van den Berghs	740	210
Vitalite sunflower	Kraft	730	207
Margherita pizza	St Michael	218	62
Marie biscuits	Tesco	441	125
Marie Rose dressing	St Michael	740	210
Mariner's bake	St Michael	107	30
Mariners pasta gratin	Birds Eye MenuMaster		per pack 370
Marmalade		261	74
	Moorhouse	250	per portion 40
all flavours	Chivers	255	per portion 40
	Roses	255	per portion 40
all other varieties	Robertson's	251	71
chunky	Safeway	251	71
coarse cut	Safeway	251	71
diabetic	Dietade	230	65
diabetic, fine cut	Boots	239	68
diabetic, thick cut	Boots	239	68
fine cut	Tesco	290	82
fresh fruit	St Michael	240	68
ginger preserve	Tesco	275	78
Golden Shred	Robertson's	251	71
lemon shred	Safeway	251	71
	Tesco	286	81
lime	Safeway	251	71
lime shred	Tesco	278	79
mature thick cut	Tesco	250	71
	Safeway	251	71
medium cut	Safeway	251	71
no added sugar	Safeway	139	39
no sugar	Whole Earth	120	34

Product	Brand	Calories per 100g/ 100ml	Calories per oz/ pack/ portion
Marmalade			
orange	Tesco	243	69
orange shred	Safeway	251	71
orange, thin cut,	Heinz Weight		
reduced sugar	Watchers	124	per 6ml
original thick cut	Robertson's	251	71
Pure Fruits, all			
flavours	Hartley's	255	per portion 40
reduced sugar	Boots	154	44
Silver Shred	Robertson's	251	71
thick cut	Tesco	279	79
	Waitrose	248	70
Marmite		179	51
	Beecham	179	51
Marrow			
canned, drained		11	3
raw		16	5
boiled		7	2
large, raw		16	5
small parwal, fresh, raw		14	4
fresh, boiled	Tesco	9	3
Marrowfat peas: see *Peas, marrowfat*			
Mars Bar		441	125
	Mars	454	129
Marshmallow	Tesco	383	109
Marvel	Cadbury's	355	per portion 10
Marzipan (almond paste)		443	126
	Safeway	408	116
	Tesco	437	124
(almond)	Whitworths	412	117
golden	Waitrose	408	116
white	Waitrose	408	116

Product	Brand	Calories per 100g/ 100ml	Calories per oz/ pack/ portion
Marzipan bars, diabetic	Boots	465	132
Mashed potatoes, old		119	34
Mashed potatoes: see also Instant			
Masur dahl: see Lentils, red			
Masur savoury snack		644	183
Matchmakers, long all flavours	Rowntree Mackintosh	485	per sweet 20
Matoki: see Plantain			
Matzo		384	109
Matzo crackers wheaten	Rakusen	347	per biscuit 17
	Rakusen	340	per biscuit 17
Mayonnaise		718	204
	Heinz	530	150
	Littlewoods	734	208
	Safeway	745	211
	St Michael	734	208
	Tesco	711	202
	Waistline	378	107
	Waitrose	734	208
French garlic	St Michael	753	213
	Hellmanns	720	204
	Safeway	745	211
	Waitrose	734	208
lemon	Hellmanns	720	204
	Safeway	745	211
	Waitrose	734	208
low calorie	Boots Shapers	382	108
	St Michael	298	84
Real reduced calorie	Hellmanns	720	204
	Hellmanns	293	83

Product	Brand	Calories per 100g/ 100ml	Calories per oz/ pack/ portion
Mayonnaise			
reduced calorie	Waitrose	734	208
Meat and potato pie	Littlewoods	280	per 177g pack 496
	Tesco	273	77
Meat paste		173	49
Meatballs			
beef gravy	Campbell's	82	23
curry sauce	Campbell's	114	32
onion gravy	Campbell's	84	24
spicey, in tomato sauce	Waitrose	150	per 350g pack 525
tomato sauce	Campbell's	96	27
Meatballs and pasta			
in barbecue sauce	Tyne Brand	133	38
in tomato sauce	Tyne Brand	130	37
Meatless savoury cuts	Granose	88	25
Meatloaf style soya mix	Hera	480	136
Mediterranean juice	St Ivel Real	35	10
Mediterranean vegetable soup	St Michael	37	10
Medium curry cooking sauce	St Michael	41	12
Medium curry Cooking-in Sauce	Baxters	91	per 425g can 387
Medlars		42	12
Megabars	Peek Frean	376	per biscuit 97
Megabite			
banana and chocolate	Wall's		per megabite 120
toffee and chocolate	Wall's		per megabite 120
Mela Menthe	Bertorelli	306	per 70g pack 213

Product	Brand	Calories per 100g/ 100ml	Calories per oz/ pack/ portion
Mela Parisienne	Bertorelli	302	per 70g pack 211
Mela Stregata	Bertorelli	298	per 70g pack 208
Melba toast	Buitoni	382	108
Melbury cheese	Dairy Crest	320	91
Mellora	Carnation	425	per 9g sachet 40
Melon			
cantaloupe, raw		24	7
cantaloupe, raw (with skin)		15	4
honeydew, raw		21	6
honeydew yellow, raw		21	6
honeydew yellow, raw (with skin)		13	4
musk, raw		24	7
Galia	Tesco	24	7
honeydew	Tesco	21	6
Ogen	Tesco	24	7
rock	Tesco	24	7
Melon seeds		581	165
Melon yogurt			
low calorie	Diet Ski	55	per 150g pack 83
Melt in the Bag cake covering			
milk chocolate	Lyons	549	156
plain chocolate	Lyons	572	162
Melton Mowbray pie	Tesco	358	101
Melton Mowbray pork pie	St Michael	402	114
	Waitrose	403	114
individual	Waitrose	377	per 127g pie 479
large	St Michael	353	100
Menthol Eucalyptus	Boots	363	per 33g stick pack 120
Menthol fruits	Trebor	362	per sweet 25

Product	Brand	Calories per 100g/ 100ml	Calories per oz/ pack/ portion
Menthol mints	Boots	363	per 33g stick pack 120
MenuMaster meals (Birds Eye): *see flavours*			
Meringue nests	Littlewoods	311	88
	Safeway	312	per meringue 17
	St Michael	380	108
	Tesco	371	105
Meringues		380	108
fresh cream	St Michael	338	96
Merlin's Brew	Lyons Maid		each 65
Mexican bean stew	Granose	130	37
Mexican chilli (dry)	Beanfeast	292	83
Mexican honey, set	Safeway	300	85
Mexican mix vegetables	Bejam	55	per 85g portion boiled 47
Mighty white bread			
medium	Sunblest	237	per slice 78
thick	Sunblest	237	per slice 95
Milanese sauce	Buitoni	47	per 283g can 133
	Tesco	76	22
	Waitrose	62	per 425g can 264
Milanese souffle	Young's	245	69
Mild chicken curry (canned)	St Michael	112	32
Mild creamy curried chicken soup	Heinz Classic Soups	52	15
Mild curry (dry)	Beanfeast	282	80
Mild curry dressing	Heinz All Seasons	276	78
Mild curry rice, frozen, cooked	Uncle Ben's	136	39

Product	Brand	Calories per 100g/ 100ml	Calories per oz/ pack/ portion
Mild curry Saucy Noodles	Batchelors	326	per 115g pack as sold 375
Mild curry savoury rice	Batchelors	338	per 137g sachet as sold 463
Mild Curry Super Noodles	Batchelors	465	per pack as sold 460
Mild mustard Dish of the Day	Crosse & Blackwell	394	112
Mild mustard pickle	Heinz Ploughman's	114	32
Mild mustard relish	Tesco	128	36
Milk			
evaporated, whole, unsweetened		158	45
skimmed		33	9
skimmed, dried		355	101
sterilised		65	18
whole, fresh		65	18
whole, dried		490	139
whole, Channel Islands, fresh		76	22
	St Michael	66	19
Channel Island	Waitrose	76	1 pint 440
dried, skimmed	Littlewoods	514	146
	Tesco	341	97
dried, skimmed, low fat	Waitrose	355	101
evaporated	Carnation	160	45
	Libby	158	45
	Safeway	159	45
	Waitrose	159	per 170g can 270
fresh skimmed	Waitrose	40	1 pint 240
full cream	Waitrose	65	2 pints 760
full cream, long life	Safeway	67	litre pack 670

Product	Brand	Calories per 100g/ 100ml	Calories per oz/ pack/ portion
Milk			
goat's	Holland and Barrett	70	21
instant	Country Maid	355	101
instant dried	Safeway	350	per 198g can 693
pasteurised	Tesco	65	18
pasteurised, longlife	Tesco	64	18
pasteurised, semi-skimmed	Littlewoods	50	14
	Waitrose	47	1 pint 280
pasteurised, skimmed	Waitrose	34	1 pint 200
semi-skimmed	Tesco	48	14
skimmed	St Michael	33	9
	Tesco	33	9
sterilised, skimmed	Safeway	34	500ml pack 170
whole, pasteurised	Littlewoods	66	per litre pack 660
Milk, dried			
powder, skimmed		355	101
Fivepints (as sold)	St Ivel	470	133
Fivepints (made up)	St Ivel	46	per pint 270
instant skimmed	Boots	355	101
Makes Five Pints	Tesco	485	137
Milquik (made up)	St Ivel	34	per pint 200
Milquik (powder)	St Ivel	355	101
Milk, UHT			
longlife		65	18
full cream	Waitrose	65	500ml pack 325
semi-skimmed	Waitrose	46	500ml pack 230
skimmed	Waitrose	34	500ml pack 170
skimmed, long life	Safeway	35	litre pack 350
	Tesco	34	10

Product	Brand	Calories per 100g/ 100ml	Calories per oz/ pack/ portion
Milk, UHT **skimmed, with vegetable fat**	Waitrose	500	142
Milk assorted biscuits	Cadbury's	495	per biscuit 60
Milk caramel wafers	Safeway	567	161
Milk choc ices	Waitrose	290	86
Milk chocolate		529	150
caramel filled	Littlewoods	495	140
diabetic	Boots	512	145
mint filled	Littlewoods	480	136
orange filled	Littlewoods	480	136
pineapple filled	Littlewoods	505	143
raspberry filled	Littlewoods	505	143
Milk chocolate bar	Boots Shapers Meal	532	151
	Tesco	541	153
with hazelnuts	St Michael	550	156
with strawberry and creme	St Michael	572	162
Milk chocolate Bounty	Mars	483	137
Milk chocolate brazil nuts	Littlewoods	553	157
Milk chocolate Brazils	Tesco	565	160
Milk chocolate breaktime biscuit	Waitrose	590	167
Milk chocolate buttons	St Michael	510	145
Milk chocolate caramel wafers	St Michael	455	129
Milk chocolate coated rings	Tesco	503	143

Product	Brand	Calories per 100g/ 100ml	Calories per oz/ pack/ portion
Milk chocolate coronet creams	Safeway	539	153
Milk chocolate covered roll	Waitrose	428	121
Milk chocolate crunch biscuits	St Michael	483	137
Milk chocolate currant topped caramel wafer	St Michael	481	136
Milk chocolate digestive biscuits	Cadbury's	490	per biscuit 50
	Safeway	505	143
	St Michael	500	142
	Tesco	504	143
Milk chocolate digestives	Waitrose	499	141
Milk chocolate drops diabetic	Tesco	507	144
	Boots	512	145
Milk chocolate eclairs	Cadbury's	450	each pocket pack 20, standard pack 40
	St Michael	445	126
Milk chocolate finger wafers	St Michael	518	147
Milk chocolate fingers	Safeway	528	150
Milk chocolate fruit and nut cereal bars	St Michael	494	140
Milk chocolate fudge bars	St Michael	447	127
Milk chocolate hazelnut caramel bar	St Michael	467	132
Milk chocolate hazelnut crunch bar	St Michael	520	147

Product	Brand	Calories per 100g/ 100ml	Calories per oz/ pack/ portion
Milk chocolate honeycomb gemini	Littlewoods	428	121
Milk chocolate mint sandwich biscuits	Littlewoods	509	144
Milk chocolate orange sandwich bar	St Michael	494	140
	Waitrose	517	147
Milk chocolate orange sandwich biscuits	Littlewoods	506	143
Milk chocolate orange wafer fingers	Waitrose	470	133
Milk chocolate peanut crunch bars	St Michael	509	144
Milk chocolate petit beurre biscuits	Waitrose	468	133
Milk chocolate Polka Dots	Lyons	493	140
Milk chocolate rolls with raspberry filling	Waitrose	365	103
with vanilla filling	Waitrose	453	128
Milk chocolate sandwich bar	Waitrose	516	146
Milk chocolate sandwich biscuits	Littlewoods	506	143
	St Michael	507	144
Milk chocolate snack fingers	Tesco	556	158
Milk chocolate sunota biscuits (half-coated)	Safeway	500	142
Milk chocolate tea cakes	St Michael	440	125

Product	Brand	Calories per 100g/ 100ml	Calories per oz/ pack/ portion
Milk chocolate toffee cups	St Michael	490	139
Milk chocolate truffle	Rowntree Mackintosh		per sweet 40
Milk chocolate wafer bar	Boots Shapers Meal	520	147
Milk chocolate wafer fingers	Waitrose	480	136
Milk chocolate wafers	Littlewoods	530	per wafer 104
Milk chocolate, diabetic filled with coffee cream	Boots	574	163
filled with **strawberry cream**	Boots	552	156
filled with yogurt **cream**	Boots	556	158
hazelnut	Boots	518	147
Milk chocolates	Nestle	534	151
Milk Club biscuits	Jacobs	510	per biscuit 117
Milk coated mallows	Peek Frean	433	per biscuit 52
Milk drink	St Ivel Shape	45	13
Milk half coated digestive biscuits	Huntley & Palmer	502	per biscuit 65
Milk orange fingers	Safeway	487	138
Milk pudding		131	37
rice		91	26
Milk, soya	Granose	50	15
carob	Granose	59	17
coconut	Granose	70	21
strawberry	Granose	64	19
sugar free	Granose	42	12

Product	Brand	Calories per 100g/ 100ml	Calories per oz/ pack/ portion
Milk, goats'		71	20
Milk, human			
mature		69	20
transitional		67	19
Milky bar chocolates	Nestle	540	153
Milky Way	Mars	433	123
Millet	Holland and Barrett	380	108
Millet flakes	Holland and Barrett	381	108
Milquik	St Ivel	34	per pint made up 200
powder	St Ivel	355	101
Mince beef and onion pie	Littlewoods	320	per pie 453
Mince Bolognese	Tyne Brand	122	35
Mince pies		435	123
	Littlewoods	369	105
	Tesco	394	112
	Waitrose	369	105
deep	Safeway	380	108
puff pastry	Waitrose	391	111
wholemeal	Waitrose	401	114
Minced beef and onion	Tesco	163	46
	Tyne Brand	118	34
Minced beef and onion pie			
canned	Tyne Brand	193	55
family (frozen)	Ross	290	82
	Tesco	277	79
frozen	Safeway	294	83
individual	Waitrose	287	81

Product	Brand	Calories per 100g/ 100ml	Calories per oz/ pack/ portion
Minced beef and onion pie			
individual (frozen)	Tesco	315	89
large oval	Waitrose	282	80
Minced beef and onion roll (chilled)	Tesco	295	84
Minced beef and vegetable pie			
value	Birds Eye		per pie for one 410
	Birds Eye		per pie for 2/3 1070
Minced beef and vegetable plate pie	St Michael	265	75
Minced beef and vegetables (canned)	Campbell's	99	28
Minced beef and vegetables	Boots Baby Foods	63	18
Minced beef in rich gravy (canned)	St Michael	150	43
Minced beef lattice roll with cheese, tomato and herb filling	Waitrose	293	83
Minced beef pancakes	Birds Eye Snacks		each shallow-fried 130
	Findus	159	45
Minced beef pie	Waitrose	267	per 142g pie 380
	Waitrose	298	per 454g pie 1344
topcrust	St Michael	210	60
traditional, small	St Michael	336	95
Minced beef roll	St Michael	297	84
savoury	Bejam		per half roll 529
Minced beef rolls with mustard	Waitrose	333	94

Product	Brand	Calories per 100g/ 100ml	Calories per oz/ pack/ portion
Minced beef savoury toasts	Findus	199	56
Minced beef with vegetables in gravy	Birds Eye MenuMaster		per pack 150
Minced lamb rolls	Waitrose	341	97
Minced soya and onion	Protoveg Menu	359	102
Minced steak and onion pie filling	Fray Bentos	196	56
Mincemeat		235	67
	Moorhouse	285	per portion 45
	Safeway	271	77
	Waitrose	275	78
luxury	Safeway	267	76
	Tesco	272	77
luxury, with brandy cherries and almonds	Waitrose	275	78
ordinary	Tesco	338	96
Pure Fruit	Hartley's	285	per portion 45
standard	Robertson's	266	75
traditional	Robertson's	266	75
Minestrone soup			
dried		298	84
dried, as served		23	7
canned	Baxters	32	per 425g can 136
	Campbell's Bumper Harvest	43	12
	Crosse & Blackwell	48	14
	Heinz Ready to Serve	31	9
	Tesco	50	14

Product	Brand	Calories per 100g/ 100ml	Calories per oz/ pack/ portion
Minestrone soup	Waitrose	47	per 425g can 200
dried	Batchelors	275	per 48g pint pack as sold 132
	Hera	384	109
	Knorr	312	88
	Littlewoods	339	per 37g pint packet 125
	Tesco	362	103
	Waitrose	307	per 68g pack 209
	Safeway	323	92
dried, instant	Tesco	338	96
dried, instant, special (made up)	Safeway	39	11
dried, made up	Chef Box	28	8
dried, with croutons	Batchelors Cup-a-Soup Special	339	per 23g pack as sold 78
	Knorr Quick Soup	359	102
Minestrone soup mix	Bejam		1/6 serving boiled 108
	St Michael	350	99
Mini Milk ice cream			
strawberry	Wall's		per portion 40
vanilla	Wall's		per portion 35
Mini pizza	St Michael	282	80
Mini waffles	Birds Eye		per pack baked or grilled 22, fried 27
Ministick chocolate bars			
fruits of the forest	St Michael	473	134
hazelnut	St Michael	550	156
Ministicks			
mint	St Michael	476	135
Mocca	St Michael	554	157

Product	Brand	Calories per 100g/ 100ml	Calories per oz/ pack/ portion
Minstrels	Mars	500	142
Mint and crispy choc bar	Wall's		per bar 185
Mint assortment	St Michael	375	106
	Waitrose	377	107
Mint carob bar	Kalibu	413	per 75g bar 310
Mint chews	St Michael	370	105
Mint choc chip Cornetto	Wall's		per cone 235
Mint choc chip dessert	Birds Eye Supermousse		per tub 140
Mint choc chip ice cream	Bejam Lyons Maid	169	48
	Gold Seal Lyons Maid	196	56
	Napoli	224	64
scooping	Wall's Italiano	120	per 1/40 4-litre pack 120
Mint choc ices	Waitrose	290	86
Mint choc King Cone	Lyons Maid		per cone 202
Mint choc ice cream Sweet Trolley	Wall's Italiano	125	per 1/10 litre pack 125
Mint chocolate chip ice cream, American style	Waitrose	199	59
Mint chocolate dessert	Waitrose	432	122
Mint Club biscuits	Jacobs	495	per biscuit 113
Mint creams	Trebor	342	per sweet 32
Mint Crisp	Lyons Maid		each 158
Mint Crisp block	Needlers	508	per 45g pack 229
Mint crisp chocolates	Waitrose	489	139

Product	Brand	Calories per 100g/ 100ml	Calories per oz/ pack/ portion
Mint filled milk chocolate	Littlewoods	480	136
Mint Granymels	Itona	370	105
Mint humbugs	Boots	371	per 33g stick pack 122
	Littlewoods	352	100
	Waitrose	362	103
soft centre	Needlers	356	101
Mint imperials	Littlewoods	373	106
	Needlers	389	110
	Tesco	379	107
diabetic	Boots	380	108
	Boots	371	105
Mint jelly	Baxters	257	per 175g jar 449
	Colman's	265	75
	Safeway	265	75
	Tesco	266	75
Mint ministicks	St Michael	476	135
Mint relish, spicy	Branston	113	32
Mint sauce	Baxters	121	per 145g jar 175
	Safeway	17	5
	Tesco	100	28
	Waitrose	80	23
fresh garden	Colman's	10	3
garden	Safeway	10	3
sweet, concentrated	O.K.	40	11
Mint sensations	Needlers	435	123
Mint sticks	Tesco	519	147
Mint toffees	Trebor	456	per sweet 31
Mint truffles	St Michael	605	172
Mint whip dessert	Wall's		per dessert 190

Product	Brand	Calories per 100g/ 100ml	Calories per oz/ pack/ portion
Minted peas (frozen)	Safeway	80	23
Mintola	Rowntree Mackintosh	450	per sweet 25
Mints			
Extra strong	Needlers	364	103
extra strong roll	Trebor	378	per sweet 10
Minute steak (frozen), grilled	Bejam	173	49
Miracle whip dressing	Kraft	440	125
Miso sauce	Sunwheel	161	46
Mr Juicy			
apple	St Ivel	39	12
grapefruit	St Ivel	31	9
orange	St Ivel	38	11
pineapple	St Ivel	40	12
Mr Men			
all flavours	Lyons Maid	45	each 20
Mr Men Cartoons cake mix (as sold)	Green's	409	made up per portion 64
Mr Men fruit gums	Bassett's	308	87
Mr Men yogurt (Raines): *see flavours*			
Mr Softee soft ice cream	Lyons Maid	139	39
Mivvi			
pineapple super	Lyons Maid		each 82
raspberry Fun Size	Lyons Maid	120	34
strawberry	Lyons Maid		each 77
Mixed cereal breakfast	Boots Baby Foods	375	106

Product	Brand	Calories per 100g/ 100ml	Calories per oz/ pack/ portion
Mixed cereal with wholewheat and wheatgerm	Boots Baby Foods	420	119
Mixed fruit dried	Waitrose	243	69
	Safeway	247	70
	Tesco	306	87
Mixed fruit	Heinz Baby Foods	53	per 128g can or jar 68
Mixed fruit bar	Granose	384	per 50g bar 192
Mixed fruit dessert	Boots Baby Foods	55	16
Mixed fruit drink	Tesco	48	14
Mixed fruit drops	Boots	363	per 33g stick pack 120
Mixed fruits in natural syrup, chunky	Libby	52	15
Mixed fruit jam	Safeway	248	70
Mixed fruit pickle, spiced	Baxters	159	per 305g jar 484
Mixed fruit salad	Boots Baby Foods	55	16
Mixed fruit sponge pudding	Heinz	298	84
Mixed fruit trifle, individual	Young's	150	43
Mixed fruit yogurt dessert	Cow and Gate	60	per 110g jar 66
Mixed grain kasha	Bewell Amazing Grains	364	103
Mixed nuts chopped	Whitworths	564	160

Product	Brand	Calories per 100g/ 100ml	Calories per oz/ pack/ portion
Mixed nuts			
raw	Tesco	611	173
salted	Tesco	641	182
	Waitrose	655	186
salted/roasted	Safeway	532	151
Mixed nuts and fruit	Safeway	536	152
Mixed nuts and raisins	Sooner	488	per 25g pack 122
	Waitrose	535	152
bag	Tesco	464	132
no salt	Tesco	566	160
tub	Tesco	516	146
Mixed nuts, raisins and chocolate chips	Tesco	489	139
Mixed peel	Whitworths	244	69
cut	Safeway	252	71
	Tesco	249	71
	Waitrose	212	60
Mixed peppers			
chopped	Waitrose	20	6
dried	Tesco	205	58
	Whitworths	212	60
frozen	Ross	20	6
	Safeway	14	4
Mixed peppers frozen, sliced	Bejam	30	per 57g portion boiled 17
Mixed pickle	Haywards	9	3
	Waitrose	21	6
clear	Safeway	8	2
Continental	Safeway	19	5
in mild vinegar	Haywards New Seasons	33	9

Product	Brand	Calories per 100g/ 100ml	Calories per oz/ pack/ portion
Mixed salad			
in French dressing	Littlewoods	75	21
	Tesco	71	20
in French dressing, other recipes	Tesco	52	15
with sweetcorn	Haywards New Seasons	38	11
Mixed salad and beansprouts	Safeway	56	16
Mixed spice	Safeway	367	104
	Tesco	281	80
Mixed toffees		430	122
Mixed vegetable and spice soup	Boots Second Nature	338	96
Mixed vegetable curry		181	51
Mixed vegetable savoury	Boots Baby Foods	63	18
Mixed vegetable savoury rice	Batchelors	333	per 125g sachet as sold 416
	Safeway	333	per 125g pack 416
	Whitworths	310	88
special	Batchelors	326	per 119g sachet as sold 388
Mixed vegetables	Safeway	37	per 284g pack 105
	Waitrose	68	per 454g pack 304
	Waitrose	35	per 907g pack 320
canned	Hartley's	55	per 109g can 60
canned	Tesco	44	12
canned	Waitrose	43	per 300g can 129
casserole mix	Ross	20	6
casserole mix	Tesco	34	10
Casserole vegetables	Birds Eye	35	10

Product	Brand	Calories per 100g/ 100ml	Calories per oz/ pack/ portion
Mixed vegetables			
Cauliflower, peas and carrots	Birds Eye	35	10
Chicken Provencale	Ross	70	20
chilli bean mix	Bejam	105	per 142g stir-fried 149
Chinese chicken	Ross	80	23
Chinese prawns	Ross	50	14
Continental	Safeway	57	16
Continental mix	Bejam	36	per 113g portion boiled 41
Continental vegetable mix	Tesco	313	89
Country mix	Findus	55	16
Country mix	Ross	30	9
dried	Batchelors Surprise	231	per 88g sachet as sold 203
	Tesco	360	102
	Whitworths	258	73
farmhouse	Ross	30	9
farmhouse-style mix	Bejam	22	per 113g portion boiled 25
French vegetable mix	Ross	25	7
frozen	Bejam	58	per 57g portion boiled 33
	Findus	59	17
	Safeway	55	16
in spiced vinegar	Haywards New Seasons	45	13
Indian chicken	Ross	90	26
Italian Beef Bolognaise	Ross	85	24
macedoine of	Waitrose	57	16

Product	Brand	Calories per 100g/ 100ml	Calories per oz/ pack/ portion
Mixed vegetables			
Mexican mix	Bejam	55	per 85g portion boiled 47
Oriental mix	Bejam	32	per 113g portion boiled 36
Oriental vegetable			
mix	Ross	40	11
original	Birds Eye	53	15
pasta mix	Bejam	68	per 85g portion boiled 58
peas and baby			
carrots	Birds Eye	35	10
petits pois, button			
sprouts baby carrots	Birds Eye	42	12
ratatouille	Bejam	49	per 113g portion 56
ratatouille mix	Ross	15	4
rice, peas and			
mushrooms, boiled	Birds Eye	123	35
rice, sweetcorn peas			
and carrots, boiled	Birds Eye	123	35
special	Tesco	68	19
special Chinese			
vegetables	Bejam	29	per 113g portion boiled 33
special mix	Ross	40	11
spring vegetable			
mix	Bejam	35	per 113g portion boiled 40
stewpack	Bejam	16	per 113g portion boiled 18
stewpack	Ross	20	6
stir fry chili bean			
mix	Bejam	105	per 142g portion boiled 149
stir fry mix	Ross	50	14
summer (canned)	Tesco	50	14

Product	Brand	Calories per 100g/ 100ml	Calories per oz/ pack/ portion
Mixed vegetables			
summer harvest mix	Findus	72	20
sweet and sour pork	Ross	70	20
Sweet corn, peas and carrots	Birds Eye	53	15
veg 'n' rice mix	Bejam	48	per 113g portion boiled 54
vegetable pasta	Birds Eye	141	40
Mocca ministicks	St Michael	554	157
Mocha almond ice cream	Safeway	248	73
Mocha cake mix (as sold)	Green's	396	made up per portion 258
Moghulai Korma curry sauce	Sharwood	190	54
Molasses	Holland and Barrett	200	57
Molasses snack bar carob coated	Sunwheel Kalibu	437	per 30g bar 131
Monkey nuts	Tesco	615	174
Montelimar	Rowntree Mackintosh		per sweet 45
Mooli: see Radish, white			
Moong dahl chilki		83	24
Moong gram, whole		66	19
Morello cherry and apple juice	Copella	35	10
Morello cherry and cream cheesecake	Young's	240	68
Morello cherry conserve	Safeway	248	70
	Waitrose	250	71

Product	Brand	Calories per 100g/ 100ml	Calories per oz/ pack/ portion
Morello cherry Fruit For-All	Chivers	110	per portion 85
Morello cherry jam, reduced sugar	Waitrose	124	35
Morello cherry juice	Copella	34	10
Morello cherry yoghurt, low fat	Waitrose	90	per 150g pack 135
Morning coffee biscuits	Tesco	471	134
Mortadella	Waitrose	371	105
Moules bonne femme	St Michael	97	27
Moussaka		195	55
	Findus	190	54
	St Michael	144	41
	Waitrose	180	51
canned	St Michael	110	31
Mousse: see flavours			
Muesli		368	104
	Holland and Barrett	370	105
"Eight" fruit	Granose	408	116
barley kernels	Sunwheel	366	104
Bircher	Granose	379	107
bran	Prewetts	320	91
country	Jordans	345	98
de-luxe	Sunwheel	390	111
	Prewetts	360	102
fruit and fibre	Waitrose	293	83
fruit and nut	Sunwheel	364	103
	Waitrose	354	100
fruit and nut sugar free	Sunwheel	360	102

Product	Brand	Calories per 100g/ 100ml	Calories per oz/ pack/ portion
Muesli			
fruit and nut, 35%	Safeway	326	92
high fibre	Holland and Barrett	340	96
honey	Boots Second Nature	417	118
no added sugar	Boots Second Nature	362	103
special recipe	Jordans	330	94
sugar free	Holland and Barrett	380	108
	Prewetts	340	96
traditional	St Michael	362	103
tropical	Prewetts	340	96
unsweetened	St Michael	340	96
wholegrain fruit	Granose	408	116
wholewheat	Tesco	346	98
Muesli and fruit biscuits	Boots Second Nature	461	131
Muesli bar			
apple	Granose	416	per 25g bar 104
chocolate chip	Granose	484	per 25g bar 121
chocolate coated	Tesco	510	145
fruit	Prewetts	310	per 42g bar 130
hazelnut	Granose	476	per 25g bar 119
hazelnut and almond	Granose	460	per 25g bar 115
Swiss style	Boots	350	99
Muesli bar square snack	Holly Mill		per bar 216
Muesli base	Prewetts	340	96
	Sunwheel	370	105
Muesli biscuits	Holland and Barrett		per biscuit 60

Product	Brand	Calories per 100g/ 100ml	Calories per oz/ pack/ portion
Muesli biscuits			
diabetic	Boots	437	124
Muesli breakfast	Cow and Gate	63	per 110g jar 69, 150g jar 95
Muesli cereal	Boots Second Nature	361	102
Muesli cookies	St Michael	476	135
	Tesco	464	132
	Waitrose	448	127
Muesli snack bar carob coated	Sunwheel Kalibu	397	per 30g bar 119
Muesli stuffing mix	Knorr	385	109
Muesli tub	Allinson	380	108
banana and brazil	Jordans	430	122
coconut and sultana	Jordans	366	104
Muesli yoghurt	Safeway	101	per 150g pack 152
	St Ivel Shape	45	13
Muffins	Sunblest Muffin Man	233	per muffin 158
plain	Tesco	225	64
wholemeal	Sunblest Muffin Man	214	per muffin 154
Mulberries		36	10
Mulligatawny soup	Heinz Ready to Serve	48	14
Munch biscuits	Moorlands		per biscuit 50
wholewheat fruit	Moorlands		per biscuit 60
Munch Bunch yogurts (Eden Vale): see flavours			
Munchies	Rowntree Mackintosh	505	per sweet 25

Product	Brand	Calories per 100g/ 100ml	Calories per oz/ pack/ portion
Mung (moong) beans			
raw		231	65
dahl, cooked		106	30
green gram, raw		231	65
	Boots	231	65
cooked	Tesco	161	cooked
dried	Holland and		
	Barrett	230	65
raw	Tesco	336	95
Mung (moong) beansprouts			
fresh, raw		35	10
canned		9	3
Murray Fruits	Cadbury's	390	per Fruit 25
Murray Mints	Cadbury's	400	per mint pocket pack 25, others 20
Muscovado sugar	Safeway	394	112
dark	Waitrose	360	102
light	Waitrose	378	107
Mushroom			
straw, canned, drained		30	9
Mushroom and bacon pizza	St Michael	232	66
Mushroom and bacon Toast Topper	Heinz	131	37
Mushroom and pasta italienne	Birds Eye MenuMaster		per pack 303
Mushroom and peppers savoury rice	Safeway	341	per 125g pack 426
Mushroom cream soup	Knorr "No Simmer"	484	137
Mushroom flan, creamy	St Michael	195	55

Product	Brand	Calories per 100g/ 100ml	Calories per oz/ pack/ portion
Mushroom pancakes in beer batter	St Michael	171	48
Mushroom Pasta Choice	Crosse & Blackwell	349	99
Mushroom pate	Vessen	256	per 45g pack 115
Mushroom Pour Over sauce mix	Colman's	335	95
Mushroom quiche	St Michael	277	79
Mushroom sandwich cream	Granose	360	102
Mushroom savoury rice	Batchelors	346	per 130g sachet as sold 450
Mushroom snack pizza	Tesco	222	63
Mushroom soup	Batchelors Cup-a-Soup	415	per 26g sachet as sold 108
	Campbell's Bumper Harvest	42	12
dried	Safeway	355	101
	Tesco	382	108
	Waitrose	340	per 41g pack 139
	Prewetts Soup in Seconds	302	86
dried, made up instant special (made up)	Chef Box	28	8
low calorie	Safeway	45	13
	Heinz Weight Watchers	24	per 292g can 70
	Waitrose	16	per 295g pack 47
Mushroom Super Noodles	Batchelors	465	per pack as sold 460

Product	Brand	Calories per 100g/ 100ml	Calories per oz/ pack/ portion
Mushrooms			
Chinese, dried		284	81
raw		13	4
fried		210	60
	Littlewoods	13	4
button, whole	Safeway	13	200g/7oz pack
	Waitrose	20	6
canned	Tesco	32	9
chopped	Waitrose	20	6
creamed (canned)	Tesco	87	25
dried	Tesco	325	92
dried, sliced	Whitworths	133	38
fresh, fried	Tesco	210	60
fresh, raw	Tesco	13	4
sliced	Bejam	11	per 113g portion 13
	Safeway	13	4
	Waitrose	20	6
stir fry	Safeway	80	23
whole	Bejam	15	per 113g portion boiled 17
Mushrooms sandwich spread	Granose	337	96
Mushy peas: see Peas, mushy			
Mussels			
raw		66	19
boiled		87	25
boiled (with shells)		26	7
cooked	Dan Maid	75	21
frozen, raw	Tesco	82	23
Mustard			
American	Colman's	110	31
Burger mild	Colman's	110	31

Product	Brand	Calories per 100g/ 100ml	Calories per oz/ pack/ portion
Mustard			
chive	Colman's	170	48
Dijon	Colman's	170	48
English	Colman's	180	51
	Safeway	95	27
French	Colman's	115	33
	Safeway	75	21
German	Colman's	135	38
horseradish	Colman's	140	40
sage and onion	Colman's	175	50
whole grain	Colman's	145	41
Mustard and cress, raw		10	3
Mustard and vinaigrette dressing	Tesco	503	143
Mustard leaves, raw		34	10
Mustard oil dressing	Safeway	440	130
Mustard powder		452	128
English DSF	Colman's	480	136
whole grain	Colman's	505	143
Mustard relish	Safeway	118	33
mild	Tesco	128	36
Mustard seeds		469	133
Mutton biriani		249	71
Mutton, boneless diced, casseroled	Bejam	194	55
Mutton curry		376	107
My Little Pony Cartoons cake mix (as sold)	Green's	412	made up per portion 64
Naan bread mix	Sharwood	360	102
Nachips	Old El Paso	550	156

Product	Brand	Calories per 100g/ 100ml	Calories per oz/ pack/ portion
Napoletana sauce	St Michael	34	10
	Tesco	40	11
	Waitrose	35	10
Napoli dairy ice cream (Lyons Maid): *see flavours*			
Napolitan sauce	Buitoni	24	per 283g can 68
	Waitrose	27	per 424g can 114
Natch cider	Taunton	34	per pint 200
Natural Complan	Farley	444	per 57g sachet 253
Natural cottage cheese	Eden Vale	97	27
	St Ivel	94	27
Natural country bran	Jordans	167	47
Natural flavour vegetarian chunks	Direct Foods	251	71
Natural flavour vegetarian mince	Direct Foods	250	71
Natural original crunchy	Jordans	405	115
Natural seed bar			
poppy	Boots	439	124
sesame	Boots	464	132
sunflower	Boots	464	132
Natural set yogurt	Safeway	47	per 150g pack 71
low fat	Waitrose	59	per 150g pack 89
low fat, unsweetened	Waitrose	59	per 500g pack 295
whole milk	Waitrose	75	per 150g pack 113
Natural water, still or sparkling	Safeway		
Natural wheatgerm	Jordans	325	92
Natural yogurt	Eden Vale	70	per 150g pack 105
	Safeway	47	per 150g pack 71

Product	Brand	Calories per 100g/ 100ml	Calories per oz/ pack/ portion
Natural yogurt			
	St Ivel	60	17
	St Michael	69	20
	St Ivel Shape	50	14
low fat	Littlewoods	45	per 150g pack 68
	Tesco	64	18
	Waitrose	47	per 150g pack 71
unsweetened	Raines	55	16
whole milk, French	St Michael	68	19
Neapolitan chequers ice cream	Bejam	162	46
Neapolitan choc ice	Bejam		each 119
Neapolitan ice cream	Bejam	166	47
	Lyons Maid	179	51
	Tesco	179	51
	Waitrose	157	46
	Wall's		per 1/5 pack 85
sliceable	Wall's		per 1/10 litre pack 95
soft scoop	Lyons Maid	178	50
Neapolitan vegetable sauce	Prewetts	304	86
Neapolitan wafers	Peek Frean	504	per biscuit 36
Nectarines			
raw		50	14
raw (*with stones*)		46	13
without skin	Littlewoods	50	14
Nectarines and orange yogurt	St Michael	98	28
New York style cheesecake (frozen)	St Michael	399	113
Nice biscuits	Boots	476	135
	Peek Frean	449	per biscuit 44

Product	Brand	Calories per 100g/ 100ml	Calories per oz/ pack/ portion
Nice biscuits			
	Rakusen	452	128
	Tesco	466	132
	Waitrose	457	130
Nice creams	Peek Frean	484	per biscuit 57
Nice fingers	Safeway	478	136
Night cap	Boots	359	102
Nik Naks, spicy	St Michael	540	153
Nik-Naks	Sooner	497	per 30g pack 149
90% beefburgers	Findus	283	80
No bake egg custard dessert mix (as sold)	Green's	380	per portion made up 148
No Simmer soups (Knorr): see flavours			
Noiseberry fruits: see Sapota			
Noisette pate	Rowntree Mackintosh		per sweet 40
Noisettes	Ross	180	51
	St Michael	323	92
Non-dairy cream	Tesco	253	72
Non-dairy ice cream		165	47
Non-dairy vanilla ice cream	Tesco	179	51
Noodle Doodles spaghetti shapes in tomato sauce	Heinz	59	17
Noodles			
egg, dried, raw		391	111
wheat, dried, raw		388	110
medium	Sharwood	352	100
Noots	Itona	420	119

Product	Brand	Calories per 100g/ 100ml	Calories per oz/ pack/ portion
Norfolk Punch fruit juice	Marlet	37	11
Norwegian prawns	Raider	70	20
Nottingham pie	Tesco	326	92
Nougat	Barratt	355	101
Number 7 cider	Bulmer	35	per half pint 100
Nut and raisin carob bar	Kalibu	453	per 75g bar 340
Nut and raisin confectionery bar, no added sugar	Sunwheel Kalibu	500	per 42g bar 210
Nut burger mix	Tomorrow Foods	353	100
Nut loaf	Granose	176	50
Nut luncheon	Mapletons	380	per 142g pack 540
Nut roast	Granose	488	138
Nut toffee creme	Rowntree Mackintosh		per sweet 45
Nutbrawn	Granose	212	60
Nutmeg			
powder		525	149
	Tesco	456	129
ground	Safeway	556	158
whole	Safeway	556	158
Nutrigrain			
brown rice and rye with raisins	Kellogg's Nutrigrain	342	97
rye and oats with hazelnuts	Kellogg's Nutrigrain	368	104
wholewheat with raisins	Kellogg's Nutrigrain	326	92

Product	Brand	Calories per 100g/ 100ml	Calories per oz/ pack/ portion
Nuts and fruit, yogurt coated	Waitrose	570	162
Nuts and raisins	Whitworths	462	131
Nuttolene	Granose	298	84
Nutty bar	Rowntree Mackintosh	495	per bar 255
Nutty choc choc bar	Wall's		per bar 190
Nutty toffee dairy ice cream	Lyons Maid Napoli	205	30
Oat and honey crunch bar	Boots Second Nature	432	122
Oat breakfast	Boots Baby Foods	420	119
Oat cereal, instant	Tesco	382	108
Oatcakes		441	125
	Safeway	440	125
bran	Allinson		per biscuit 50
Oatcakes and bran biscuits	Mitchellhill		per biscuit 50
Oaten crunch biscuits	Safeway	459	130
Oatmeal			
raw		401	114
medium	Whitworths	401	114
Oatmeal/oats	Holland and Barrett	400	113
Oatmeal and raisin cookies	Barbaras		per biscuit 220
Oatmeal biscuits	Holland and Barrett		per biscuit 60
carob coated	Holland and Barrett		per biscuit 70

Product	Brand	Calories per 100g/ 100ml	Calories per oz/ pack/ portion
Oatmeal cookies, mini	Tesco	474	134
Ocean pie (frozen)	Ross	120	34
	St Michael	107	30
Octopus, raw		68	19
Oil-free French dressing	Waistline	13	4
OJ ice cream	Wall's		per portion 50
Okra (lady's fingers)			
raw		17	5
canned, drained		15	4
Okra curry		259	73
Old English ginger beer	Idris	35	10
with lemonade	Idris	37	11
Olde English chutney	Pan Yan	176	50
Old fashioned mixture drops	Boots	363	per 33g stick pack 120
Olive oil		900	255
	Boots	899	255
	Crosse & Blackwell	900	255
	Holland and Barrett	720	213
	Safeway	887	263
	Tesco	875	248
	Waitrose	900	266
extra virgin first cold pressed, unrefined	Safeway	887	263
	Sunwheel	900	255
Olive sandwich cream	Granose	340	96
Olives			
in brine		103	29

Product	Brand	Calories per 100g/ 100ml	Calories per oz/ pack/ portion
Olives			
in brine (with stones)		82	23
stuffed	Tesco	160	45
Olives sandwich spread	Granose	308	87
100% beefburgers	Birds Eye Steakhouse		each, grilled or fried 120
	Ross	330	94
Onion and cheddar cottage cheese	St Ivel	113	32
	St Ivel Shape	85	24
Onion and chives cottage cheese	Eden Vale	95	27
	St Ivel	85	24
	St Ivel Shape	72	20
	Waitrose	85	24
Onion and pepper cottage cheese	Safeway	92	26
Onion and watercress spreading cheese	Medley	284	81
Onion bhajia mix	Sharwood	310	88
Onion bhajjis	St Michael	211	60
	Waitrose	226	64
Onion chutney	Waitrose	154	44
Onion flavour Chinese noodles, instant	Sharwood	487	138
Onion kites	St Michael	463	131
Onion relish	Branston	126	36
	Crosse & Blackwell	135	38
	Tesco	135	38
Onion ring crisps	Littlewoods	500	per 50g pack 250
Onion Ringers	Ross	230	65

Product	Brand	Calories per 100g/ 100ml	Calories per oz/ pack/ portion
Onion rings	Safeway	516	per 50g pack 258
	Tesco	494	140
	Waitrose	483	137
Onion rings, battered (frozen)	Bejam	125	per 85g portion baked 106
Onion sauce		99	28
Onion sauce mix	Knorr	343	97
	Safeway	364	per 30g pack 109
	Tesco	317	90
Pour Over	Colman's	330	94
Onion soup, thick (dried), made up	Chef Box	29	8
Onion sour cream dressing	St Michael	385	109
Onions			
raw		23	7
boiled		13	4
fried		345	98
fresh	Littlewoods	23	7
fresh, boiled	Tesco	13	4
fresh, fried	Tesco	339	96
frozen, cooked	Tesco	19	5
sliced (frozen)	Bejam	11	per 113g portion boiled 12
	Safeway	23	per 227g pack 56
whole, small (frozen)	Bejam	39	per 57g portion boiled 22
Onions, cocktail	Tesco	13	4
	Waitrose	27	8
Onions, dried sliced	Tesco	280	79
	Whitworths	294	83
	Batchelors Surprise	242	per 88g sachet 213

Product	Brand	Calories per 100g/100ml	Calories per oz/pack/portion
Onions, pickled	Haywards	16	5
	Littlewoods	19	5
	Safeway	37	10
	St Michael	23	7
	Tesco	18	5
	Waitrose	19	5
silverskin	Haywards	20	6
	Heinz	13	4
	Littlewoods	27	8
	Safeway	21	6
	Tesco	18	5
sweet	Haywards	25	7
	Safeway	36	10
	Tesco	28	8
	Waitrose	38	11
Onions, spring **raw**		35	10
	Littlewoods	35	10
Onions and white sauce, small	Birds Eye	134	per 142g/4oz pack
Opals	Mars	391	111
Orange and apricot drink	Safeway	90	27
chilled	Safeway	43	13
	Waitrose	41	12
long life	Safeway	45	13
Orange and banana dessert	Boots Baby Foods	405	115
Orange and cointreau yogurt	St Ivel Cabaret	101	29

Product	Brand	Calories per 100g/100ml	Calories per oz/pack/portion
Orange and ginger sherry Chinese barbecue sauce	Sharwood	140	40
Orange and grapefruit drink low calorie,	Quosh	5	1
undiluted	Quosh	94	28
Orange and lemon cup cakes	Lyons	361	102
Orange and lemon slices	Littlewoods	349	99
	Tesco	320	91
Orange and passionfruit drink concentrated	Kia-Ora	97	29
sparkling	Schweppes	35	10
	Tango	44	13
Orange and peach drink	Safeway	85	25
	Waitrose	86	25
undiluted	Tesco	115	34
Orange and pineapple drink	Britvic	40	per 330ml can 133
	Quosh	32	9
	Quosh	93	28
concentrated	Kia-Ora	105	31
sparkling	Tango	44	13
sparkling, low calorie	Diet Tango	2	1
undiluted	Corona	93	28
Orange and pineapple fruit juice	Del Monte	46	14
Orange and pineapple juice, longlife	Tesco	45	13
Orange and pineapple whole fruit drink	Robinsons Special R	23	7

Product	Brand	Calories per 100g/ 100ml	Calories per oz/ pack/ portion
Orange and rosehip drink	Boots Baby Drinks	287	81
Orange/strawberry Woppas	Wall's		per woppa 40
Orange, banana and lemon juice	Prewetts	37	11
Orange bar	Granose	376	per 50g bar 188
Orange barley crush, sparkling	Lucozade	72	21
Orange barley drink	Boots	130	38
	Robinsons	30	9
Orange barley water	Robinsons	110	33
	Safeway	90	27
Orange 'C'			
reduced calories	Libby	28	8
sweetened	Libby	51	14
Orange C drink, long life	Safeway	35	10
Orange cakes, chocolate topped	Waitrose	381	108
Orange carob bar			
no added sugar	Sunwheel Kalibu	493	per 60g bar 296
with raw sugar	Sunwheel Kalibu	518	per 60g bar 311
Orange chocolate coated wafers, diabetic	Boots	555	157
Orange chocolate wafer bar	Boots Shapers Meal	519	147
Orange Club biscuits	Jacobs	497	per biscuit 113

Product	Brand	Calories per 100g/ 100ml	Calories per oz/ pack/ portion
Orange coated mallows	Peek Frean	433	per biscuit 52
Orange cream			
(Black Magic)	Rowntree Mackintosh		per sweet 45
(Quality Street)	Rowntree Mackintosh		per sweet 40
Orange creams	Peek Frean	473	per biscuit 57
	Rakusen	469	133
	Tesco	455	129
Orange creme biscuits	Cadbury's	500	per biscuit 80
Orange crisp block	Needlers	508	144
Orange crunch breakfast cereal	Whole Earth	400	113
Orange crush	St Michael	43	12
50% juice	St Michael	53	15
low calorie	St Michael	3	1
	Slimsta	5	per 180ml pack 9
Orange dessert with vitamin C	Heinz Baby Foods	73	per 128g jar 93
Orange drink undiluted		107	30
	Britvic	44	per 330ml can 145
	Littlewoods	29	per 330ml pack 96
	Quosh	34	10
	Robinsons	35	10
	Safeway	50	per 330ml can 165
	St Michael	49	14
	Waitrose	104	31
concentrated	Kia-Ora	97	29
dilutable	Safeway	99	29
Jaffa	St Michael	110	33

Product	Brand	Calories per 100g/ 100ml	Calories per oz/ pack/ portion
Orange drink			
Jaffa, colour free	St Michael	110	33
long life	Waitrose	40	per 250ml carton 100
low calorie	Littlewoods	4	1
	Littlewoods	4	1
	Quosh	5	1
	Quosh	5	1
	Safeway	17	5
	Tesco	24	7
	Waitrose	15	4
	Waitrose	15	4
low calorie, sparkling	Diet Tango	3	1
no added colour	St Michael	104	29
original, ready to drink	Robinsons	40	12
sparkling	St Michael	45	13
	Schweppes	40	12
	Tango	46	14
	Waitrose	48	14
sparkling, low calorie	Schweppes Slimline	2	1
Special R	Robinsons	3	1
undiluted	Tesco	107	32
whole	Boots	102	30
	Corona	90	27
	Quosh	90	27
	Sqeez	34	10
	Tesco	38	11
whole, diabetic	Boots	7	2
Orange-filled bars, chocolate coated	Tesco	503	143

Product	Brand	Calories per 100g/ 100ml	Calories per oz/ pack/ portion
Orange filled milk chocolate	Littlewoods	480	136
Orange flavour dessert mix	Dietade	264	75
Orange flavour jelly crystals	Waitrose	272	77
	Dietade	290	82
Orange-flavoured concentrate	Safeway	196	58
Orange fruit drink undiluted	Baby Ribena	316	94
Orange fruit juice canned	Del Monte	42	12
	Heinz	46	14
Orange Frutie	Wall's		per portion 60
Orange ice lolly, sugar-free	Bejam		each 35
Orange jelly	Littlewoods	260	74
	Safeway	268	76
	Tesco	57	16
Orange jelly crystals, diabetic	Boots	365	103
Orange jelly marmalade, fine cut	Waitrose	248	70
Orange juice sweetened, canned		51	14
unsweetened, canned		33	9
Orange juice	Boots	33	10
	Britvic	44	per 133ml pack 49
	Hycal	243	72
	Prewetts	33	10
	Safeway	40	12
	St Ivel Mr Juicy	38	11
	St Ivel Real	38	11

Product	Brand	Calories per 100g/ 100ml	Calories per oz/ pack/ portion
Orange juice	Tesco	42	12
	Volonte	40	12
concentrated	Tesco	136	40
concentrated (frozen)	Waitrose	40	12
freshly squeezed	Tesco	42	12
	Waitrose	31	9
Jaffa	St Michael	35	10
Jaffa, concentrated	St Michael	38	11
long life	Waitrose	37	11
	Tesco	42	12
natural	Schweppes	47	14
pure	St Michael	38	11
	Waitrose	35	10
pure, chilled	Waitrose	35	10
pure, long life	Safeway	42	12
sparkling	Orangina	38	per half pint 109
sweetened	Hunts	52	15
	Libby	51	14
	Schweppes	56	17
unsweetened	Hunts	38	11
	Libby	33	9
Orange juice bar	Lyons Maid	70	each 39
Orange, lemon and pineapple drink	Tesco	38	11
dilutable	Safeway	104	31
Orange, lemon and pineapple whole fruit drink	Robinsons	95	28
Orange Liga rusks	Cow and Gate	381	per rusk 27
Orange lollies	Bejam		per lolly 20
Orange Maid	Lyons Maid		each 43

Product	Brand	Calories per 100g/ 100ml	Calories per oz/ pack/ portion
Orange, mango and passion fruit drink	Quosh	29	9
undiluted	Quosh	92	27
Orange marmalade	Tesco	243	69
fine shred	Baxters	253	72
fresh, thick cut	Waitrose	248	70
matured, thick cut	Waitrose	248	70
reduced sugar, thin cut	Heinz Weight Watchers	124	35
reduced sugar, thin cut	Waitrose	124	35
vintage	Baxters	248	70
Orange marmalade preserve reduced sugar	Robertson's	150	43
Orange, pineapple and lemon drink	Robinsons	35	10
Orange pure fruit spread, fine cut	Robertson's	120	34
Orange Quick-Set Jel	Tesco	365	103
Orange ripple yogurt	St Michael	126	36
Orange segments in orange juice (canned)	St Michael	45	13
Orange shred marmalade	Safeway	251	71
Orange sorbet ice cream	Tesco	62	18
	Wall's Alpine		per 1/10 pack 85
Orange souffle	St Ivel	163	46
Orange squash concentrated	St Michael	169	48
	Rose's High Juice	160	47
	Schweppes	111	33
diluted	Britvic	22	6

Product	Brand	Calories per 100g/100ml	Calories per oz/pack/portion
Orange squash			
diluted	Britvic High Juice	26	7
	Quosh	48	14
low calorie	Dietade	10	3
real, undiluted	Quosh	143	42
undiluted	Britvic	108	31
	Britvic High Juice	129	37
Orange squash drink			
Jaffa	St Michael	104	31
Orange squosh	Waitrose	134	40
Orange Surprise	Bertorelli	220	per 80g pack 176
Orange water ice	Bertorelli	110	31
Orange whole fruit drink	Robinsons	95	28
	Robinsons Special R	20	6
original	Robinsons	155	46
Orange yogurt	St Ivel Real	81	23
	Ski	82	per 150g pack 123
whole milk	Safeway	63	per 150g pack 95
Orange yogurt dessert	Heinz Baby Foods	80	per 128g jar 102
Orangeade	Corona	27	8
	Safeway	33	9
	Tesco	18	5
	Whites	23	7
diabetic	Boots	-1	per 100ml 0.6
low calorie	Canada Dry Slim	3	per 175ml pack 5
Orangeade sparkles	Wall's		per portion 30
Oranges			
raw		35	10

Product	Brand	Calories per 100g/ 100ml	Calories per oz/ pack/ portion
Oranges			
raw (with peel and pips)		26	7
juice, fresh		38	11
fresh, without skin	Littlewoods	35	10
Orangina sparkling orange juice	Bulmer	38	per half pint 109
Orbit Nutra sweet chewing gum	Wrigley		per stick 7
Orchard apple pudding	Boots Baby Foods	56	16
Oregano powder		306	87
Oriental mix vegetables	Bejam	32	per 113g portion boiled 36
Oriental prawn stir-fry meal	Bejam		per serving stir-fried 350
Oriental prawns (chilled)	Young's	110	31
Oriental vegetable mix	Ross	40	11
Original beefburgers	Birds Eye Steakhouse		each grilled or fried 130
Original cheesecake mix (as sold)	Green's	425	made up per portion 236
Original cider	Bulmer	37	per half pint 104
Original Cookies	Cadbury's	480	per biscuit 50
Original crunchy	Jordans	416	118
bran and apple	Jordans	369	105
honey, almond and raisins	Jordans	396	112
natural	Jordans	405	115
original	Jordans	416	118

Product	Brand	Calories per 100g/ 100ml	Calories per oz/ pack/ portion
Original crunchy bar			
apple and bran	Jordans	394	per bar 132
coconut and honey	Jordans	416	per bar 138
honey and almond	Jordans	412	per bar 135
Original Dolmio (as sold)	Dolmio	41	11
Original Liga rusks	Cow and Gate	381	per rusk 27
Original mixed vegetables	Birds Eye	53	15
Original pickle	Pan Yan	133	38
Original Ready Brek	Lyons	391	111
Ortaniques, raw		49	14
fresh	Tesco	57	16
OsterRusks	Farley	404	per rusk 34
Outline dairy spread, low fat	Van den Berghs	370	105
Ovaltine		378	107
	Wander	378	107
instant	Wander	392	111
Ovaltine drinking chocolate	Wander	387	110
instant	Wander	400	113
Oven Bake chicken	Ross	215	61
Oven chips	Ross	140	40
	Safeway	150	43
	Tesco	150	43
	Waitrose	158	45
baked or grilled	Birds Eye	194	55
cooked	Tesco	235	67
Oven cod, battered	Ross	200	57

Product	Brand	Calories per 100g/ 100ml	Calories per oz/ pack/ portion
Oven crispy cod steaks	Birds Eye		each baked or grilled 215
Oven crispy fish 'n' chips	Birds Eye		per pack baked 470
Oven crispy haddock steaks	Birds Eye		each baked or grilled 215
Oven Crunches	Ross	160	45
Oven Stars			
baked or grilled	Birds Eye	229	65
fried	Birds Eye	300	85
Ox tongue	Waitrose	143	41
sliced	St Michael	170	48
	Tesco	280	79
Oxford cheese	Safeway	412	117
Oxo beef drink	Brooke Bond		
	Oxo	100	28
Oxo cubes		229	65
chicken	Brooke Bond		
	Oxo	210	60
red	Brooke Bond		
	Oxo	245	69
Oxtail			
raw		171	48
stewed		243	69
stewed (with bones)		92	26
Oxtail and vegetable soup	Crosse & Blackwell	38	11
low calorie	Waistline	23	7
Oxtail soup			
canned		44	12
dried		356	101
dried, as served		27	8

Product	Brand	Calories per 100g/ 100ml	Calories per oz/ pack/ portion
	Baxters	42	
	Campbell's		per 425g can 179
	Bumper Harvest	44	12
	Crosse & Blackwell	49	14
	Heinz Ready to Serve	43	12
	Littlewoods	44	425g/15oz can
	Safeway	43	per 425g can 183
	Tesco	48	14
	Waitrose	38	per 425g can 162
condensed	Campbell's	86	24
dried	Knorr	329	93
	Knorr Quick Soup	363	103
	Littlewoods	349	per 37g pint packet 129
	Safeway	350	99
	Tesco	330	94
	Waitrose	349	per 39g packet 136
	Batchelors	360	per 52g pint pack 187
	Batchelors Cup-a-Soup	388	per 24g sachet 93
dried, made up	Chef Box	29	8
low calorie	Heinz Weight Watchers	26	per 288g can 75
Oyster Chinese pouring sauce	Sharwood	66	19
Oyster crackers	Safeway	431	per biscuit 3
Oyster sauce		80	23
Oysters raw		51	14

Product	Brand	Calories per 100g/ 100ml	Calories per oz/ pack/ portion
Oysters			
raw (with shell)		6	2
Pacific drink (chilled)	Tesco	49	15
Pacific pilchards in tomato sauce	Armour	126	per 227g can
Pack-a-Pie (Batchelors): see flavours			
Paella	Vesta	399	per 160g pack for two as served 638
low calorie	Batchelors Slim-a-Meal	346	per 66.5g pack 230
Paella, seafood and chicken	Birds Eye MenuMaster		each as sold 320, cooked with butter 340
Paella style	Beanfeast	309	88
Paglia-e-fieno (as sold)	Signor Rossi	271	77
Pakoras (bhajia)		183	52
	Waitrose	226	64
Pale ale, bottled		32	9
Pan: see Betel leaves			
Pancake mix	Whitworths	348	99
Pancake roll, Chinese crispy	St Michael	178	50
Pancakes		307	87
plain	Tesco	247	70
Pancakes: see also flavours			
Pancho peanuts	Trebor	545	per sweet 6
Pancho raisins	Trebor	545	per sweet 6
Papadums, raw		272	77
Papaya: see Paw-paw			

Product	Brand	Calories per 100g/ 100ml	Calories per oz/ pack/ portion
Papaya chunks in syrup	Del Monte	57	16
Papri beans			
fresh, raw		40	11
canned, drained		26	7
Paprika		289	82
Hungarian	Safeway	377	107
Paradise cake	Waitrose	347	98
Paradise fruits	Trebor	342	per sweet 25
Paradise slice	Lyons	426	121
Parkin cut cake	St Michael	329	93
Parmesan cheese	Buitoni	498	141
	Safeway	444	126
	St Ivel	500	142
grated	Tesco	390	111
Italian	Waitrose	408	116
wedge	Tesco	370	105
Parsley			
dried		276	78
raw		21	6
fresh	Littlewoods	21	6
	Tesco	21	6
Parsley and thyme stuffing mix	Safeway	350	per 85g pack 297
	Tesco	366	104
	Whitworths	355	101
Parsley sauce mix	Knorr	348	99
	Safeway	356	101
	Tesco	355	101
Pour Over	Colman's	360	102
Parsley, thyme and lemon stuffing mix	Waitrose	325	227g/8oz pack

Product	Brand	Calories per 100g/ 100ml	Calories per oz/ pack/ portion
Parsnips			
raw		49	14
boiled		56	16
fresh, boiled	Tesco	56	16
whole, small	Bejam	67	per 113g portion boiled 76
Partridge			
roast		212	60
roast (with bone)		127	36
fresh	Waitrose	400	per 250g bird 1000
Party rings	Littlewoods	430	per biscuit 27
	Safeway	443	126
Party Twigs	Waitrose	399	113
Parwal: see Marrow			
Passata	Waitrose	21	per 400g pack 84
Passion Splitz	Canada Dry	45	per 250ml pack 113
Passionfruit			
raw		34	10
raw (with skin)		14	4
Passionfruit and melon yogurt	Safeway	89	per 150g pack
low fat	Waitrose	89	per 150g pack 134
Passionfruit and peach ice cream	Bejam	180	51
Passionfruit and raspberry yogurt	Ski	83	per 150g pack 125
Passionfruit sorbet	Waitrose	125	per 500ml pack 625
Pasta	Waitrose	378	107
bows	Buitoni	340	96

Product	Brand	Calories per 100g/ 100ml	Calories per oz/ pack/ portion
Pasta			
bows	Safeway	344	98
	Waitrose	378	107
cooked (typical figures)	Tesco	138	39
quills	Buitoni	340	96
	Safeway	344	98
shells	Buitoni	340	96
	Buitoni Country Harvest	318	90
	Safeway	344	98
	St Michael	359	102
	Waitrose	378	107
shells, cooked	Tesco	150	cooked
shells, green and white	Signor Rossi	309	88
shells, uncooked	Tesco	348	99
spirals, wholewheat	Signor Rossi	275	as sold
tubes	Waitrose	378	107
twists	Buitoni	340	96
	Buitoni Country Harvest	318	90
	Safeway	344	98
	Waitrose	378	107
uncooked (typical figures)	Tesco	348	99
wheels	Waitrose	378	107
whirls	Buitoni Country Harvest	318	90
Pasta Bolognese	Branston		
	Snackatak	365	103
Pasta Choice (Crosse & Blackwell): see flavours			
Pasta florentine	St Michael	176	50

Product	Brand	Calories per 100g/ 100ml	Calories per oz/ pack/ portion
Pasta mix vegetables	Bejam	68	per 85g portion boiled 58
Pasta salad	Eden Vale	197	56
Pasta shells, wholewheat, in spicy tomato sauce	Heinz	65	18
Pasties			
chicken	Ross	270	77
Cornish	Ross	270	77
jumbo traditional	Ross	275	78
Pasties with fresh vegetables			
mini	St Michael	258	73
Pastilles		253	72
	Bassett's	322	91
Pastrami	Waitrose	143	41
Pastry: see also Puff pastry, Shortcrust pastry			
choux		214	61
choux, cooked		330	94
flaky, raw		427	121
flaky, cooked		565	160
choux, baked	Bejam	335	95
vol au vent cases	Birds Eye		per case 70
vol au vents	Jus-Rol	393	111
vol au vents, cocktail	Bejam		each 43
vol au vents, medium	Bejam		each 69
Pastry mix	Whitworths	484	137
flaky	Tesco	558	158
short	Safeway	495	140
shortcrust (dry)	Tesco	484	137

Product	Brand	Calories per 100g/ 100ml	Calories per oz/ pack/ portion
Pastry mix			
shortcrust (made up)	Tesco	450	128
Pate			
with herbs	Vessen	244	per 45g pack 110
with peppers	Vessen	211	per 45g pack 95
Pate en croute	Waitrose	221	63
Patent cornflour	Brown and Polson	330	94
Patra leaves		26	7
Pavlova: see flavours			
Paw-paw (Papaya)			
fresh, raw		45	13
canned, whole contents		65	18
Pea (fresh) curry		350	99
Pea (tinned) and potato curry		142	40
Pea and ham soup	Baxters	58	per 425g can 247
	Granny's	52	as served 35
	Heinz Ready to Serve	56	16
	St Michael	60	17
	Waitrose	56	per 425g can 238
condensed	Campbell's	123	35
Pea soup	Campbell's Bumper Harvest	55	16
dried	Tesco	384	109
thick, dried (made up)	Chef Box	26	7
Pea with ham soup (dried)	Knorr	327	93
	Knorr Quick Soup	354	100
made up	Chef Box	29	8

Product	Brand	Calories per 100g/ 100ml	Calories per oz/ pack/ portion
Peach and papaya yogurt	Safeway	93	per 150g pack 140
Peach and passionfruit harvest ice cream	Lyons Maid	152	43
Peach and passionfruit Pavlova	Young's	290	82
Peach and redcurrant yogurt	Safeway	91	per 150g pack 137
Peach blancmange mix	Brown and Polson	330	94
Peach chutney	Sharwood	173	49
	Tesco	146	41
	Waitrose	221	63
Peach halves	Safeway	87	per 411g can 358
in fruit juice	Del Monte	46	13
in natural syrup	Libby	47	13
in syrup	Del Monte	69	20
	Waitrose	62	per 411g can 255
Peach jelly	Tesco	57	16
Peach melba	Cow and Gate	56	per 110g jar 62, 150g jar 84
Peach melba dairy ice cream	Lyons Maid Napoli	172	49
Peach melba ice cream	Lyons Maid	177	50
soft scoop	Lyons Maid	180	51
Peach Melba sundae	Bejam		per sundae 164
Peach melba tub dessert	Birds Eye		per tub 130
Peach melba yogurt	Mr Men	93	26
	Raines	96	27
	Safeway	103	per 150g pack 155

Product	Brand	Calories per 100g/ 100ml	Calories per oz/ pack/ portion
Peach melba yogurt	St Ivel Rainbow	71	20
	St Michael	90	26
	Ski	82	per 150g pack 123
	Diet Ski	54	per 150g pack 81
	St Ivel Shape	41	12
low fat	Littlewoods	87	per 150g pack 131
	Tesco	102	29
	Waitrose	103	per 150g pack 155
whole milk	Safeway	62	per 150g pack 93
Peach melba yogurt dessert	Cow and Gate	65	per 110g jar 72
Peach slices	Safeway	87	per 411g can 358
diabetic	Boots	20	6
in fruit juice	Del Monte	46	13
in juice	Waitrose	35	per 220g can 77
in natural syrup	Libby	49	14
in syrup	Del Monte	69	20
	Waitrose	62	per 411g can 255
Peach trifle	St Ivel	145	41
Peach yogurt	Ski	83	per 150g pack 125
Peaches			
fresh, raw		37	10
canned		87	25
dried, raw, stewed with sugar		93	26
dried, raw, stewed without sugar		79	22
fresh, raw (weighed with stones)		32	9
dried, raw		212	60
	Libby	69	20
dried	Holland and Barrett	200	57
fresh, without stones	Littlewoods	37	10
in natural juice	Tesco	42	12

Product	Brand	Calories per 100g/ 100ml	Calories per oz/ pack/ portion
Peaches			
in syrup	Tesco	78	22
in water	Dietade	23	7
low calorie	Boots Shapers	21	6
Peaches and pears	Safeway	82	per 411g can 337
in syrup	Waitrose	95	per 411g can 390
Peanut and almond cluster	Lyons	463	131
Peanut butter			
smooth		623	177
	Whole Earth	580	164
crunchy	Boots Second Nature	605	172
	Gales	600	170
	Safeway	600	170
	Sun-Pat	607	172
	Tesco	610	173
	Waitrose	600	170
natural	Prewetts	620	176
smooth	Boots Second Nature	605	172
	Gales	600	170
	Safeway	600	170
	Sun-Pat	607	172
	Tesco	610	173
	Waitrose	600	170
	Waitrose	600	170
Peanut butter cookies	Waitrose	300	85
Peanut butter/ crumble	Granose	586	166
Peanut butter spread	Sunwheel	559	158
Peanut carob bar no added sugar	Sunwheel Kalibu	507	per 60g bar 304

Product	Brand	Calories per 100g/ 100ml	Calories per oz/ pack/ portion
Peanut carob bar			
with raw sugar	Sunwheel Kalibu	528	per 60g bar 317
Peanut cluster	Lyons Maid		each 190
Peanut crackle	Tesco	487	138
Peanut crisp block	Needlers	513	145
Peanut crunch biscuits	Tesco	485	137
Peanut M & Ms	Mars	500	142
Peanut nougat	Rowntree Mackintosh		per sweet 45
Peanut, raisin and chocolate chips	Waitrose	480	136
Peanut Sunsnack	Sunwheel	622	176
Peanuts			
(*weighed with shells*)		394	112
fresh		570	162
roasted and salted		570	162
	Holland and Barrett	560	159
	St Michael	600	170
blanched	Tesco	605	172
chocolate covered	Littlewoods	497	141
crunchy coated	Sooner	490	per 40g pack 196
dry roast	St Michael	544	154
	Sooner	602	per 50g pack 301
dry roasted	Safeway	570	162
	Tesco	616	175
	Waitrose	625	177
kernels	Littlewoods	570	162
	Whitworths	570	162
roast salted	St Michael	600	170
roasted salted	Waitrose	610	173

Product	Brand	Calories per 100g/ 100ml	Calories per oz/ pack/ portion
Peanuts			
roasted salted large	Waitrose	650	184
salted	Sooner	572	per 25g pack 143
	Sun-Pat	615	174
	Tesco	627	178
salted snacks	Littlewoods	570	162
salted, large	Waitrose	598	170
salted/roasted	Safeway	570	162
shelled	Safeway	570	162
	Waitrose	610	173
yogurt coated, no added sugar	Sunwheel	559	158
Peanuts and raisins	Safeway	495	140
	St Michael	410	116
	Waitrose	495	140
blanched	Tesco	500	142
carob coated	Sunwheel Kalibu	503	143
chocolate	Tesco	489	139
plain	Sooner	476	per 25g pack 119
yogurt coated, no added sugar	Sunwheel	477	135
Pear 'n' apple fruit spread	Sunwheel	239	68
Pear 'n' apple jam	Whole Earth	280	79
Pear and apple juice	Copella	40	12
Pear 'n' apricot fruit spread	Sunwheel	264	75
Pear 'n' black cherry fruit spread	Sunwheel	258	73
Pear and cherry fruity juice dessert	Heinz Baby Foods	61	per 128g jar 78

Product	Brand	Calories per 100g/ 100ml	Calories per oz/ pack/ portion
Pear and chocolate Regale dessert	St Ivel	138	39
Pear and peach pure juice	Cow and Gate	40	per 125g jar 50
concentrated	Cow and Gate	227	per 130ml jar 295
Pear and raspberry yogurt	Safeway	89	per 150g pack 134
Pear 'n' strawberry fruit spread	Sunwheel	242	69
Pear chews	Trebor	375	per sweet 15
Pear dessert	Boots Baby Foods	62	18
	Heinz Baby Foods	56	per 128g can 72
Pear drops	Trebor	366	per sweet 15
roll	Trebor	351	per sweet
Pear flan, continental style	St Michael	233	66
Pear flavour drops	Littlewoods	366	104
Pear fruit cream trifle	Safeway	135	38
Pear halves	Libby	69	20
	Safeway	77	per 411g can 316
dried	Tesco	308	87
in fruit juice	Del Monte	48	14
in juice	Waitrose	50	per 425g can 213
in natural syrup	Libby	49	14
in syrup	Del Monte	63	18
	Waitrose	71	per 411g can 292
Pear Helene slice	Waitrose	215	61
Pear Helene sundae	Eden Vale	132	per 125g pack 165
Pear quarters			
diabetic	Boots	21	6

Product	Brand	Calories per 100g/ 100ml	Calories per oz/ pack/ portion
Pear quarters			
in juice	Waitrose	50	per 220g can 110
in syrup	Safeway	77	per 227g can 175
	Waitrose	71	per 220g can 156
Pear treat dessert	Boots Baby Foods	62	18
Pear yogurt	Ski	80	per 150g pack 120
Pear yogurt dessert	Cow and Gate Heinz Baby Foods	62	per 110g jar 68
		77	per 128g jar 99
Pearl barley: see Barley, pearl			
Pearl drink	St Michael	45	13
Pears			
cooking		36	10
cooking, canned		77	22
cooking, stewed with sugar		65	18
cooking, stewed without sugar		30	9
eating		41	12
eating (weighed with skin and core)		29	8
conference, fresh	Tesco	29	8
dessert, without skin, fresh	Littlewoods	41	12
dried	Holland and Barrett	268	76
in natural juice	Tesco	34	10
in syrup	Tesco	67	19
in water	Dietade	23	7
low calorie	Boots Shapers	21	6
Peas: see also mange tout, petits pois			
Peas			
fresh, boiled		52	15
fresh, raw		67	19

Product	Brand	Calories per 100g/ 100ml	Calories per oz/ pack/ portion
Peas			
frozen, boiled		41	12
frozen, raw		53	15
dried, boiled		103	29
dried, raw		286	81
dried	Holland and Barrett	286	81
	Safeway	286	81
frozen	Birds Eye	53	15
	Findus	53	15
	Littlewoods	53	per 454g pack 241
	Ross	50	14
	Safeway	80	per 227g pack 184
	Tesco	70	20
mint	Waitrose	53	per 454g pack 240
mint (frozen)	Tesco	70	20
minted (frozen)	Safeway	80	per 454g pack 368
Peas, blackeye			
dried	Holland and Barrett	340	96
Peas, chick			
Bengal gram, raw		320	91
chana dahl		97	27
dahl, cooked		144	41
	Waitrose	75	21
dried	Holland and Barrett	300	85
Peas, garden			
canned		47	13
canned	Del Monte	71	20
	Hartley's	45	per 111g can 50
	Littlewoods	65	per 300g can 195
	Morton	58	16
	Safeway	47	per 284g can 133

Product	Brand	Calories per 100g/ 100ml	Calories per oz/ pack/ portion
Peas, garden			
canned	Tesco	60	17
	Waitrose	47	per 300g pack 141
dried (as sold)	Batchelors		per 40g standard
	Surprise	193	pack 77
frozen	Waitrose	53	per 454g pack 240
frozen, economy	Bejam	90	per 57g portion boiled 51
frozen, grade A	Bejam	76	per 57g portion boiled 43
minted (frozen)	Bejam	69	per 57g portion boiled 39
no salt added	Del Monte	69	20
Peas, marrowfat	Morton	90	26
	Safeway	78	per 284g can 222
	Tesco	314	89
	Waitrose	95	per 300g can 285
canned	Tesco	78	22
dried	Waitrose	286	81
dried, boiled	Whitworths	103	29
dried, raw	Whitworths	286	81
Peas, mushy	Morton	80	23
canned	Batchelors	84	24
Chip Shop (canned)	Batchelors	76	22
mint flavour (canned)	Batchelors	83	24
Peas, processed			
canned		80	23
	Safeway	80	per 284g can 227
all varieties (canned)	Batchelors	80	23
canned	Del Monte	92	26
	Hartley's	80	per 113g can 90
	Tesco	117	33

Product	Brand	Calories per 100g/ 100ml	Calories per oz/ pack/ portion
Peas, processed			
processed	Waitrose	95	per 300g can 285
Peas, red pigeon, raw		301	85
Peas, split			
boiled		118	33
dried, raw		310	88
dried	Safeway	310	88
	Waitrose	310	88
green, cooked	Tesco	128	36
green, uncooked	Tesco	330	94
yellow, boiled	Whitworths	118	33
yellow, cooked	Tesco	137	39
yellow, raw	Whitworths	310	88
yellow, uncooked	Tesco	335	95
Peas and baby carrots	Birds Eye	35	10
Peas, corn and peppers	Waitrose	68	per 454g pack 304
Pease pudding (canned)	Batchelors	103	29
Pecan nuts	Holland and Barrett	680	193
Peking Classic Chinese sauce			
aromatic	Homepride	91	per 383g pack 348
barbecue	Homepride	94	per 383g pack 360
Penny Pets	Trebor	542	per sweet 26
Pepper		308	87
black ground	Tesco	275	78
black whole	Tesco	275	78
white	Tesco	275	78
Pepper and onion relish	Branston	137	39
Pepper salami	Waitrose	427	per 99g pack (appr) 423

Product	Brand	Calories per 100g/ 100ml	Calories per oz/ pack/ portion
Peppered mackerel			
(chilled)	Young's	333	94
hot (frozen), cooked	Tesco	363	103
Peppermint carob bar			
no added sugar	Sunwheel Kalibu	493	per 60g bar 296
with raw sugar	Sunwheel Kalibu	518	per 60g bar 311
Peppermint chewing gum	PK Wrigley		per pellet 6
	Freedent		per stick 9
Peppermint cordial			
diluted	Britvic	18	5
non-alchoholic, concentrated	Schweppes	104	31
undiluted	Britvic	92	26
Peppermint cream bar	Cadbury's	420	per 50g bar 210
Peppermint creams	Littlewoods	350	99
Peppermint lumps	Littlewoods	380	108
Peppermint pastilles, diabetic	Boots	99	28
Peppermint sweet chewing gum	Wrigley Orbit Nutra		per stick 7
Peppermints		392	111
Pepperoni luxury pizza (frozen)	Safeway	205	58
Peppers			
green, boiled		14	4
green, raw		15	4
green fresh	Littlewoods	15	4
mixed (frozen)	Ross	20	6

Product	Brand	Calories per 100g/ 100ml	Calories per oz/ pack/ portion
Peppers			
mixed (frozen)	Safeway	14	per 227g pack 32
red, sweet	Waitrose	18	per 185g pack 33
yellow, fresh	Tesco	35	10
Peppers, red/chilli, raw		116	33
Perry	Bulmer	43	per half pint 122
Petit beurre biscuits	Waitrose	468	133
Petits pois	Waitrose	61	198g/7oz pack
canned	Morton	58	16
	Safeway	99	per 198g can 196
	Tesco	89	25
frozen	Findus	63	18
	Safeway	53	per 907g pack 480
	Tesco	73	21
	Waitrose	53	per 454g pack 240
Petits pois and baby carrots	Waitrose	65	per 397g pack 258
quality choice	Bejam	41	per 57g portion boiled 23
Petits pois and carrots (bottled)	Tesco	55	16
Petits pois, button sprouts and baby carrots	Birds Eye	42	12
Petits pois quality choice (frozen)	Bejam	76	per 57g portion boiled 43
Petticoat shortbread biscuits	Tesco	502	142
Petticoat tails	Safeway	465	132
	Waitrose	515	146
Pheasant roast		213	60

Product	Brand	Calories per 100g/ 100ml	Calories per oz/ pack/ portion
Pheasant			
roast (with bone)		134	38
hen (fresh)	Waitrose	400	600g/21@oz bird
hen (frozen)	Waitrose	400	113
Philadelphia soft			
cheese	Kraft	322	per 85g pack 274
light	Kraft	198	56
with chives	Kraft	322	per 85g pack 274
with garlic and herbs	Kraft	322	per 85g pack 274
Phosferine Tonic Wine	Beecham	137	41
Piccalilli		33	9
	Haywards	29	8
	Heinz		
	Ploughman's	85	24
	Littlewoods	47	13
	Pan Yan	68	19
	Safeway	35	10
	Tesco	56	16
	Waitrose	48	14
chunky sweet	Safeway	98	28
sweet	Haywards	75	21
	Tesco	103	29
	Waitrose	48	14
Pickle			
chilli		271	77
chow chow, sour		29	8
chow chow, sweet		116	33
lime		178	50
mango		177	50
sweet		134	38
	Heinz		
	Ploughman's	120	34

Product	Brand	Calories per 100g/ 100ml	Calories per oz/ pack/ portion
Pickle			
original	Pan Yan	133	38
sweet	Branston	131	37
	Littlewoods	160	45
	Safeway	91	26
	Tesco	172	49
	Waitrose	215	61
sweet, low calorie	Boots Shapers	66	19
Pickle crisps, natural	Hedgehog	407	per 27g pack 110
Pickled beetroot			
baby	Waitrose	35	10
sliced	Littlewoods	37	10
	Waitrose	37	10
sliced, in sweet vinegar	Waitrose	55	16
Pickled dill cucumber	Tesco	14	4
Pickled gherkins	Safeway	6	2
Pickled Jalapenos	Old El Paso	32	per 283g can 91
Pickled onion crisps	Hunters	520	per 26g bag 130
Pickled onions	Haywards	16	5
	Littlewoods	19	5
	Safeway	37	10
	St Michael	23	7
	Tesco	18	5
	Waitrose	19	5
silverskin	Littlewoods	27	8
sweet	Haywards	25	7
	Tesco	28	8
	Waitrose	38	11
Pickled red cabbage	Waitrose	21	6
Pickles			
gherkin		13	4
mixed, clear	Safeway	8	2

Product	Brand	Calories per 100g/ 100ml	Calories per oz/ pack/ portion
Pickles			
mixed, Continental	Safeway	19	5
Picnic	Cadbury's	495	per 46g bar 230
Picnic eggs	St Michael	293	83
Pie filling mixes: *see flavours*			
Piermont soft drink	Taunton	18	per pint 100
Pigeon			
roast		230	65
roast (*with bone*)		101	29
fresh	Waitrose	400	per 240g bird (min) 960
frozen	Waitrose	400	113
Pigeon peas/Red gram, raw		301	85
Pilchard and tomato paste	Shippams	169	per 75g pack 127
Pilchards			
canned in tomato sauce		126	36
in tomato sauce	Shippams	162	per 425g can 689
Pacific, in tomato sauce	Armour	126	per 156g can 197
Pina colada cocktail	Lyons Maid		each 60
Pina colada cup	Lyons Maid		each 105
Pina colada dairy ice cream	Safeway	225	67
Pina colada yogurt	St Ivel Cabaret	105	30
Pine kernels	Holland and Barrett	580	164
Pineapple			
canned in syrup		77	22
fresh, raw		46	13
in juice, crushed	Del Monte	61	17
in juice, sliced	Del Monte	61	17

Product	Brand	Calories per 100g/ 100ml	Calories per oz/ pack/ portion
Pineapple			
in juice, sliced	St Michael	61	17
in natural juice	Tesco	52	15
in syrup	Tesco	67	19
in syrup, sliced	Del Monte	78	22
in water	Dietade	29	8
pieces in juice	Waitrose	59	per 439g pack 259
pieces in syrup	Waitrose	76	per 439g pack 334
rings in natural juice	Safeway	50	per 227g can 112
slices (canned)	Libby	57	16
slices in juice	Waitrose	58	per 227g pack 132
slices in natural syrup	Libby	54	15
slices in syrup	Waitrose	76	per 227g pack 184
without skin	Littlewoods	46	13
Pineapple and banana dessert	Boots Baby Foods	390	111
Pineapple and coconut choc ices	Waitrose	288	85
Pineapple and coconut drink	Safeway	90	27
Pineapple and coconut ice cream	Bejam	166	47
Pineapple and coconut yoghurt, low fat	Waitrose	87	per 150g pack 131
Pineapple and grapefruit drink, low calorie	St Michael	4	1
Pineapple and grapefruit juice	Appella	42	12
	Del Monte	46	14
Pineapple and grapefruit yogurt	St Michael	106	30

Product	Brand	Calories per 100g/ 100ml	Calories per oz/ pack/ portion
Pineapple and ham cottage cheese	Waitrose	96	27
Pineapple 'C'	Libby	44	12
Pineapple Chunks	Trebor	354	per sweet 17
Pineapple chunks in juice	Del Monte	61	17
Pineapple cottage cheese	Eden Vale	98	28
	Safeway	98	28
	St Ivel	91	26
	St Ivel Shape	74	21
Pineapple crush, low calorie	Slimsta	5	1
Pineapple dessert with vitamin C	Cow and Gate	50	per 150g jar 75
	Heinz Baby Foods	61	per 128g jar 78
Pineapple filled milk chocolate	Littlewoods	505	per 50g pack 253
Pineapple fruit filling	Morton	64	18
Pineapple fruit harvest ice cream	Lyons Maid	150	43
Pineapple fruit juice	Del Monte	50	15
	Heinz	57	17
Pineapple, grapefuit and lemon fruit drink	Del Monte Island Blend	46	14
Pineapple jam	Waitrose	248	70
Pineapple juice canned		53	15
Pineapple juice	Britvic	50	per 113ml pack 57
	Libby	53	15
	St Ivel Mr Juicy	40	12
	St Ivel Real	40	12
	Schweppes	48	14

Product	Brand	Calories per 100g/ 100ml	Calories per oz/ pack/ portion
Pineapple juice	Volonte	49	15
chilled	Safeway	43	13
	Tesco	42	12
longlife	Tesco	42	12
	Waitrose	44	13
pure	St Michael	49	14
pure, chilled	Waitrose	43	13
pure, longlife	Safeway	49	15
sweetened	Hunts	54	16
Pineapple juice bar	Lyons Maid		each 42
Pineapple, lemon and lime fruit drink	Del Monte Island Blend	41	12
Pineapple, orange and mandarin fruit drink	Del Monte Island Blend	46	14
Pineapple pancakes	St Michael	161	46
Pineapple Pavlova	Ross	290	82
Pineapple preserve	Tesco	255	72
Pineapple split	Wall's		per split 81
Pineapple Super Mivvi	Lyons Maid		each 82
Pineapple sweet and sour chutney	Sharwood	61	17
Pineapple tidbits	Libby	58	16
Pineapple yogurt	Safeway	90	per 150g pack 135
	St Ivel Real	82	23
	Ski	83	per 150g pack 125
low fat	Littlewoods	86	per 150g pack 129
	Tesco	83	24
Pinto beans, dried	Holland and Barrett	263	75
Pistachio nuts		626	177

Product	Brand	Calories per 100g/ 100ml	Calories per oz/ pack/ portion
Pistachio nuts	Holland and		
	Barrett	600	170
	St Michael	594	168
	Tesco	625	177
salted	Waitrose	630	179
Pitta bread			
white		265	75
white	Tesco	242	69
Pizza: see also flavours			
Pizza			
American style	Tesco	233	66
American style, with cheese and tomato	St Michael	212	60
American style, with pepper and mushroom	St Michael	209	59
crusty bun	Findus	231	65
French bread	Birds Eye MenuMaster		per pizza 330
	Ross	270	77
luxury	Tesco	226	64
Margherita	St Michael	218	62
mini	St Michael	282	80
premier	Tesco	195	55
Pizza a la mare	Tesco	181	51
Pizza base mix			
(as sold)	Granny Smiths	248	per 240g pack made up 595
(as sold)	Tesco	363	103
(made up)	Tesco	250	71
Pizza bites snacks	Littlewoods	547	per 50g pack 274
Pizza bits Italian style	St Michael	473	134

Product	Brand	Calories per 100g/ 100ml	Calories per oz/ pack/ portion
Pizza bologna	Buitoni	866	246
Pizza Compagnola	Waitrose	164	46
Pizza crackers	Tesco	472	134
Pizza fingers	Tesco	250	71
Pizza Italiana	Tesco	275	78
Pizza Marinara	Waitrose	179	51
Pizza Napoli	Buitoni	760	215
Pizza Pepperoni	Waitrose	189	54
Pizza provencal	Tesco	195	55
Pizza roma	Buitoni	834	236
Pizza style cheese	St Ivel	405	115
Pizza topping Prego sauce	Campbell's	76	22
Pizza Venezia	Buitoni	870	247
Pizza wedges	Tesco	235	67
Pizzaiola Prego sauce	Campbell's	37	10
PK chewing gum			
arrowmint	Wrigley		per pellet 6
licorice	Wrigley		per pellet 6
peppermint	Wrigley		per pellet 6
Plaice			
fried in batter		279	79
fried in crumbs		228	65
raw		91	26
steamed		93	26
steamed (with bones and skin)		50	14
	Waitrose	91	26
breaded	Waitrose	110	31
breaded boneless	St Michael	132	37
breaded, in white sauce	Tesco	242	69

Product	Brand	Calories per 100g/ 100ml	Calories per oz/ pack/ portion
Plaice			
crispy whole, fried	Birds Eye	229	65
filled with butter sauce (chilled)	Young's	158	45
filled with mornay sauce (chilled)	Young's	158	45
fresh	Littlewoods	91	26
fresh, in breadcrumbs (chilled)	Young's	249	71
frozen	Safeway	105	30
goujons, breaded	Waitrose	150	43
in a butter sauce	Waitrose	200	57
in a mornay sauce	Waitrose	190	54
in breadcrumbs (frozen)	Safeway	165	47
in ovencrisp crumb	St Michael	132	37
stuffed	St Michael	109	31
whole	Waitrose	91	26
	Young's	81	23
whole boneless breaded	St Michael	132	37
whole breaded	Waitrose	132	37
whole in breadcrumbs	Findus	116	33
Plaice and prawn veronique	Waitrose	83	482g/17oz pack
Plaice fillets			
breaded, deep-fried	Bejam	254	72
chilled	Young's	81	23
crispy, shallow-fried	Birds Eye	247	70
frozen	Ross	80	23

Product	Brand	Calories per 100g/ 100ml	Calories per oz/ pack/ portion
Plaice fillets			
in golden breadcrumb, baked or grilled	Birds Eye	229	65
in golden breadcrumb, shallow-fried	Birds Eye	300	85
prime, poached	Bejam	106	30
supercrumb, baked	Bejam	258	73
Plaice			
whole, breaded boneless, deep-fried	Bejam	236	67
whole, breaded, with prawn and mushroom	Bejam		each deep-fried 414
Plain cake mix, diabetic (as sold)	Boots	459	130
Plain carob bar			
no added sugar	Sunwheel Kalibu	493	per 60g bar 296
with raw sugar	Sunwheel Kalibu	518	per 60g bar 311
Plain chocolate		525	149
	Waitrose	530	150
diabetic	Boots	500	142
Plain chocolate bar	Boots Shapers		
	Meal	506	143
	St Michael	531	151
	Tesco	540	153
Plain chocolate biscuit thins	St Michael	470	133
Plain chocolate Bounty	Mars	485	137

Product	Brand	Calories per 100g/ 100ml	Calories per oz/ pack/ portion
Plain chocolate Brazils	Tesco	581	165
Plain chocolate breaktime biscuit	Waitrose	588	167
Plain chocolate crunch biscuits (half-coated)	Safeway	478	136
Plain chocolate digestive biscuits	Safeway	500	142
	St Michael	505	143
	Tesco	508	144
	Waitrose	505	143
half-coated	Huntley & Palmer	496	per biscuit 65
Plain chocolate drops	Tesco	516	146
Plain chocolate fingers	Safeway	562	159
Plain chocolate ginger biscuits	St Michael	490	139
Plain chocolate Melt in the Bag cake covering	Lyons	572	162
Plain chocolate mint sandwich bar	St Michael	491	139
	Waitrose	519	147
Plain chocolate petit beurre biscuits	Waitrose	470	133
Plain chocolate Polka Dots	Lyons	507	144
Plain chocolate wafer fingers	Waitrose	504	143
Plain chocolate with hazelnuts	Waitrose	554	157

Product	Brand	Calories per 100g/ pack/ 100ml	Calories per oz/ pack/ portion
Plain Club biscuits	Jacobs	494	per biscuit 112
Plain confectionery bar, no added sugar	Sunwheel Kalibu	517	per 42g bar 217
Plain digestive biscuits		471	134
Plain fruit cake		354	100
Plain luxury cheesecake mix (as sold)	Green's	430	made up per portion 236
Plain M & Ms	Mars	483	137
Plain mint wafer fingers	Waitrose	510	145
Plain peanuts and raisins	Sooner	476	per 25g pack 119
Plain superfine chocolates	Nestle	546	155
Plantain			
boiled		122	35
green, raw		112	32
ripe, fried		267	76
Plantain (Green banana, matoki)		89	25
Plate apple pie	Waitrose	314	89
PLJ lemon juice less sharp, undiluted	Beecham	25	7
original sharp, undiluted	Beecham	25	7
Ploughman's Ideal sauce	Heinz	106	30
Ploughman's mild mustard pickle	Heinz	114	32
Ploughman's piccalilli	Heinz	85	24

Product	Brand	Calories per 100g/ 100ml	Calories per oz/ pack/ portion
Ploughman's pickle	Heinz	120	34
Ploughman's tangy pickle spread	Heinz Ploughman's	118	33
Ploughman's tomato pickle	Heinz	95	27
Plum and walnut yoghurt	Safeway	106	per 150g pack 159
Plum jam	Safeway	251	71
Plum preserve	Tesco	255	72
Plum yoghurt	Safeway	96	per 150g pack 144
Plums			
cooking, raw		26	7
cooking, raw (with stones)		23	7
cooking, stewed with sugar		59	17
cooking, stewed with sugar (with stones)		55	16
cooking, stewed without sugar		22	6
cooking, stewed without (with stones)		20	6
Victoria dessert, raw		38	11
Victoria dessert, raw (with stones)		36	10
dessert, without stones, fresh	Littlewoods	38	11
golden	Waitrose	58	16
Victoria	Waitrose	80	23
Poacher's broth	Baxters	35	per 425g can 149
Polar mints	Trebor	365	per sweet 19
Polka Dots			
milk chocolate	Lyons	493	140
plain chocolate	Lyons	507	144
Polo fruits	Rowntree Mackintosh	380	per sweet 8

Product	Brand	Calories per 100g/ 100ml	Calories per oz/ pack/ portion
Polo peppermints	Rowntree Mackintosh	395	per sweet 6
Polony		281	80
Pomagne			
medium dry	Bulmer	52	per half pint 148
medium sweet	Bulmer	65	per half pint 185
Pomegranate, raw, fresh		72	20
Pomegranate juice, fresh		44	12
Pomelo, fresh	Tesco	36	10
Pommia cider, dry	Taunton	54	per pint 310
sweet	Taunton	65	per pint 370
Pontefract cakes	Bassett's	296	84
Popcorn			
Butterkist	Tesco	390	111
chocolate	Tesco	414	117
Popping corn	Holland and Barrett	375	106
Poppy and sesame crackers	Tesco	511	145
Poppy seed bar			
natural	Boots	439	124
Popular pies			
apple	Lyons	349	99
apple and blackcurrant	Lyons	353	100
apricot	Lyons	361	102
Pork			
lean, raw		147	42
leg, raw, lean and fat		269	76
trotters and tails, salted		280	79
belly rashers, grilled, lean and fat		398	113
belly rashers, raw, lean and fat		381	108

Product	Brand	Calories per 100g/ 100ml	Calories per oz/ pack/ portion
Pork			
dressed carcase, raw		338	96
fat, cooked		619	175
fat, raw		670	190
lean, raw		147	42
leg, raw, lean and fat		269	76
leg, roast, lean and fat		286	81
leg, roast, lean only		185	52
barbecue spare ribs	St Michael	239	68
barbeque ribs	Waitrose	340	96
belly slices, grilled	Bejam	303	86
cooked	Littlewoods	201	57
diced, casseroled	Bejam	201	57
escalopes	St Michael	147	42
half leg (knuckle), roasted	Bejam	236	67
joint, cooked	Tesco	174	49
leg (fillet), roasted	Bejam	215	61
leg cured	Waitrose	179	51
leg of, roast	Waitrose	189	54
leg roast, boneless, roasted	Bejam	254	72
leg steaks	St Michael	329	93
leg steaks, seasoned	Waitrose	262	74
loin joint with herb, cured	St Michael	360	102
loin roast, sliced	St Michael	159	45
loin steaks, boneless, grilled	Bejam	198	56
rib, loin and leg steaks	St Michael	329	93
rib-steaks	Bejam		per steak grilled 228
rib-steaks, Chinese style	Bejam		per steak grilled 201

Product	Brand	Calories per 100g/ 100ml	Calories per oz/ pack/ portion
Pork			
roast	Waitrose	189	54
roast loin	Waitrose	156	44
roast, sliced	Tesco	193	55
savoury roast, roasted	Bejam	282	80
shoulder roast, boneless, roasted	Bejam	187	53
shoulder steaks, boneless, grilled	Bejam	222	63
shoulder, cured, sliced	St Michael	95	27
smoked loin	St Michael	180	51
smoked loin steak, cured, Danish	St Michael	180	51
smoked loin, sliced	Tesco	167	47
spare ribs in a barbecue sauce	Waitrose	453	454g/16oz pack
spare ribs, grilled	Bejam	236	67
tongue	Waitrose	176	50
tongue, pressed, sliced	St Michael	152	43
Pork chops			
loin, grilled, lean and fat		332	94
loin, grilled, lean and fat (with bone)		258	73
loin, grilled, lean only		226	64
loin, grilled, lean (with fat and bone)		133	38
loin, raw		329	93
	St Michael	329	93
chump, grilled	Bejam	265	75
loin, cured	St Michael	350	99
loin, grilled	Bejam	205	58
spare rib, grilled	Bejam	250	71

Product	Brand	Calories per 100g/ 100ml	Calories per oz/ pack/ portion
Pork chops			
unsmoked cured			
Danish	St Michael	350	99
Pork and beef chipolatas	Tesco	314	89
	Waitrose	335	227g/8oz pack
Pork and beef luncheon sausage	Waitrose	256	73
Pork and beef sausages	Ross	285	81
	St Michael	370	105
	Waitrose	335	95
jumbo	Bejam		per sausage grilled 281
	Ross	285	81
skinless	St Michael	250	71
thick	Bejam		per sausage grilled 150
	Littlewoods	265	75
	Littlewoods	265	per sausage 150
thick economy	Bejam		per sausage grilled 115
thin	Bejam		per sausage grilled 75
	Littlewoods	265	75
	Littlewoods	265	75
Pork and chicken pie	Waitrose	226	64
Pork and egg pie	Tesco	370	105
large	St Michael	324	92
sliced	St Michael	385	109
Pork and ham roulade with cheese	Waitrose	262	74
Pork and herb sausages	Tesco	379	107

Product	Brand	Calories per 100g/ 100ml	Calories per oz/ pack/ portion
Pork and herb sausages			
thick	Bejam		per sausage grilled 135
Pork and pepper kebab	Waitrose	150	43
Pork brochettes	Waitrose	207	59
Pork buffet pie	Bejam		per pie as sold 351
	Littlewoods	395	per pie 320
Pork casserole cooking mix	Colman's	295	84
Pork chipolatas	Tesco	338	96
	Waitrose	358	101
Cumberland	Waitrose	320	91
premium	Tesco	343	97
	Waitrose	310	88
skinless	Waitrose	326	92
Pork crackling crisps	Hunters	520	per 26g bag 130
Pork crunchies	Tesco	462	131
Pork, ham and egg pie			
gala	Waitrose	221	63
Pork lattice pie			
individual	Littlewoods	351	per 115g pie 404
large	Littlewoods	321	per 336g pie 1079
Pork luncheon meat	Waitrose	356	113g/4oz pack
Pork luncheon meat, Chinese		288	82
Pork mixed grill	Waitrose	207	59
Pork parisien Ready Meal	Tesco	129	37
Pork pie			
individual		376	107
	St Michael	348	99
	Waitrose	355	454g/16oz pie

Product	Brand	Calories per 100g/ 100ml	Calories per oz/ pack/ portion
Pork pie			
crisp bake	St Michael	349	99
crisp bake, individual	St Michael	339	96
cured	St Michael	348	99
cured, individual	St Michael	348	99
farmhouse	Waitrose	237	67
hand raised	Littlewoods	380	108
individual	Littlewoods	390	per 142g pie 554
	Waitrose	377	107
Melton Mowbray	St Michael	402	114
	Waitrose	444	126
Melton Mowbray, individual	Waitrose	377	per 127g pie 479
Melton Mowbray, large	St Michael	353	100
mini	Waitrose	378	107
slicing	Littlewoods	365	103
traditional (as sold)	Bejam		per pie 626
traditional, cured	Tesco	411	117
Pork provencale (canned)	St Michael	110	31
Pork roll			
stuffed (canned)	Tyne Brand	153	43
stuffed, sliced	Tesco	316	90
with egg, sliced	Tesco	294	83
Pork, sage and onion stuffing	St Michael	200	57
Pork sate stick	Waitrose	160	45
Pork sausage	Waitrose	358	101
premier	Tesco	353	100
smoked	Tesco	344	98
	Waitrose	328	93
smoked, cooked	Littlewoods	320	91

Product	Brand	Calories per 100g/ 100ml	Calories per oz/ pack/ portion
Pork sausage			
with garlic, quality	Tesco	296	84
with herbs, premium	Tesco	308	87
with onion	Tesco	349	99
Pork sausage meat	Tesco	317	90
	Waitrose	270	77
grilled	Bejam	307	grilled
premium	Tesco	329	93
Yorkshire	Waitrose	285	81
Pork sausage rings			
Cumberland	Waitrose	358	101
Pork sausages	Ross	340	96
	Waitrose	287	81
butcher's	Littlewoods	251	71
	Littlewoods	277	per sausage 79
cocktail	St Michael	350	99
	Tesco	378	107
	Tesco	378	107
	Waitrose	287	81
Cotswold, low fat	Waitrose	240	68
Cumberland	Waitrose	320	91
economy	Tesco	291	82
large	Waitrose	179	51
low fat	St Michael	180	51
premium	Bejam		per sausage grilled 198
	Waitrose	310	88
prize-winning	St Michael	268	76
skinless	Tesco	321	91
	Tesco	316	90
spiced	Waitrose	292	83
thick	Bejam		per sausage grilled 144

Product	Brand	Calories per 100g/ 100ml	Calories per oz/ pack/ portion
Pork sausages			
thick	Littlewoods	277	per sausage 157
	Waitrose	270	77
thick economy	Bejam		per sausage grilled 148
thick low-fat	Bejam		per sausage grilled
thin	Bejam		per sausage grilled 72
	Littlewoods	277	per sausage 79
	Waitrose	275	78
Yorkshire	Waitrose	285	81
Pork, chopped slices, cured	St Michael	194	55
Pork, cured (canned)	St Michael	270	77
Porridge		44	12
Porridge oats	Tesco	366	104
	Waitrose	355	101
cooked	Whitworths	44	12
uncooked	Whitworths	401	114
with bran	Tesco	370	105
Porridge oats with malt	Boots Baby Foods	415	118
Port		157	45
Port Salut cheese	Tesco	310	88
wedge	St Michael	313	89
Potato and chive salad	Eden Vale	163	46
Potato and leek soup, homestyle	Heinz Ready to Serve	36	10
Potato and onion salad	Waitrose	141	per 227g pack 320
Potato Bake country	Birds Eye		per pack 435

Product	Brand	Calories per 100g/ 100ml	Calories per oz/ pack/ portion
Potato cake Swiss style	Findus	80	23
Potato, celery and dill salad	Littlewoods	153	per 227g pack 347
Potato, cheese and asparagus pancakes	Waitrose	156	44
Potato crisps: *see also Crisps and flavours*		533	151
all flavours	Littlewoods	520	per 25g pack 130
Potato Crispy Crosses	Ross	180	51
Potato croquettes	Bejam		each deep-fried 41
	Findus	91	26
	Ross	100	28
	St Michael	216	61
Potato curry		167	47
Potato dauphinoise	Waitrose	144	per 311g pack 448
Potato fritters crispy, grilled, fried or baked	Birds Eye	212	60
Potato lamb cutlet	Waitrose	226	64
Potato leek soup	Granny's	44	as served 29
Potato mix, instant	Tesco	327	93
Potato pancakes: see also flavours	Bejam		each grilled 97
	Ross	210	60
Potato rings	St Michael	510	145
	Tesco	532	151
	Waitrose	516	146
Potato salad	Heinz	168	48
	Safeway	209	59
	St Michael	322	91

Product	Brand	Calories per 100g/ 100ml	Calories per oz/ pack/ portion
Potato salad	Tesco	114	32
in reduced calorie dressing	Tesco	85	24
in reduced calorie dressing, others	Tesco	90	26
mild	Eden Vale	224	64
other recipes	Tesco	150	43
spicy	Safeway	184	52
Potato Saucery (Batchelors): *see flavours*			
Potato scones	St Michael	210	60
	Tesco	235	67
Potato shells	Tesco	563	160
Potato sticks	Waitrose	508	144
ready salted	Safeway	505	143
	St Michael	505	143
Potato thins, ready salted	St Michael	472	134
Potato triangle biscuits	Tesco	467	132
Potato twirls, salt and vinegar	Waitrose	423	120
Potato waffles	Birds Eye		per pack baked or grilled 115
	Birds Eye		per pack fried
	Ross	190	54
	St Michael	463	131
crispy	Bejam		each, grilled 95
mini	Birds Eye		per pack baked or grilled 22, fried 27
Potato, instant mashed			
made up		70	20
powder		318	90

Product (as sold)	Brand	Calories per 100g/ 100ml	Calories per oz/ pack/ portion
(as sold)	Littlewoods	265	75
	Safeway	265	75
(made up)	Safeway	60	17
made up with full cream milk	Yeoman	52	15
made up with water	Yeoman	49	14
made up, complete mix	Yeoman	52	15
with chopped onion, made up	Yeoman	53	15
without added salt, made up	Yeoman	49	14

Potatoes			
new, boiled		76	22
new, canned		53	15
old, baked		105	30
old, baked (with skins)		85	24
old, boiled		80	23
old, chips		253	72
old, chips, frozen		109	31
old, chips, frozen, fried		291	82
old, mashed		119	34
old, raw		87	25
old, roast		157	45
	Waitrose	64	18
croquette, baked or grilled	Birds Eye	71	20
croquette, fried	Birds Eye	159	45
duchesse	Ross	110	31
Jersey	Waitrose	80	23
Jersey (canned)	Tesco	56	16
Jersey peeled (canned)	St Michael	48	14

Product	Brand	Calories per 100g/ 100ml	Calories per oz/ pack/ portion
Potatoes			
Jersey royal (canned)	Safeway	53	per 150g can 283
new (canned)	Del Monte	33	9
	Hartley's	60	per 117g can 70
	Tesco	49	14
new small (canned)	Safeway	53	per 425g can 225
new, fresh, boiled old crop, fresh,	Tesco	77	22
boiled	Tesco	80	23
roast	Ross	100	28
saute	Findus	97	27
traditional roast (frozen)	Tesco	155	44
Potted beef (canned)	St Michael	170	48
Potted salmon with butter (canned)	St Michael	166	47
Pouch batter mix (as sold)	Green's	348	99
Pour Over sauce (Crosse & Blackwell): *see flavours*			
Pour Over sauce mix (Colman's): *see flavours*			
Pouring syrup	Tate and Lyle	284	81
Poussin	Waitrose	232	66
Praline and apricot gateau	Safeway	365	103
Praline and toffee dairy ice cream	Safeway	230	68
Praline dairy ice cream	Bertorelli	210	60
Praline truffles, diabetic	Boots	582	165
Prawn and marie rose sandwich	Waitrose	212	60

Product	Brand	Calories per 100g/ 100ml	Calories per oz/ pack/ portion
Prawn and mayonnaise sandwich	St Michael	250	71
Prawn cocktail crisps	Christies	520	per 26g bag 130
	Hunters	520	per 26g bag 130
	Tesco	550	156
Prawn cocktail sauce	O.K.	380	108
Prawn cocktail snacks	St Michael	486	138
	Tesco	492	139
	Waitrose	520	147
Prawn crackers	St Michael	435	123
	Sharwood	350	99
Prawn curry	Findus	84	24
	Vesta	349	per 211g pack for two as served 736
Chinese-style meal	Bejam		per serving baked 85
with rice	Birds Eye MenuMaster		per pack 350
Prawn mayonnaise sandwiches	Tesco	260	74
Prawn mayonnaise with lettuce sandwich	Waitrose	285	81
Prawn quiche (chilled)	Young's	240	68
Prawn salad	Eden Vale	155	44
	Littlewoods	146	41
	St Ivel	155	44
	Tesco	119	34
	Waitrose	144	41
other recipes	Tesco	155	44
Prawn salad meal	St Michael	110	31

Product	Brand	Calories per 100g/ 100ml	Calories per oz/ pack/ portion
Prawn, smoked salmon, tuna and salad bap	Waitrose	211	60
Prawnaise			
blue cheese	Lyons Seafoods	200	57
curry	Lyons Seafoods	200	57
garlic	Lyons Seafoods	185	52
thousand islands	Lyons Seafoods	150	43
Prawns			
boiled		107	30
boiled (*with shell*)		41	12
dried		362	103
raw, fresh		87	25
battercrisp, deep-fried	Dan Maid	240	68
cooked and peeled	Waitrose	107	30
cooked, shell-on (chilled)	Young's	103	29
frozen	Littlewoods	84	per 114g pack 96
garlic (chilled)	Young's	75	21
Icelandic, raw (frozen)	Tesco	80	23
Indian	Dan Maid	45	13
Indian, raw (frozen)	Tesco	55	16
Norwegian	Raider	70	20
Norwegian	Waitrose	75	per 198g pack 147
peeled, as sold	Bejam	71	20
peeled, cooked	St Michael	107	30
Prawns cottage cheese	Waitrose	112	32
Prego sauce (Campbell's): *see flavours*			
Premier pizza (chilled)	Tesco	195	55
Premium tea, infused	Safeway	1	

Product	Brand	Calories per 100g/ 100ml	Calories per oz/ pack/ portion
Preserves	Thursday Cottage	280	79
diabetic	Thursday Cottage	140	40
Preserving sugar	Tate and Lyle	394	112
Prizesteak	Birds Eye Steakhouse		each grilled or shallow-fried 235
Processed cheese	Waitrose	260	74
Cheddar slices	Kraft	326	92
Cheshire slices	Kraft	335	95
Family Favourites (average)	St Ivel	280	79
Gold Spinner	St Ivel	280	79
singles slices	Kraft	302	86
slices	Safeway	300	85
slices, reduced fat	Heinz Weight Watchers	195	per slice 40
with walnut	Tesco	344	98
Processed cheese spread			
dairy	St Michael	300	85
soft, with butter	St Michael	360	102
walnut	St Michael	310	88
Processed peas: see Peas, processed			
Profiteroles	Waitrose	425	120
and chocolate sauce	Young's	330	94
Protein baby cereal	Boots Baby Foods	410	116
Protein bar square snack	Holly Mill		per bar 184
Protose	Granose	159	45
Provamel soya dessert	Provamel	94	28
Provencal Ready Meal	Tesco	89	25

Product	Brand	Calories per 100g/ 100ml	Calories per oz/ pack/ portion
Provencale Cooking-in Sauce	Baxters	116	per 425g can 493
Prune juice	Leisure Drinks	82	24
Prunes			
dried, raw		161	46
dried, raw (with stones)		134	38
dried, stewed with sugar		104	29
dried, stewed with sugar (with stones)		95	27
dried, stewed without sugar		82	23
dried, stewed without sugar (and stones)		74	21
canned	Del Monte	117	33
	Hartley's	95	per 111g can 105
canned in syrup	Tesco	109	31
	Waitrose	117	per 425g can 497
dried	Safeway	161	46
	Whitworths	119	34
dried, breakfast	Whitworths	147	42
dried, jumbo	Tesco	279	79
dried, no need to soak	Tesco	127	36
dried, ready cooked	Whitworths	114	32
dried, stoned	Holland and Barrett	160	45
	Tesco	272	77
	Whitworths	136	39
extra large	Waitrose	239	68
large	Waitrose	239	68
pitted	Waitrose	239	68
Pudding mix, steamed/baked	Creamola	352	100
Pudding rice, cooked	Tesco	153	43

Product	Brand	Calories per 100g/ 100ml	Calories per oz/ pack/ portion
Puff pastry (frozen)	Birds Eye	423	120
	Jus-Rol	393	111
	Safeway	425	120
	Waitrose	400	113
baked	Bejam	473	134
Puff pastry sausage rolls	St Michael	409	116
Puff pastry (frozen) sheets	Birds Eye		per sheet 360
Puffed Wheat		325	92
Pumpkin			
raw		15	4
fresh, boiled	Tesco	21	6
Pumpkin seeds	Holland and Barrett	400	113
Pure fruit jam, all flavours	Hartley's	255	per portion 40
Pure Fruit jelly jam, all flavours	Hartley's	260	per portion 40
Pure Fruit lemon cheese	Hartley's	295	per portion 45
Pure Fruit mincemeat	Hartley's	285	per portion 45
Pure fruit spread (Robertson's): *see flavours*			
Pure Fruits marmalade, all flavours	Hartley's	255	per portion 40
Quality Street assortment			
caramel	Rowntree Mackintosh		per sweet 30
coconut eclair	Rowntree Mackintosh		per sweet 45

Product	Brand	Calories per 100g/ 100ml	Calories per oz/ pack/ portion
Quality Street assortment			
coffee cup	Rowntree		
	Mackintosh		per sweet 40
cracknel	Rowntree		
	Mackintosh		per sweet 40
dairy toffee	Rowntree		
	Mackintosh		per sweet 30
fudge	Rowntree		
	Mackintosh		per sweet 45
gooseberry cream	Rowntree		
	Mackintosh		per sweet 40
milk chocolate truffle	Mackintosh		per sweet 40
noisette pate	Rowntree		
	Mackintosh		per sweet 40
nut toffee creme	Rowntree		
	Mackintosh		per sweet 45
orange cream	Rowntree		
	Mackintosh		per sweet 40
peanut nougat	Rowntree		
	Mackintosh		per sweet 45
strawberry cream	Rowntree		
	Mackintosh		per sweet 45
toffee cup	Rowntree		
	Mackintosh		per sweet 40
toffee de luxe	Rowntree		
	Mackintosh		per sweet 45
toffee finger	Rowntree		
	Mackintosh		per sweet 30
toffee pat	Rowntree		
	Mackintosh		per sweet 30
Quarter pound beefburgers	Bejam		each grilled 209
Quarter pounders	Birds Eye Steakhouse		per piece grilled 260, fried 290

Product	Brand	Calories per 100g/ 100ml	Calories per oz/ pack/ portion
Quarter pounders			
all beef	Findus	283	80
jumbo	Ross	265	75
Queen of puddings		216	61
Quenchers	Bassett's	326	92
Quiche: *see also flavours*			
Quiche lorraine		391	111
	St Michael	300	85
(as sold)	Bejam		per quiche 338
large	St Michael	300	85
Quiche with cheese and onion	St Michael	300	85
Quiche with tomato and cheese	St Michael	270	77
Quick batter mix	Whitworths	338	96
Quick chilli sauce mix			
Cook In	Colman's	335	95
Pour Over	Colman's	335	95
Quick Cook (Tesco): *see flavours*			
Quick cooking oats	Safeway	377	107
Quick custard	Batchelors	424	per 90g jar/sachet 382
Quick grills	Ross	320	91
Quick Jel dessert mix, all flavours (as sold)	Green's	360	made up per portion 22
Quick macaroni (as sold)	Buitoni	340	96
Quick Snacks (Campbell's): *see flavours*			
Quick Soups (Knorr): *see flavours*			
Quick-Cook egg lasagne			
cooked	Tesco	135	38
uncooked	Tesco	343	97

Product	Brand	Calories per 100g/ 100ml	Calories per oz/ pack/ portion
Quick-Cook macaroni			
cooked	Tesco	152	43
uncooked	Tesco	348	99
Quick-Cook spaghetti	Tesco	355	101
Quick-Set Jel (Tesco): see flavours			
Quinces, raw		25	7
Rabbit			
raw		124	35
stewed		179	51
stewed (with bone)		91	26
Radish			
red, raw		15	4
white/mooli, raw		24	7
fresh	Littlewoods	15	4
	Tesco	15	4
red, fresh, cooked	Tesco	28	8
Rainbow bright biscuits	St Michael	511	145
Rainbow trout	Bejam		each grilled 196
	St Michael	135	38
large	Bejam		each grilled 249
smoked	St Michael	135	38
whole	Waitrose	130	37
with mushrooms and onion stuffing	Waitrose	244	69
Rainbow yogurt (St Ivel): see flavours			
Raisin and lemon pancakes	Tesco	306	87
Raisin biscuits	Huntley & Palmer	454	per biscuit 59
Raisin bran buns	Vitbe	313	per bun 166
Raisin fudge	Trebor	425	per sweet 40

Product	Brand	Calories per 100g/ 100ml	Calories per oz/ pack/ portion
Raisin snack bar, yogurt coated	Sunwheel Kalibu	340	per 30g bar 102
Raisins			
dried		246	70
	Holland and Barrett	240	68
	Safeway	246	70
California seedless	Waitrose	301	85
	Safeway	246	70
	Tesco	249	71
	Waitrose	246	70
	Whitworths	246	70
stoned	Whitworths	246	70
yoghurt coated (canned or dried)	Tesco	451	128
yogurt coated	Tesco	451	128
yogurt coated, no added sugar	Sunwheel	396	112
Rapeseed oil	Boots	899	255
Raspberries			
canned		87	25
raw		25	7
stewed with sugar		68	19
stewed without sugar		26	7
	Littlewoods	25	7
canned	Hartley's	70	per 114g can 80
in syrup	St Michael	82	23
	Tesco	89	25
Scottish, in apple juice	Waitrose	48	per 400g can 192
Scottish, in syrup	Waitrose	87	per 383g can 333
Raspberry and melon yoghurt, creamy	Waitrose	146	per 125g pack 183

Product	Brand	Calories per 100g/ 100ml	Calories per oz/ pack/ portion
Raspberry and passionfruit yogurt	Safeway	91	per 150g pack 137
	St Michael	105	30
Raspberry and redcurrant brulee	Young's	310	88
Raspberry and redcurrant cheesecake	St Michael	285	81
Raspberry and redcurrant fruit crunch	Young's	255	72
Raspberry and redcurrant oat crunch	Young's	250	71
Raspberry and redcurrant pies	St Michael	341	97
Raspberry and strawberry cup ice cream ice cream	Wall's Italiano		per cup 110
Raspberry and vanilla Swiss roll	Lyons	338	96
Raspberry baked roll	Waitrose	356	101
Raspberry blancmange	Brown and Polson	330	94
Raspberry charlotte	St Michael	168	48
Raspberry cheesecake individual	Eden Vale	194	55
	Young's	250	71
Raspberry conserve	Safeway	248	70
	Tesco	268	76
	Waitrose	250	71
Raspberry cream dessert	Young's	200	57
Raspberry cream gateau	Waitrose	263	75

Product	Brand	Calories per 100g/ 100ml	Calories per oz/ pack/ portion
Raspberry dessert sauce	Lyons Maid	266	75
Raspberry drink	Safeway	140	41
Raspberry filled milk chocolate	Littlewoods	505	143
Raspberry flan filling	Armour	119	per 795g pack 946
Raspberry flavour dessert mix	Dietade	264	75
Raspberry flavour jelly	Waitrose	272	77
crystals	Dietade	290	82
Raspberry fruit cream trifle	Safeway	127	36
Raspberry fruit harvest ice cream	Lyons Maid	174	49
Raspberry fruit spread	Waitrose	124	35
Raspberry ice cream tub	Tesco	430	122
Raspberry jam	Robertson's	251	71
	Safeway	251	71
	Waitrose	248	70
diabetic	Boots	240	68
	Dietade	234	66
no added sugar	Safeway	139	39
reduced sugar	Heinz Weight Watchers	124	35
	Waitrose	124	35
seedless	Safeway	251	71
	Waitrose	248	70
Raspberry jam sponge pudding	Heinz	285	81

Product	Brand	Calories per 100g/ 100ml	Calories per oz/ pack/ portion
Raspberry jelly	Safeway	268	76
	Tesco	57	16
crystals, diabetic	Boots	365	103
table	Littlewoods	260	74
Raspberry juice	Hycal	243	72
Raspberry madeleines	Lyons	333	94
Raspberry Mivvi, Fun Size	Lyons Maid	120	34
Raspberry mousse	Ross	170	48
	Safeway	159	47
tub dessert	Birds Eye		per tub 110
wizard	St Ivel	183	52
Raspberry preserve	Baxters	242	69
	Tesco	255	72
reduced sugar	Robertson's	150	43
Raspberry pure fruit spread	Robertson's	120	34
Raspberry ring dessert	St Michael	136	39
Raspberry ripple ice cream	Bejam	169	48
	Lyons Maid	173	49
	Ross	170	48
	Safeway	164	49
	Tesco	176	50
	Waitrose	193	57
	Wall's		per 1/5 pack 95
	Wall's Blue Ribbon	100	per 1/20 2-litre pack 100
dairy	St Michael	174	49
sliceable	Wall's	105	per 1/10 litre pack 105
soft scoop	Safeway	172	51

Product	Brand	Calories per 100g/ 100ml	Calories per oz/ pack/ portion
Raspberry ripple ice cream soft serve	Ross	180	51
Raspberry ripple mousse	Bejam		per tub as sold 77
	Findus	171	48
	Tesco	173	49
	Waitrose	157	45
Raspberry ripple yogurt	St Michael	126	36
Raspberry Romano ice cream, scooping	Wall's Italiano		per 1/40 4-litre
Raspberry royale dessert, individual	St Michael	134	38
Raspberry ruffles	Tesco	385	109
Raspberry sauce	Tesco	323	92
Raspberry sorbet and vanilla ice cream, scooping	Wall's Italiano	90	per 1/40 4-litre pack 90
Raspberry split lolly	Bejam		per lolly 61
Raspberry sponge roll	St Michael	342	97
Raspberry sponge sandwich cake	Lyons	314	89
Raspberry sponge with buttercream	Safeway	380	108
Raspberry sundae cups	Lyons Maid		each 89
Raspberry Swiss roll	Lyons	295	84
Raspberry Topsy Turvy	Ambrosia	103	29
Raspberry trifle	Eden Vale	153	43
	Littlewoods	134	38
	St Ivel	144	41
	Waitrose	129	37

Product	Brand	Calories per 100g/ 100ml	Calories per oz/ pack/ portion
Raspberry trifle			
real	Young's	150	43
Raspberry water ice	Bertorelli	101	29
Raspberry yogurt	Mr Men	94	27
	Munch Bunch	99	per 125g pack 124
	Raines	89	25
	Safeway	94	per 150g pack 141
	Ski	83	per 150g pack 125
	St Ivel Rainbow	69	20
	St Ivel Real	82	23
French style low fat	Littlewoods	102	per 150g pack 153
	Diet Ski	55	per 150g pack 83
	Littlewoods	83	per 150g pack 125
	St Ivel Shape	41	12
	St Michael Lite	39	11
	Tesco	96	27
	Waitrose	90	per 150g pack 135
whole milk	Safeway	62	per 150g pack 93
Raspberry yogurt dessert	Cow and Gate	62	per 110g jar 68
Raspberry yogurt snack bar, carob coated	Sunwheel Kalibu	410	per 30g bar 123
Raspbree chews	Trebor	373	per sweet 28
Ratatouille	Bejam	49	per 113g portion 56
	Boots Ready Meal	30	9
	St Michael	62	18
	Tesco	36	10
	Waitrose	35	10
canned	Buitoni	37	per 375g can 139
	Safeway	46	per 390g can 179
	St Michael	39	11

Product	Brand	Calories per 100g/ 100ml	Calories per oz/ pack/ portion
Ratatouille			
canned	Tesco	47	13
	Waitrose	46	per 390g can 179
Ratatouille mix	Ross	15	4
Ratatouille vegetables, fresh	Safeway	56	16
Ravioli	Granose	64	18
	St Michael	120	34
as sold	Signor Rossi	277	78
canned	Buitoni	82	per 200g can 164
in beef and tomato sauce	Heinz	76	22
in meat and tomato sauce	Waitrose	83	per 400g can 332
in tomato sauce	Heinz	75	21
pomodoro (as sold)	Signor Rossi	230	65
wholewheat (canned)	Buitoni	84	per 400g can 336
Raw sugar marzipan snack bar, carob coated	Sunwheel Kalibu	433	per 30g bar 130
Ready Brek		390	111
Coco	Lyons	388	110
Golden	Lyons	391	111
Original	Lyons	391	111
Ready Meals: *see flavours*			
Ready salted chips	Tesco	524	149
Ready salted crisps	Christies	520	per 26g bag 130
	Hunters	520	per 26g bag 130
	Littlewoods	561	per 25g pack 140
	Nature's Snack	530	per 50g pack 265
	Safeway	500	per 25g pack 125
	St Michael	545	155

Product	Brand	Calories per 100g/ 100ml	Calories per oz/ pack/ portion
Ready salted crisps	Tesco	547	155
	Waitrose	520	per 75g pack 390
crinkle cut	Littlewoods	534	per 75g pack 401
	Safeway	543	per 75g pack 407
lower-fat	St Michael	485	137
Ready salted crispy squares	Safeway	472	per 50g pack 236
Ready salted crunchy sticks	Safeway	481	per 75g pack 361
	Tesco	442	125
Ready salted potato sticks	Safeway	505	per 75g pack 379
	St Michael	505	143
Ready salted potato thins	St Michael	472	134
Real fruit gums	Bassett's	293	83
	St Michael	340	96
Real fruit jellies	Trebor	320	per sweet 31
Real fruit pastilles	Bassett's	303	86
Real fruit teddy bear gums	St Michael	340	96
Real juice, squash, yogurt, etc: *see also flavours*			
Real mayonnaise	Hellmanns	720	204
Real milk ice			
strawberry	Lyons Maid		each 49
vanilla	Lyons Maid		each 50
Red cabbage: *see also Cabbage, red*			
Red cabbage with apple	Bejam		per 5 mini portions 61
	Haywards New Seasons	37	10
Red cheese and pineapple salad	Littlewoods	172	49

Product	Brand	Calories per 100g/ 100ml	Calories per oz/ pack/ portion
Red cherries in syrup	Waitrose	78	per 425g pack 332
Red cherry and brandy yogurt	St Ivel Cabaret	102	29
Red cherry cheesecake	Young's	235	67
Red cherry fruit filling	Morton	82	23
	Waitrose	82	per 400g pack 328
Red cherry luxury cheesecake mix (as sold)	Green's	266	made up per portion 243
Red cubes	Oxo	245	69
Red gram: see Peas, red			
Red grape juice	Schloer	49	15
	Waitrose	55	16
Red kidney beans: see Kidney beans, red			
Red Leicester cheese	Safeway	400	113
	Waitrose	390	111
farmhouse	Waitrose	390	111
Red palm oil		875	248
Red peppers	Tesco	24	7
Red peppers sweet	Waitrose	18	5
Red Quick-Set Jel	Tesco	365	103
Red snapper/malabar, raw		99	28
Red sockeye salmon, canned	Waitrose	163	per 213g can 347
Red wine		68	19
Red wine Cook in Sauce	Homepride	76	per 376g pack 286
Red wine cooking sauce	St Michael	55	16

Product	Brand	Calories per 100g/ 100ml	Calories per oz/ pack/ portion
Red wine sauce mix	Knorr	355	101
Redcurrant and raspberry fruit filling	Morton	56	16
Redcurrant and raspberry Pack-A-Pie	Batchelors	72	per 385g jar/ sachet 279
Redcurrant jelly	Crosse & Blackwell	259	73
	Tesco	290	82
Redcurrant sauce	O.K.	290	82
Redcurrants			
raw		21	6
stewed without sugar		18	5
stewed with sugar		53	15
Reduced calorie dressing	Heinz Weight Watchers	148	42
Reduced fat spread	Heinz Weight Watchers	360	102
Refreshers	Trebor	375	per sweet 6
Refried beans	Old El Paso	92	per 453g can 417
Regale desserts (St Ivel): see flavours			
Revels	Mars	478	136
Rhubarb			
raw		6	2
stewed with sugar		45	13
stewed without sugar		6	2
fresh, stems only	Littlewoods	6	2
fresh, stewed without sugar	Tesco	6	2
in syrup	Tesco	60	17
	Waitrose	51	per 539g can 275

Product	Brand	Calories per 100g/ 100ml	Calories per oz/ pack/ portion
Rhubarb and ginger preserve	Baxters	246	70
Rhubarb fruit fool	St Michael	133	38
Rhubarb yogurt	Raines	81	23
	Safeway	95	per 150g pack 143
	St Michael	95	27
low fat	Diet Ski	52	per 150g pack 78
	Littlewoods	81	per 150g pack 122
	St Ivel Shape	39	11
	Tesco	89	25
Ribena			
undiluted		229	65
Baby, undiluted	Beecham	316	94
concentrated	Beecham	293	87
Ribena juice drinks (Beecham): *see flavours*			
Rice			
boiled		123	35
polished, raw		361	102
brown, raw		357	101
flakes, raw		346	98
glutinous, raw		359	102
long grain, boiled		123	35
long grain, polished, raw		361	102
raw, parboiled		364	103
red, raw		354	100
	Safeway	361	102
	Waitrose	360	102
American, long grain	St Michael	349	99
American, parboiled	Whitworths	364	103
Basmati	Safeway	363	103
	Sharwood	355	101

Product	Brand	Calories per 100g/ 100ml	Calories per oz/ pack/ portion
Rice			
Basmati	St Michael	349	99
	Whitworths	359	102
Basmati, cooked	Tesco	158	45
Basmati, raw	Tesco	338	96
boil in bag, cooked	Tesco	125	35
boil in the bag	Kellogg's	333	94
brown	Boots Second		
	Nature	350	99
	Holland and		
	Barrett	360	102
	Safeway	360	102
	Tesco	341	97
	Whitworths	357	101
brown, cooked	Tesco	130	37
brown, natural			
wholegrain	St Michael	349	99
Chinese style	St Michael	151	43
cooked	Tesco	153	43
easy cook	Safeway	364	103
	Waitrose	360	102
easy cook, American	Waitrose	360	102
easy cook, cooked	Tesco	120	34
easy cook, raw	Tesco	353	100
flaked	Safeway	346	98
	Waitrose	360	102
ground	Safeway	314	89
	Whitworths	361	102
ground, cooked	Tesco	104	29
ground, raw	Tesco	339	96
long brown,			
American	Waitrose	360	102
long grain	Safeway	361	102
	Whitworths	361	102

Product	Brand	Calories per 100g/ 100ml	Calories per oz/ pack/ portion
Rice			
long grain (frozen, cooked)	Uncle Ben's	131	37
long grain (frozen, cooked), cooked	Uncle Ben's	115	32
long grain and wild, made with butter	Uncle Ben's	112	32
long grain, American	Waitrose	360	102
long grain, cooked	Tesco	99	28
long grain, raw	Tesco	356	101
long grain, three minute (canned)	Uncle Ben's	113	32
long-grain, ready cooked	Bejam	91	per 142g portion boiled 129
pilau	Waitrose	453	128
risotto	Waitrose	360	102
	Whitworths	359	102
risotto, cooked	Tesco	180	51
short grain	Tesco	356	101
	Whitworths	361	102
Special Chinese	Sharwood	350	99
special Chinese	Sharwood	350	99
special fried	Waitrose	226	64
stir fry	Waitrose	88	25
whole grain (frozen cooked)	Uncle Ben's	127	36
whole grain (frozen cooked), cooked	Uncle Ben's	114	32
whole grain, three minute (canned)	Uncle Ben's	117	33
Rice and vegetable salad	Tesco	135	38

Product	Brand	Calories per 100g/ 100ml	Calories per oz/ pack/ portion
Rice cakes	La Source de Vie	384	109
carob original	Newform		per cake 133
carob, sugar free	Newform		per cake 130
Rice, creamed	Ambrosia	91	26
	Libby	89	25
Rice creamola	Creamola	357	101
Rice crisp with raisins cake	St Michael	321	91
Rice crunchies	Safeway	352	100
	Waitrose	350	440g/15*oz pack
Rice dessert and apricot puree	St Michael	178	50
Rice Krispies		372	105
	Kellogg's	351	100
Rice, peas and mushrooms, boiled	Birds Eye	123	35
Rice pudding	Itona	70	per 425g can 297
	Tesco	87	25
light	Ambrosia	76	22
low fat, no added sugar	Heinz Weight Watchers	70	per 220g can 154
traditional	Ambrosia	102	29
Rice pudding with rosehip	Boots Baby Foods	385	109
Rice, sweetcorn, peas and carrots, boiled	Birds Eye	123	35
Rice, basmati raw		359	102
Rich beef casserole	St Michael	69	20
Rich chocolate ripple Napoli ice cream	Lyons Maid	178	50
Rich fruit cake		332	94

Product	Brand	Calories per 100g/ 100ml	Calories per oz/ pack/ portion
Rich fruit cake			
iced		352	100
	Waitrose	354	100
with marzipan	Tesco	389	110
Rich fruit Christmas cake	Safeway	375	106
and marzipan	Safeway	389	110
Rich fruit loaf	St Michael	245	69
Rich Osborne biscuits	Peek Frean	437	per biscuit 35
Rich oxtail with sherry soup	Heinz Classic Soups	35	10
Rich shortie biscuits	Tesco	499	141
Rich table water biscuits	Jacobs	411	per biscuit 30
Rich tea biscuits	Littlewoods	450	per biscuit 43
	Peek Frean	438	per biscuit 25
	Safeway	451	128
	St Michael	460	130
	Tesco	451	128
	Waitrose	460	130
Rich tea finger biscuits	St Michael	459	130
Rich tea finger creams	St Michael	479	136
Rich tea fingers	Waitrose	458	130
Rich tomato soup, dried	Crosse & Blackwell Pot Soup		per sachet made up 78
Ricicles	Kellogg's	354	100
Ripple	Mars	547	155
Risotto Ready Meal, vegetarian	Boots	133	38
Risotto rice: see Rice, risotto			

Product	Brand	Calories per 100g/ 100ml	Calories per oz/ pack/ portion
Rissoles, savoury	Birds Eye Snacks		each grilled or fried 190
Rissolnut	Granose	376	107
Rissotto style pot meal	Boots Shapers	318	90
Ritz crackers	Nabisco	495	per biscuit 16
cheese	Nabisco	480	per biscuit 16
Roast almond bar	Cadbury's	540	153
Roast beef and tomato sandwich	St Michael	149	42
Roast beef crisps	Christies	520	per 26g bag 130
	Hunters	520	per 26g bag 130
Roast beef dinner	Birds Eye MenuMaster		per tray 360
Roast beef in gravy	Findus	82	23
Roast beef platter	Birds Eye MenuMaster		per meal 375
Roast chicken, prepared	St Michael	124	35
Roast chicken and gravy	Birds Eye MenuMaster	84	per 227g pack 190
Roast chicken and salad sandwich	St Michael	209	59
Roast chicken meal	St Michael	124	35
Roast chicken plate pie	St Michael	254	72
Roast chicken platter	Birds Eye MenuMaster		per meal 360
Roast chicken sandwich	St Michael	201	57

Product	Brand	Calories per 100g/ 100ml	Calories per oz/ pack/ portion
Roast pork loin, sliced	St Michael	159	45
Roast potatoes (frozen)	Ross	100	28
Roast turkey and ham plate pie	St Michael	220	62
Roast turkey and salad sandwich	Waitrose	209	59
Rock around the Choc	Lyons Maid		each 129
Rock cake mix	Tesco	354	100
made up	Tesco	411	117
Rock cakes		394	112
Roe			
cod (hard), raw		113	32
cod, fried		202	57
herring (soft), raw		80	23
herring, fried		244	69
Rogan Josh curry sauce	Sharwood	117	33
Classic	Homepride	85	per 383g pack 326
Rolled brisket, roasted	Bejam	190	54
Rolls: see Bread rolls			
Rolo	Rowntree Mackintosh	450	per sweet 25
Romagna Prego sauce	Campbell's	64	18
Romero	Wall's		per portion 165
Rose coco beans, dried	Holland and Barrett	271	77
Rose wine, medium		71	20
Rosehip and raspberry yogurt dessert	Boots Baby Foods	380	108

Product	Brand	Calories per 100g/ 100ml	Calories per oz/ pack/ portion
Rosehip bar	Granose	382	per 50g bar 191
Rosehip drink	Boots Baby Drinks	287	81
Rosehip syrup, undiluted		232	66
Rosemary, dried		331	94
Rose's lime juice cordial, concentrated	Rose's	101	30
Roses marmalade, all flavours	Roses	255	per portion 40
Roule cheese	Tesco	383	109
	Waitrose	335	95
Round shorties	St Michael	494	140
Rounders	Sooner		per packet 102
Royal Game soup	Baxters	37	per 425g can 157
Royale Brie cheese	Tesco	356	101
Royale King Cone	Lyons Maid		per cone 203
Royale truffles	St Michael	553	157
Rum and raisin crunch mix (as sold)	Royal	264	per 480g pack made 1266
Rum and raisin ice cream	Lyons Maid Gold Seal	184	52
	Wall's		per 1/5 pack 95
	Wall's Blue Ribbon	100	per 1/20 2-litre pack 100
sliceable	Wall's	100	per 1/10 litre pack 100
Rum baba cake, fresh cream	Tesco	256	73
Rum babas, mini	St Michael	240	68
Runner beans, raw		26	7
boiled		19	5

Product	Brand	Calories per 100g/ 100ml	Calories per oz/ pack/ portion
Ruskmen	Boots Baby Foods	394	112
Rusks			
original	Farley	397	per rusk 67
OsterRusks	Farley	404	per rusk 34
round	Boots Baby Foods	401	114
with wholemeal	Farley	396	per rusk 67
Rusks, low sugar	Boots Baby Foods	401	114
	Farley	408	per rusk 69
apricot	Boots Baby Foods	400	113
Russchian	Stchweppes	23	7
Rydal biscuits	Safeway	475	135
Rye and oats with hazelnuts	Kellogg's Nutrigrain	368	104
Rye crispbread			
light	St Michael	375	106
whole	Boots Shapers	391	111
	Tesco	375	106
Rye flakes	Holland and Barrett	316	90
Rye flour	Holland and Barrett	335	95
Rye flour (100%)		335	95
Shape yogurts (St Ivel): *see flavours*			
Saccharin tablets	Boots		per tablet negl.
Safflower oil	Holland and Barrett	720	213
	Sunwheel	900	255
	Waitrose	900	266

Product	Brand	Calories per 100g/ 100ml	Calories per oz/ pack/ portion
Saffron (Kaisar)		310	88
Sag, cooked dish		100	28
Sage and onion mustard	Colman's	175	50
Sage and onion stuffing mix	Safeway	350	99
	Tesco	359	102
	Waitrose	325	92
	Whitworths	342	97
Sage Derby cheese mini	Waitrose	399	113
	Safeway	406	115
Sage, onion and bacon stuffing mix	Knorr	404	115
Sago			
raw		355	101
	Whitworths	355	101
cooked	Tesco	137	39
raw	Tesco	328	93
Sago, creamed	Ambrosia	81	23
Sago pudding	Whitworths	131	37
St Clements ice cream			
sliceable	Wall's	90	per 1/10 litre pack 90
twinpack	Wall's	85	per 1/20 2-litre 85
Saithe			
raw		73	21
steamed		99	28
steamed (with bones and skin)		84	24
Salad cream		311	88
	Crosse & Blackwell	346	98
	Heinz	342	97
	Littlewoods	330	94

Product	Brand	Calories per 100g/ 100ml	Calories per oz/ pack/ portion
Salad cream	Safeway	310	88
	Tesco	387	110
	Waitrose	324	92
Salad dressing, herb	St Michael	105	30
Salami		491	139
Danish	Waitrose	520	147
Danish, sliced	Tesco	529	150
German	Waitrose	427	121
German spiced	Waitrose	422	120
German, sliced	Tesco	405	115
Hungarian	Waitrose	520	147
Italian	Waitrose	411	117
Italian thin sliced	St Michael	491	139
Land	Waitrose	436	124
pepper	Waitrose	427	121
Salmon			
canned		155	44
raw		182	52
smoked		142	40
steamed		197	56
steamed (with bones and skin)		160	45
Cryovac (frozen)	Marine Harvest		35-55 per oz
fish cakes	Birds Eye		each grilled 100, fried 160
pink (canned	Waitrose	141	per 440g can 620
pink or red (canned)	Armour	155	per 107g can 166
red sockeye (canned)	Waitrose	163	per 213g can 347
Scottish fillets, fresh	St Michael	182	52
Scottish joints, fresh	St Michael	182	52
smoked	St Michael	142	40

Product	Brand	Calories per 100g/ 100ml	Calories per oz/ pack/ portion
Salmon			
smoked kosher, Scottish	Waitrose	262	74
smoked Lochinvar Scottish	Marine Harvest	141	40
smoked Pacific (chilled)	Young's	142	40
smoked Scotch (chilled)	Young's	142	40
smoked Scottish	Waitrose	204	per 113g pack 231
smoked Tamdhu Scottish	Marine Harvest	141	40
smoked, sliced (frozen)	Bejam	141	40
steaks	Waitrose	180	51
steaks (chilled)	Young's	148	42
steaks, Scottish, fresh	St Michael	182	52
Salmon and broccoli mornay	Birds Eye MenuMaster		per pack 320
Salmon and cucumber cottage cheese	Eden Vale	110	31
	Safeway	129	37
Salmon and cucumber sandwich	St Michael	204	58
	Tesco	165	47
Salmon and shrimp paste	Littlewoods	128	per 35g pack 45
	Safeway	206	per 75g pack 155
	Shippams	173	per 35g pack 61
	Tesco	150	43
Salmon en croute	Young's	270	77
Salmon joints, Scottish	Young's	148	42
Salmon spread	Littlewoods	126	per 35g pack 44
	Shippams	159	per 35g pack 56

Product	Brand	Calories per 100g/ 100ml	Calories per oz/ pack/ portion
Salmon with butter, potted (canned)	St Michael	166	47
Salsify			
boiled		18	5
fresh, cooked	Tesco	73	21
Salt		0	
Salt substitute	Boots	0	
Salt and pepper fries	Littlewoods	440	per 50g pack 221
Salt and pepper Super Fries	Hunters	441	per 24g pack 106
Salt and vinegar chiplets	St Michael	487	138
Salt and vinegar chips	Tesco	466	132
Salt and vinegar crisps	Christies	520	per 26g bag 130
	Hunters	520	per 26g bag 130
	Safeway	500	per 25g pack 125
	St Michael	525	149
	Tesco	520	147
	Waitrose	520	147
Salt and vinegar crispy squares	Safeway	472	per 50g pack 236
Salt and vinegar crunchy sticks	Safeway	487	per 75g pack 365
	Tesco	466	132
Salt and vinegar potato twirls	Waitrose	423	120
Salt and vinegar savoury sticks	Waitrose	483	137
Salt and vinegar twirls	Safeway	444	per 50g pack 222
Salted cashew nuts: *see Cashew nuts*			

Product	Brand	Calories per 100g/ 100ml	Calories per oz/ pack/ portion
Salted fish, Chinese, steamed, bone removed		155	44
Salted mixed nuts	Waitrose	655	186
Salted peanuts: see Peanuts			
Samosas			
minced lamb (Asian)		578	164
chicken	Waitrose	226	64
lamb	Waitrose	226	64
six vegetable	Waitrose	191	54
vegetable	Waitrose	226	64
Samsoe cheese, Danish	Waitrose	344	98
Sandwiches: see flavours			
Sandwich bar biscuits, chocolate coated	Tesco	512	145
Sandwich biscuits		513	145
cheese	Nabisco	528	per biscuit 48
cheese and onion	Nabisco	522	per biscuit 47
Sandwich biscuits: see also flavours			
Sandwich cakes: see flavours			
Sandwich cake mixes: see flavours			
Sandwich cream			
mushroom	Granose	360	102
olive	Granose	340	96
Sandwich spread	Heinz	206	58
cereals	Granose	225	64
cucumber	Heinz	183	52
herbs	Granose	263	75
mushrooms	Granose	337	96
olives	Granose	308	87

Product	Brand	Calories per 100g/ 100ml	Calories per oz/ pack/ portion
Sandwich wafer biscuits, chocolate flavour filling	Waitrose	571	162
Sandwichmaker (Shippams): see flavours			
Sapota (sapodilla, noiseberry fruits), raw		76	22
Sardine and tomato paste	Littlewoods	125	per 35g pack 44
	Tesco	160	45
Sardine and tomato spread	Shippams	183	per 35g pack 64
Sardines			
canned in oil, fish only		217	62
canned in oil, fish plus oil		334	95
canned in tomato sauce		177	50
in edible oil	Waitrose	198	per 120g can 238
in oil	Armour	332	per 120g can 398
in oil (fish only)	Armour	222	per 120g can 266
in olive oil	St Michael	248	70
	Waitrose	198	per 120g can 238
in tomato sauce	Armour	182	per 120g can 218
	Waitrose	177	per 120g can 212
Sata pastries, assorted		538	153
Sate sauce	Waitrose	165	47
Satsumas in syrup	Tesco	63	18
Sauce au poivre	Nestle Bonne Cuisine	383	109
Sauce basquaise	Nestle Bonne Cuisine	360	102
Sauce chasseur	Nestle Bonne Cuisine	345	98
Sauce hollandaise	Nestle Bonne Cuisine	384	109

Product	Brand	Calories per 100g/ 100ml	Calories per oz/ pack/ portion
Sauce tartare: *see Tartare sauce*			
Sauces: *see also flavours*			
Saucy Noodles (Batchelors): *see flavours*			
Sausage			
Scottish lorne, sliced	St Michael	355	101
sliced round	Littlewoods	396	per slice 140
smoked, sliced	Tesco	339	96
top quality	St Michael	400	113
Sausage and bacon plait	Waitrose	314	89
Sausage and bacon rissole	Waitrose	232	66
Sausage casserole Cook in the Pot	Crosse & Blackwell	353	100
Sausage casserole cooking mix	Colman's	345	98
Sausage roll pie	Littlewoods	546	155
Sausage rolls			
flaky pastry		479	136
short pastry		463	131
	Littlewoods	296	each, pack of 10, 139
	Littlewoods	450	each, pack of 2, 135
	Ross	350	99
	Tesco	398	113
	Waitrose	355	101
cocktail	Birds Eye Snacks		each baked 65
	Littlewoods	425	per roll 106
	Waitrose	430	122

Product	Brand	Calories per 100g/ 100ml	Calories per oz/ pack/ portion
Sausage rolls			
jumbo	Ross	350	99
kingsize	Bejam		each baked 179
	Birds Eye Snacks		each baked 190
lattice	St Michael	396	112
party size	Bejam		each baked 78
puff pastry	St Michael	409	116
Sausagemeat	St Michael	350	99
Sausages	St Michael	350	99
Bierwurst, sliced	Tesco	254	72
butcher style	St Michael	350	99
butcher's choice	Tesco	285	81
chestnut stuffing	St Michael	358	101
cocktail	Bejam		each grilled 34
	St Michael	350	99
country recipe	Wall's Light and Lean	198	each 99
English recipe	Wall's Light and Lean	190	each 95
pork and beef	St Michael	370	105
Suffolk	Waitrose	254	72
turkey recipe	Wall's Light and Lean	199	each 99
Sausages and chips snack, battered	Bejam		per serving baked 563
Sausages and mash	Waitrose	140	per 283g pack 400
Sausages: see also Beef, Pork, etc			
Sausages, beef			
fried		269	76
grilled		265	75
raw		299	85
Sausages, pork			
fried		317	90

Product	Brand	Calories per 100g/ 100ml	Calories per oz/ pack/ portion
Sausages, pork			
grilled		318	90
raw		367	104
Sausalatas	Granose	137	per 284g pack 390
Sausfry	Granose	492	139
Saute potatoes	Findus	97	27
with eggs, onion and bacon	Waitrose	170	per 500g pack 850
with onion and smoked bacon	Waitrose	135	per 400g pack 540
with onion, sausages and cheese	Waitrose	120	per 500g pack 600
Saveloy		262	74
Saviand	Granose	199	56
Savoury barbecue French bread pizza	Findus	223	63
Savoury beef noodles	Boots Baby Foods	390	111
Savoury beef rice	Tesco	345	98
Savoury chicken and rice	Boots Baby Foods	415	118
Savoury chicken casserole	Boots Baby Foods	400	113
Savoury chicken rice	Tesco	350	99
Savoury cocktail biscuit assortment	St Michael	575	163
Savoury Complan	Farley	436	per 57g sachet 249
Savoury crackers	Waitrose	495	140
Savoury curried rice	Crosse & Blackwell	105	30
Savoury curry rice hot	Tesco	334	95

Product	Brand	Calories per 100g/ 100ml	Calories per oz/ pack/ portion
Savoury curry rice			
mild	Tesco	327	93
Savoury cuts, meatless	Granose	88	25
Savoury eggs	Bejam		each as sold 205
Savoury mince	Tyne Brand	86	25
Savoury minced beef pasties	Waitrose	264	75
Savoury minced beef roll	Bejam		per 1/2 roll 529
Savoury minced beef with onions in gravy	Fray Bentos	168	48
Savoury mixed vegetables	Boots Baby Foods	395	112
Savoury mixed vegetables rice	Tesco	249	71
Savoury onion Potato Saucery (as sold)	Batchelors	338	per 98g pack 331
Savoury pudding	Granose	207	59
country style	Granose	167	47
Savoury puffs	Safeway	600	per 50g pack 300
cheese flavoured	Waitrose	526	149
Savoury rice			
and mushrooms	Crosse & Blackwell	106	30
and peppers	Crosse & Blackwell	106	30
and vegetables	Crosse & Blackwell	105	30
Savoury rice: see also flavours			
Savoury rissoles	Birds Eye Snacks		each grilled or fried 190

Product	Brand	Calories per 100g/ 100ml	Calories per oz/ pack/ portion
Savoury roast pork, roasted	Bejam	282	80
Savoury Scotch eggs	Tesco	298	84
Savoury snaps	St Michael	490	139
Savoury spread	Boots	205	58
	Safeway	194	per 113g pack 220
Savoury sticks	Tesco	422	120
	Waitrose	483	137
Savoury toasts (Findus): *see flavours*			
Savoury tomato rice	Tesco	329	93
Savoury twigs	Safeway	391	per 50g pack 196
Savoury vegetable casserole	Boots Baby Foods	63	18
Savoury vegetables and spaghetti meal	Prewetts	308	87
Savoury vinegar crunchy sticks	Tesco	466	132
Savoury white sauce mix	Knorr	360	102
Savoy cabbage			
raw		26	7
boiled		9	3
Scalloped potatoes au gratin	Whitworths	355	101
	Whitworths		per pack 531, made up 813
with savoury white sauce	Whitworths		per pack 544, made up 826
with sour cream and chives	Whitworths		per pack 565, made up 847
Scallops			
steamed		105	30

Product	Brand	Calories per 100g/ 100ml	Calories per oz/ pack/ portion
	Waitrose	90	26
breaded	Waitrose	110	31
frozen, raw	Tesco	70	20
queen, frozen, raw	Tesco	157	45
sea, chilled	Young's	93	26
sea, in breadcrumbs, chilled	Young's	168	48
Scampi			
fried		316	90
breaded	Baxters	133	38
	Waitrose	120	34
breaded, deep-fried	Bejam	205	58
	Dan Maid	220	62
breaded, frozen, raw	Tesco	128	36
whole, chilled	Young's	87	25
Scampi with Patna rice			
indienne	Baxters	117	per 312g pack 365
Scampi provencale (chilled)	Young's	65	18
Scampi tails, chilled	Young's	87	25
whole, in breadcrumbs	Young's	203	58
Scampi with Patna rice			
americaine	Baxters	125	per 312g pack 390
francaise	Baxters	114	per 312g pack 356
provencale	Baxters	90	per 312g pack 280
thermidor	Baxters	114	per 312g pack 356
Scamps	St Michael	493	140
Scone mix (as sold)	Granny Smiths	330	per 202g pack made up 666
	Tesco	396	112
	Whitworths	433	123

Product	Brand	Calories per 100g/ 100ml	Calories per oz/ pack/ portion
Scone mix (as sold)			
made up	Tesco	395	112
Scones		371	105
cream	St Michael	340	96
Scotch broth	Baxters	41	per 425g can 174
	Campbell's Bumper Harvest	40	11
	Crosse & Blackwell	62	18
	Granny's	55	as served 37
	Heinz Ready to Serve	36	10
	Safeway	42	per 425g can 179
	Tesco	60	17
	Waitrose	37	per 425g can 157
condensed	Campbell's	71	20
dried	Tesco	345	98
Scotch eggs		279	79
	St Michael	315	89
	Tesco	286	81
savoury	Tesco	298	84
Scotch fritters			
with beans	Ross	240	68
with cheese	Ross	240	68
Scotch mince	Baxters	93	per 432g can 395
Scotch orange marmalade	Baxters	248	per 340g jar 843
Scotch pancakes		283	80
	St Michael	305	86
Scotch pie	St Michael	282	80
Scotch pies	Littlewoods	508	144
Scotch salmon bisque	Baxters	69	per 425g can 293
Scotch vegetable soup	Baxters	28	per 425g can 117

Product	Brand	Calories per 100g/ 100ml	Calories per oz/ pack/ portion
Scottish buns	Tesco	316	90
Scottish crumpets	Tesco	260	74
Scottish haggis	Baxters	172	per 411g can 731
Scottish lentil soup with vegetables	Crosse & Blackwell	45	13
Scottish raspberries: *see Raspberries*			
Scottish salmon: *see Salmon*			
Scottish vegetable soup with lentils	Heinz Ready to Serve	43	12
Scrambled egg breakfast	Boots Baby Foods	395	112
Sea kale		8	2
Sea-salt and cider vinegar crisps	Hedgehog	407	per 27g pack 110
Sea-salt crisps natural	Hedgehog	407	per 27g pack 110
Seafood and prawn cocktail dressing	Safeway	325	92
Seafood cottage cheese	Eden Vale	92	26
Seafood dressing	Safeway	385	109
	Tesco	301	85
Seafood flaky bake pie	Birds Eye MenuMaster		per pie 445
Seafood lasagne	Young's	110	31
Seafood pasta	St Michael	121	34
	Young's	120	34
Seafood platter	Tesco	143	41
Seafood sticks	Young's	85	24
Seafood tagliarini	St Michael	98	28
Second Nature biscuits (Boots): *see flavours*			

Product	Brand	Calories per 100g/ 100ml	Calories per oz/ pack/ portion
Semi-skimmed chocolate drink	St Michael	66	19
Semi-skimmed strawberry drink	St Michael	57	16
Semolina			
raw		350	99
	Safeway	350	99
	Waitrose	350	99
	Whitworths	350	99
cooked	Tesco	98	28
raw	Tesco	336	95
Semolina, creamed	Ambrosia	83	24
Semolina pudding	Whitworths	131	37
Sesame and sunflower biscuits	Prewetts	per biscuit 83	
Sesame crackers	Safeway	475	135
	Waitrose	465	132
Sesame nut crunch	Tesco	583	165
Sesame oil		881	250
	Holland and Barrett	900	266
	Sunwheel	900	255
Sesame oil Chinese pouring sauce	Sharwood	900	255
Sesame seed bar, natural	Boots	464	132
Sesame seeds		588	167
	Holland and Barrett	560	159
Sesame spread	Sunwheel	563	160
Sev (ganthia), savoury, Asian		485	137

Product	Brand	Calories per 100g/ 100ml	Calories per oz/ pack/ portion
Seville orange marmalade, thin cut	Waitrose	248	70
Sevyiaan (sweet), Asian		443	126
Seyshells	Sooner		per packet 47
Shakers crisps	St Michael	56	16
Shallot, raw		48	14
Shandy	Barr	26	per 330ml can 85
	Britvic	25	per 330ml can 81
	Corona	25	7
	St Michael	22	7
	Tesco	23	7
	Tesco	33	10
Shandy bass	Canada Dry	26	per 250ml can 65
Shandy cider	Canada Dry	26	per 250ml can 65
Shandy drink	Littlewoods	25	per 330ml pack 83
Shandy pilsner	Canada Dry	26	per 250ml can 65
Shanghai beef noodles	Vesta	388	per 173g pack for two as served 672
Shape cheese (wedge)	St Ivel	260	74
Shape coleslaw	St Ivel	38	11
Shape cottage cheese (St Ivel): *see flavours*			
Shape milk drink	St Ivel	45	13
Shapers (Boots): *see also products, flavours*			
Shapers Sugarlite	Boots	391	111
Shapers tablets	Boots		per tablet 0
Shawburger mix	Hera	340	96
Shepherd's pie cooked		119	34
	Safeway	109	per 227g pack 248
	Waitrose	125	per 283g pack 350

Product	Brand	Calories per 100g/ 100ml	Calories per oz/ pack/ portion
Shepherd's pie	Birds Eye MenuMaster	119	per 227g pack 270
	Findus	121	34
	Ross	110	31
	Tesco	110	31
individual	St Michael	149	42
Shepherd's pie Cook in the Pot	Crosse & Blackwell	339	96
Shepherd's pie filling	Tyne Brand	113	32
Sherbert lemon yogurt	Munch Bunch	92	per 125g pack 115
Sherbet dip dabs	Barratt	346	98
Sherbet fountain	Barratt	328	93
Sherbet lemons	Trebor	359	per sweet 23
Sherry			
dry		116	33
medium		118	33
sweet		136	39
Sherry trifle	St Michael	157	45
Short pastry mix (as sold)			per 225g pack
	Granny Smiths	497	made up 1327
	Safeway	495	140
Shortbread	Boots Second Nature	476	135
Shortbread biscuits		504	143
	Tesco	518	147
Shortbread fingers	Littlewoods	525	per finger 87
	Safeway	461	131
	Waitrose	500	142
wholemeal	Waitrose	500	142
Shortbread mix (as sold)	Granny Smiths	487	per 255g pack made up 1240

Product	Brand	Calories per 100g/ 100ml	Calories per oz/ pack/ portion
Shortbread mix	Tesco	381	108
made up	Tesco	508	144
Shortcake	Waitrose	500	142
Shortcake bar biscuits, chocolate coated	Tesco	498	141
Shortcake biscuits	Peek Frean	454	per biscuit 49
	Rakusen	479	136
	Safeway	494	140
	Tesco	501	142
Dutch	Huntley & Palmer	539	per biscuit 40
fruit	Peek Frean	443	per biscuit 36
Shortcake snack	Cadbury's	490	per biscuit 35
Shortcrust pastry, raw		455	129
cooked		527	149
	Birds Eye	441	125
	Safeway	446	369g/13oz pack
	Waitrose	440	125
baked	Bejam	494	140
Shortcrust pastry mix (as sold)	Tesco	484	137
	Waitrose	497	141
made up	Tesco	450	128
Shredded Wheat		324	92
Shrimps			
boiled		117	33
boiled (with shell)		39	11
canned		94	27
dried		245	69
frozen, shell removed		73	21
Shrimps/prawns	Armour	94	per 200g can 188
Siciliana sauce	Buitoni	74	per 283g can 209

Product	Brand	Calories per 100g/ 100ml	Calories per oz/ pack/ portion
Siciliana sauce	Waitrose	54	per 425g can 230
Siciliana spaghetti sauce	Campbell's	70	20
Silky smooth choc ice	Lyons Maid		each 132
Silver mints	Littlewoods	374	106
Silver Shred marmalade	Robertson's	251	71
Silverskin onions: see Onions, pickled			
Simply topping mix	Royal	179	per 1.85g pack made up 330
Singapore curry Chinese sauce mix	Sharwood	290	82
Six grain biscuits	Boots Second Nature	441	125
Sizzles, vegetarian	Protoveg Menu	587	166
Skate			
fried (with waste)		163	46
fried in batter		199	56
Ski yogurts (Eden Vale): see flavours			
Skippy	Cadbury's	455	per 42g bar 190
Slender (as sold)			
chocolate	Carnation	360	per sachet + 190ml milk 229
coffee, strawberry, vanilla	Carnation	350	99
lemon, raspberry, yogurt	Carnation		per sachet + 190ml milk 227
Slender bars			
chocolate and coffee	Carnation	430	per 2-bar meal 250
fruit country	Carnation	393	111

Product	Brand	Calories per 100g/ 100ml	Calories per oz/ pack/ portion
Slender bars			
natural country	Carnation	500	per 2-bar meal 250
Slender Slim chocolate drink	Carnation	365	per serving 40
Slender soup, all flavours	Carnation	335	per serving 40
Sliced sausage, round	Littlewoods	396	per slice 140
Slim-a-Meals (Batchelors): see flavours			
Slim-a-Soups (Batchelors): see flavours			
Slim drinks (Canada Dry): see flavours			
Slimlime drinks (Schweppes): see flavours			
Slippery Elm food	Lanes	337	96
Small onions and white sauce	Birds Eye	134	per 142g pack 190
Smarties	Rowntree Mackintosh	460	per small 35g tube 160
Smash	Cadbury's	265	per portion 55
Smatana, creamed	Raines	129	37
Smoked almonds	Tesco	630	179
Smoked cheese	Waitrose	305	86
Austrian	St Ivel	315	89
with ham	Waitrose	305	86
Smoked fish: see also Cod, Haddock, etc			
Smoked fish kebabs	Young's	134	38
Smoked haddock and broccoli quiche	St Michael	210	60
Smoked haddock croquettes	Young's	188	53
Smoked haddock crumble	Tesco	186	53

Product	Brand	Calories per 100g/ 100ml	Calories per oz/ pack/ portion
Smoked haddock lasagne	Bejam		per serving baked
Smoked haddock pastie	Tesco	312	88
Smoked haddock pie	Ross	200	57
Smoked haddock savoury bake	Waitrose	144	454g/16oz pack
Smoked ham	Waitrose	121	per 113g pack (appr) 136
Smoked mackerel and onion pate	Tesco	321	91
Smoked mackerel pate	St Michael	318	90
Smoked pork sausage	Tesco	344	98
	Waitrose	328	93
cooked	Littlewoods	320	91
Smoked salmon pate	St Michael	236	67
Smoked sausage, sliced	Tesco	339	96
Smoked trout	Bejam		each as sold 157
Smoked whiting fillets	Ross	80	23
Smoky bacon pancakes	Findus	140	40
Smoky cheese spread	Sun-Pat	268	76
Snack-a-Soups (Batchelors): see flavours			
Snack crackers	Tesco	445	126
Snack meals (Tesco): see flavours			
Snackbar, carob coated	Allinson	469	per 32g bar 150

Product	Brand	Calories per 100g/ 100ml	Calories per oz/ pack/ portion
Snacks			each grilled 75,
Cheesies	Birds Eye		fried 85
Chicklets	Birds Eye		each grilled 160, fried 195
Sno ice lolly	Bejam		per lolly 83
Snow White Cartoons			made up per
cake mix (as sold)	Green's	414	portion 64
Snow Ball biscuits	Peek Frean	418	per biscuit 131
	Safeway	251	71
Snowballs	Tesco	405	115
Snowballs			
coconut	Littlewoods	449	127
strawberry	Littlewoods	449	127
Snowballs	Tesco	460	130
Snowcaps	St Michael	344	98
Soda scones, plain	Tesco	286	81
Soda water			
Soft and smooth			
caramels	St Michael	485	137
Soft-centred drops	Trebor	348	per sweet 24
Soft cheese			
dairy	Tesco	271	77
dairy, with chives	Tesco	290	82
dairy, with pineapple	Tesco	358	101
full fat	Raines	288	82
	Waitrose	296	84
medium fat	Raines	173	49
skimmed milk	Raines	76	22
Soft chewy fruits	Wilkinson	360	102
Soft fruit gums	Wilkinson	319	90

Product	Brand	Calories per 100g/ 100ml	Calories per oz/ pack/ portion
Softmints	Trebor	374	per sweet 16
Sojal	Hera	45	13
Sole, breaded	Waitrose	116	33
Somerset chicken and vegetable bake	Birds Eye MenuMaster		per pack 365
Somerset pie	Waitrose	91	per 510g pie 468
Somerset soft cheese			
high fat	Eden Vale	321	91
low fat	Eden Vale	135	38
medium fat with cucumber	Eden Vale	196	56
medium fat with onion and gherkin	Eden Vale	201	57
medium fat with pineapple	Eden Vale	206	58
Somervale low fat soft cheese	Kraft	138	39
Sonata dessert log	Wall's		per 1/6 log 130
Sorbitol (fructose)	Holland and Barrett	400	113
Sosmix, vegetarian	Ranch House Meals	598	170
Soup in Seconds (Prewetts): see flavours			
Soup mix, dried	Boots	328	93
Soup mixture	Whitworths	332	94
Sour cream and chives flavour crisps	Waitrose	520	per 75g pack 390
Sour cream dressing, onion	St Michael	385	109
Southern fried Coat and cook sauce	Homepride	180	per 43g pack 77

Product	Brand	Calories per 100g/ 100ml	Calories per oz/ pack/ portion
Southern style Dish of the Day	Crosse & Blackwell	461	131
Soutsoukakia	Waitrose	226	64
Soy Chinese pouring sauce			
light	Sharwood	24	7
rich	Sharwood	60	17
Soy sauce			
dark, thick		86	24
light, thin		64	18
Soya flour			
full fat		447	127
low fat		352	100
Soya bean curd: *see Tofu*			
Soya bean flakes	Holland and Barrett	384	109
Soya bean oil	Holland and Barrett	920	272
	Waitrose	900	266
Soya bean paste	Granose	140	40
Soya beans			
raw		403	114
dried	Holland and Barrett	400	113
Soya bolognese mix	Protoveg Menu	275	78
Soya bran	Granose	100	28
	Itona	220	62
Soya chocolate dessert	Granose	72	20
Soya curd/Tofu			
canned, fried		302	86
steamed		70	20

Product	Brand	Calories per 100g/ 100ml	Calories per oz/ pack/ portion
Soya flour low fat	Holland and Barrett	350	99
Soya franks	Granose	272	77
Soya margarine	Safeway	730	207
Soya milk		39	11
	Granose	51	15
carob	Granose	59	17
coconut	Granose	70	21
concentrate	Plamil	103	30
honey and malt	Provamel	50	15
powdered	Soyagen	496	141
strawberry	Granose	64	19
sugar free	Granose	42	12
unsweetened	Granose	42	HB
Soya mince with onion, dried	Beanfeast	334	95
Soya mix, meatloaf style	Hera	480	136
Soya oil	Boots	899	255
	Safeway	900	266
Soya strawberry dessert	Granose	72	20
Soya thread (Foo-juk), dried		387	110
Soya vanilla dessert	Granose	72	20
Soya wurst, chicken flavour	Granose	300	85
Soyagen	Granose	496	141
Soyal dessert	Provamel	94	28
Soyapro slices beef	Granose	210	60
chicken	Granose	210	60

Product	Brand	Calories per 100g/ 100ml	Calories per oz/ pack/ portion
Soyapro wieners	Granose	210	60
Soybrits	Hofels	367	per 15g pack 55
Soysage mix	Hera	410	116
Soyvita	Healtheries	517	147
Spaghetti			
boiled		117	33
raw		342	97
	Boots Second Nature	354	100
	Buitoni	340	96
	Buitoni Country Harvest	318	90
	St Michael	370	105
	Tesco	348	99
cooked	Tesco	138	39
Italian	Waitrose	378	107
long	Safeway	344	96
Quick-Cook	Tesco	355	101
short	Safeway	344	96
standard	Signor Rossi	272	77
wholemeal	Holland and Barrett	350	99
wholewheat	Tesco	141	cooked
	Tesco	347	98
	Waitrose	325	92
Spaghetti, canned in tomato sauce		59	17
	Crosse & Blackwell	57	16
	Heinz	68	19
	Heinz Invaders	65	18
	Safeway	59	per 425g can 251
	Tesco	61	17
	Waitrose	55	per 439g can 241

Product	Brand	Calories per 100g/ 100ml	Calories per oz/ pack/ portion
Spaghetti, canned			
hoops	Heinz	64	18
no added sugar	Heinz Weight Watchers	53	per 220g can 117
rings	Crosse & Blackwell	61	17
	Safeway	59	per 213g can 126
	Tesco	61	17
	Waitrose	67	per 213g can 143
shapes	Heinz Haunted House	72	20
shapes	Heinz Noodle Doodles	59	17
shapes and meatballs	Heinz Invaders and Meteors	89	25
wholewheat	Crosse & Blackwell	65	18
wholewheat rings	Crosse & Blackwell	58	16
wholewheat spirals	Crosse & Blackwell	62	18
Spaghetti bolognaise (frozen)	St Michael	121	34
Spaghetti bolognaise	Cow and Gate	62	per 110g jar 68, 150g jar 93
Spaghetti bolognese	Bejam		per serving baked 256
	Birds Eye MenuMaster		per pack 370
	Findus Lean Cuisine	74	21
	Heinz	82	23
	Tyne Brand	110	per 340g pack 406

Product	Brand	Calories per 100g/ 100ml	Calories per oz/ pack/ portion
Spaghetti bolognese	Heinz Baby Foods	56	per 128g can 72
Spaghetti bolognese sauce mix			
Cook In	Colman's	370	105
Pour Over	Colman's	370	105
Spaghetti hoops with sausage supper	Heinz Baby Foods	76	per 128g can 97
Spaghetti sauce			
bolognese	Campbell's	90	26
siciliana	Campbell's	70	20
tomato and mushroom	Campbell's	68	19
Spaghetti sauce mix	Knorr	334	95
Spaghetti verdi	Tesco	338	96
	Waitrose	350	99
cooked	Tesco	110	31
Spanish fig cake	Wilcox and Lomer	556	per 45g pack 250
Spanish mandarins (canned)	Safeway	56	per 312g can 176
Spanish orange trifle	Eden Vale	155	44
Spanish salad	Eden Vale	112	32
	Safeway	170	per 227g pack 384
Spanish savoury rice	Safeway	334	95
Spanish seafood and chicken	Ross	70	20
Spanish style soup and sweet pepper	Crosse & Blackwell	45	ready to serve
Sparkles, all flavours	Wall's		per portion 30
Sparkling drinks: see flavours			
Sparkling fruits	Tesco	380	108

Product	Brand	Calories per 100g/ 100ml	Calories per oz/ pack/ portion
Sparkling mints	Tesco	380	108
Sparks bar	St Michael	480	136
Spartan apples	Tesco	46	13
Spearmint chewing gum	Wrigley		per stick 9
Freedent	Wrigley		per stick 9
sweet	Wrigley Orbit Nutra		per stick 7
Spearmint chews	Littlewoods	366	104
Special Chinese vegetables	Bejam	29	per 113g portion boiled 33
Special cream of mushroom soup	Heinz Classic Soups	40	11
Special fried rice	Waitrose	226	64
Special fried rice Chinese-style meal	Bejam		per serving baked 217
Special K		388	110
	Kellogg's	355	101
Special mix vegetables	Ross	40	11
Special mixed vegetables	Tesco	68	19
Special R drinks (Robinsons): *see flavours*			
Special recipe muesli	Jordans	330	94
Special reserve cider	Bulmer	52	per half pint 148
Special savoury rice (Batchelors): *see flavours*			
Special tea, infused	Safeway	1	
Special Vat cider	Taunton	44	per pint 250
Speciality assortment biscuits	St Michael	504	143

Product	Brand	Calories per 100g/ 100ml	Calories per oz/ pack/ portion
Specialty soup			
Consomme	Crosse & Blackwell	22	6
Vichyssoise	Crosse & Blackwell	47	13
Spiced mixed fruit pickle	Baxters	159	per 305g jar 484
Spicy barbecue fried special savoury rice	Batchelors	456	129
Spicy brown sauce	Waitrose	60	per 624g jar 374
Spicy cake mix (as sold)	Granny Smiths	324	per 370g pack made up 1199
Spicy chicken crisps	Hunters	520	per 26g bag 130
Spicy fruit crunch biscuits	Tesco	453	128
Spicy lamb/beef marinade	Knorr	279	79
Spicy meatballs in tomato sauce	Waitrose	150	per 350g can 525
Spicy mint relish	Branston	113	32
Spicy Nik Naks	St Michael	540	153
Spicy potato salad	Safeway	184	per 227g pack 416
Spicy risotto	Vesta	312	per 205g pack for two as served 640
Spicy sauce	Branston	112	32
	O.K.	95	27
	Safeway	94	27
traditional	Tesco	147	42
Spicy vegebanger	Real Eats	828	235
Spicy vegetables Ready Meal	Tesco	57	16

Product	Brand	Calories per 100g/ 100ml	Calories per oz/ pack/ portion
Spinach			
boiled		30	9
canned, drained		24	7
fresh, raw		26	7
canned	Del Monte	24	7
fresh, boiled	Tesco	30	9
frozen	Tesco	25	7
frozen, chopped	Bejam	21	per 113g portion boiled 24
	Findus	31	9
	Safeway	14	per 227g pack 32
	Waitrose	30	per 397g pack 119
frozen, creamed	Bejam		per 5 mini portions boiled 54
frozen, cut leaf	Birds Eye	18	5
frozen, leaf	Bejam	24	per 113g portion boiled 27
	Ross	30	9
	Safeway	30	per 227g pack 72
frozen, whole leaf	Findus	32	9
Spinach tortelloni with ricotta filling (as sold)	Signor Rossi	286	81
Spingapore curry Classic Chinese sauce	Homepride	95	per 383g pack 364
Spirits 70% proof		222	63
Split lentils, peas: see Lentils, Peas			
Splits chews	Trebor	385	per sweet 15
Splitz			
apple	Canada Dry	47	per 250ml bottle 118
passion	Canada Dry	45	per 250ml pack 113

Product	Brand	Calories per 100g/ 100ml	Calories per oz/ pack/ portion
Sponges: see also flavours			
Sponge bar cake, fresh			
cream	Tesco	332	94
Sponge cake			
jam filled		302	86
with fat		464	132
without fat		301	85
Sponge cake mix (as sold)			
Devon	Green's	396	made up per portion 223
traditional recipe	Green's	354	made up per portion 93
Sponge cake mixes: see also flavours			
Sponge finger biscuits	Huntley & Palmer	388	per biscuit 21
Sponge fingers	Tesco	382	108
	Waitrose	433	123
Sponge flan			
large	Littlewoods	1	per 200g flan 1
medium	Littlewoods	1	per 102g flan 1
Sponge gateau			
with buttercream			
and jam	St Michael	391	111
with chocolate and			
buttercream	St Michael	413	117
Sponge mix, luxury (as			per 355g pack
sold)	Granny Smiths	342	made up 1216
	Whitworths	425	120
Sponge pudding, steamed		344	98
Sponge puddings: see also flavours			

Product	Brand	Calories per 100g/ 100ml	Calories per oz/ pack/ portion
Sponge sandwich cake with buttercream and jam	St Michael	424	120
Sponge slice cake	Littlewoods	334	95
Sponge trifle	Lyons	308	87
Sports biscuits	Safeway	473	134
Spotted Dick	Ross	350	99
	St Michael	339	96
Sprats			
dried		168	48
fresh, raw		100	28
fried		441	125
fried (with bones)		388	110
Spread, low fat	Tesco	340	96
with cheese	Sun-Pat	176	50
with cheese and garden herbs	Sun-Pat	176	50
Spread, reduced fat	Heinz Weight Watchers	360	102
Spread with cheese and onion low fat	Sun-Pat	176	50
Spreading cheese (Medley): see flavours			
Spring cabbage, boiled		7	2
Spring greens			
boiled		10	3
fresh, boiled	Tesco	10	3
Spring onion crisps	Christies	520	per 26g bag 130
	Hunters	520	per 26g bag 130
	Littlewoods	548	per 75g pack 411
	St Michael	546	155

Product	Brand	Calories per 100g/ 100ml	Calories per oz/ pack/ portion
Spring onion dressing	Heinz All Seasons	264	75
Spring onions			
bulbs and tops, raw		28	8
flesh of bulb only, raw		35	10
fresh	Littlewoods	35	10
fresh, boiled	Tesco	35	10
Spring roll	Waitrose	226	64
Spring rolls Chinese-style meal	Bejam		per roll baked 162
Spring vegetable mix	Bejam	35	per 113g portion boiled 40
Spring vegetable soup	Heinz Ready to Serve	33	9
	Heinz Weight Watchers	22	per can 65
dried	Batchelors	268	per 38g pint pack as sold 102
	Littlewoods	320	per 37g pint packet 118
	Safeway	317	90
	Tesco	334	95
	Waitrose	286	per 40g pack 114
dried (made up)	Chef Box	16	5
dried, low calorie	Knorr Quick Soup	285	81
Spring vegetables	Heinz Baby Foods	70	per 128g can 90
Sprouts (frozen)	Tesco	35	10
button	Bejam	46	per 57g portion boiled 25
medium	Waitrose	18	per 454g pack 80

Product	Brand	Calories per 100g/ 100ml	Calories per oz/ pack/ portion
Sprouts: *see also Brussels sprouts*			
Square snack			
muesli bar	Holly Mill		per bar 216
protein bar	Holly Mill		per bar 184
Squash: *see Courgettes*			
Squid			
dried		328	93
fresh, raw		75	21
frozen, raw		66	19
St Paulin cheese	Safeway	300	85
	Tesco	289	82
	Waitrose	300	85
Stackers	Cadbury's	450	per crisp 5
Star Bar	Cadbury's	495	per 53g bar 260
Starship 4	Wall's		per portion 35
Start	Kellogg's	340	96
Steak, flash fry	St Michael	128	36
Steak and kidney, diced, casseroled	Bejam	183	52
Steak and kidney casserole	Boots Baby Foods	400	113
Steak and kidney dinner			
3-9 months	Heinz Baby Foods	75	per 128g jar 96
7-15 months	Heinz Baby Foods	66	per 128g can 84
Steak and kidney lunch	Heinz Baby Foods	68	per 170g jar 116
Steak and kidney pancakes	Findus	141	40

Product	Brand	Calories per 100g/ 100ml	Calories per oz/ pack/ portion
Steak and kidney pie			
individual		323	92
pastry top only		286	81
	Birds Eye		per pie for one 370
	Birds Eye		per pie for 2/3 1120
	Fray Bentos	220	62
	Littlewoods	326	per pie, pack of 2, 461
	Safeway	235	per 142g pie 335
	Tesco	296	84
	Tesco	285	81
	Waitrose	254	per 142g pie 360
family	Bejam		per 1/4 pie baked
	Ross	270	77
individual	Bejam	276	per 142g pie baked 391
	Littlewoods	310	per 177g pack 549
	Ross	300	85
	Waitrose	239	68
large	Littlewoods	295	per 474g pack 1398
plate pie	St Michael	296	84
rich pastry	St Michael	305	86
traditional, small	St Michael	290	82
Steak and kidney pie filling	Fray Bentos	147	42
Steak and kidney pie meal with carrots	St Michael	200	57
Steak and kidney pudding	Fray Bentos	212	60
	St Michael	157	45

Product	Brand	Calories per 100g/ 100ml	Calories per oz/ pack/ portion
Steak and kidney pudding			
individual	Waitrose	250	71
large	Tesco	274	78
small	Tesco	294	83
Steak and kidney pudding pie			
individual	Ross	215	61
Steak and kidney stew	Campbell's	64	18
Steak and mushroom flaky bake pie	Birds Eye MenuMaster		per pie 505
Steak and mushroom pie filling	Fray Bentos	106	30
Steak and onion pie filling	Fray Bentos	156	44
Steak and vegetable pie	St Michael	94	27
	Tesco	280	79
Steak burger, prime	Safeway	250	71
Steak chips	Bejam	126	per 170g baked 214
Steak fries	Bejam	150	per 170g portion deep-fried 255
Steak grills	Bejam		each grilled 203
Steak hotpot	Heinz Baby Foods	57	per 128g can 73
Steak, kidney and vegetables soup	Campbell's Main Course	55	16
Steak, mushroom and red wine pie	Waitrose	239	68
Steak pie	Littlewoods	512	145
	Littlewoods	318	per pie, pack of two, 450
	Tesco	215	61
chunky	Waitrose	282	80

Product	Brand	Calories per 100g/100ml	Calories per oz/pack/portion
Steakhouse chips	Tesco	207	59
Steaklet, ground beef	St Michael	128	36
Stem ginger in syrup	Waitrose	260	per 425g can 1105
Stem ginger biscuits	Prewetts		per biscuit 77
Stem ginger cookies	Tesco	478	136
	Waitrose	487	138
Sterilized cream	Littlewoods	240	168g/6oz can
	Tesco	227	64
Stewed steak with gravy (canned)		176	50
Stewpack vegetables	Bejam	16	per 113g portion boiled 18
	Ross	20	6
	Waitrose	35	per 454g pack 160
Stewpot pie (individual)			
beef and kidney	Ross	251	71
chicken and veg	Ross	224	64
Stilton cheese	St Michael	462	131
	Tesco	380	108
blue	Dairy Crest	405	115
	Safeway	432	122
	St Ivel	405	115
	Waitrose	405	115
blue, half	Waitrose	360	102
farmhouse blue	Waitrose	390	111
white	Dairy Crest	360	102
	St Ivel	360	102
	Waitrose	360	102
Stilton pots, blue	St Michael	405	115
Stir fry chili bean mix	Bejam	105	per 142g portion boiled 149

Product	Brand	Calories per 100g/ 100ml	Calories per oz/ pack/ portion
Stir fry meal			
Chinese	Bejam		per portion stir-fried 280
oriental prawn	Bejam		per serving stir-fried 350
Stir fry mushrooms	Safeway	80	per 340g pack 276
Stir fry rice	Waitrose	88	per 340g pack 300
Stir fry rice mix	Ross	70	20
Stir fry sweetcorn mix	Ross	70	20
Stir fry vegetables			
cauliflower, mushrooms, peas	Waitrose	39	11
continental (as sold)	Birds Eye	42	12
continental (fried)	Birds Eye	53	15
country (as sold)	Birds Eye	28	8
country (fried)	Birds Eye	35	10
courgettes, corn, mushrooms	Waitrose	36	10
mixed	Ross	50	14
rice, corn and prawns	Waitrose	101	29
Stock cubes			
vegetable and chicken	Bovril	190	54
vegetable and meat	Bovril	200	57
Stollen cakes	Tesco	371	105
Stork margarine	Van den Berghs	740	210
Special Blend	Van den Berghs	740	210
Stout			
bottled		37	10
extra		39	11
Straw mushroom: *see Mushroom*			

Product	Brand	Calories per 100g/ 100ml	Calories per oz/ pack/ portion
Strawberries			
canned		81	23
raw		26	7
	Littlewoods	26	7
canned	Hartley's	115	per 117g can 135
	Safeway	85	24
in syrup	Tesco	78	22
	Waitrose	74	per 220g pack 163
Strawberry and apple juice	Copella	39	12
Strawberry and champagne yogurt	St Ivel Cabaret	109	31
Strawberry and chocolate ice cream	Wall's	90	25
Strawberry and cream cheesecake	Young's	240	68
Strawberry and cream ice cream, American style	Waitrose	178	53
Strawberry and cream mousse	Tesco	170	48
Strawberry and orange yogurt dessert	Boots Baby Foods	390	111
Strawberry and vanilla bombes	Bejam		per bombe 193
Strawberry and vanilla ice cream	Wall's	90	25
Strawberry and wild herb yogurt	St Michael	117	33
Strawberry Arctic gateau	Birds Eye		per 1/5 gateau 105
Strawberry bar	Granose	374	per 50g bar 187

Product	Brand	Calories per 100g/ 100ml	Calories per oz/ pack/ portion
Strawberry blancmange	Brown and Polson	330	94
Strawberry Bon Bons	Trebor	403	per sweet 27
Strawberry bubble gum	Wrigley Hubba Bubba		per chunk 15/24
Strawberry champagne sundae	Eden Vale	128	125g/4*oz pack
Strawberry cheesecake	Eden Vale	196	56
	Young's	240	68
individual	Young's	255	72
Strawberry cheesecake mix (made up)	Lyons	234	66
Strawberry Complan	Farley	444	per 57g sachet 253
Strawberry conserve	Safeway	248	70
	St Michael	240	68
	Tesco	268	76
	Waitrose	250	71
Strawberry Cornetto	Wall's		per cone 205
Strawberry creams	Rowntree Mackintosh		per sweet 45
Strawberry cream cake	Birds Eye		per 1/6 cake 145
Strawberry crumble creams	Tesco	497	141
Strawberry cup	Rowntree Mackintosh		per sweet 45
Strawberry delight dessert	St Michael	116	33
Strawberry dessert	Waitrose	444	per 69g pack 306

Product	Brand	Calories per 100g/ 100ml	Calories per oz/ pack/ portion
Strawberry dessert sauce	Lyons Maid	264	75
Strawberry Devonshire cheesecake	St Ivel	250	71
Strawberry drink, semi-skimmed	St Michael	57	16
Strawberry fingers	Lyons	368	104
Strawberry flan filling	Armour	130	per 795g pack 1034
Strawberry flavour cake mix (as sold)	Green's	397	made up per portion 223
Strawberry flavour cordial, undiluted	Quosh	108	32
Strawberry flavour dessert mix	Dietade	264	75
Strawberry flavour drink	Quosh	35	10
Strawberry flavour jelly	Waitrose	272	77
crystals	Dietade	290	82
Strawberry fool	Cow and Gate	69	per 110g jar 76, 150g jar 104
Strawberry fruit cream trifle	Safeway	132	37
Strawberry fruit filling	Morton	76	22
Strawberry fruit pie filling	Tesco	84	24
Strawberry fruit softy	Eden Vale	129	37

Product	Brand	Calories per 100g/ 100ml	Calories per oz/ pack/ portion
Strawberry fruit spread	Waitrose	124	35
Strawberry Fruit Whisk mix	Green's	113	per portion made up with whole milk 124
	Green's	113	per portion made with skimmed milk 104
Strawberry gateau	Bejam		per 1/18 gateau 169
	Birds Eye		per 1/6 gateau 280
	St Ivel	236	67
	Tesco	282	80
party	Bejam		per 1/14 gateau 204
Strawberry Harlequin dessert	Wall's		per 1/5 pack 110
Strawberry ice cream	Safeway	175	52
	Waitrose	189	56
	Wall's Alpine		per 1/10 pack 120
	Wall's Italiano	90	per 1/10 litre pack 90
dairy	Bertorelli	176	per pack
	Lyons Maid Napoli	176	50
Mini Milk	Wall's		per portion 40
non-dairy	Lyons Maid	175	50
slicing	Wall's		per slice 60
Strawberry jam	Robertson's	251	71
	Safeway	251	71
	Waitrose	248	70
diabetic	Boots	239	68
	Dietade	232	66

Product	Brand	Calories per 100g/ 100ml	Calories per oz/ pack/ portion
Strawberry jam			
no added sugar	Safeway	141	40
reduced sugar	Boots	152	43
	Heinz Weight Watchers	124	35
	Waitrose	124	35
Strawberry jam sponge pudding	Heinz	286	81
Strawberry jelly	Safeway	268	76
	Tesco	57	16
diabetic crystals	Boots	365	103
table	Littlewoods	260	74
Strawberry juice, concentrated	Western Isles	325	96
Strawberry King Cone	Lyons Maid		per cone 191
Strawberry luxury cheesecake mix	Tesco	300	85
made	Tesco	245	69
Strawberry milkshake	St Michael	75	21
	Waitrose	68	20
Strawberry Mivvi	Lyons Maid		each 77
Strawberry mousse	Bejam		per tub as sold 75
	Ross	170	48
	Safeway	150	44
	Tesco	180	51
wizard	St Ivel	183	52
Strawberry mousse and cream swirl	Safeway	150	43
Strawberry mousse tub dessert	Birds Eye		per tub 110
Strawberry Pack-A-Pie	Batchelors	76	per 385g jar/ sachet 293
Strawberry preserve	Baxters	240	per 340g jar

Product	Brand	Calories per 100g/ 100ml	Calories per oz/ pack/ portion
Strawberry preserve	Tesco	255	72
reduced sugar	Robertson's	150	43
Strawberry pure fruit spread	Robertson's	120	34
Strawberry real milk ice	Lyons Maid		each 49
Strawberry Regale dessert	St Ivel	135	38
Strawberry rice dessert	Boots Baby Foods	410	116
Strawberry ripple ice cream	Tesco	173	49
slice	Wall's		per 1/5 pack 100
soft scoop	Lyons Maid	181	51
Strawberry ripple mousse	Findus	171	48
	Waitrose	149	42
Strawberry royale ice cream	St Michael	193	55
carte d'or cup	Wall's		per portion 155
Strawberry sauce	Tesco	315	89
Strawberry sherbets	Trebor	359	per sweet 23
Strawberry snowballs	Littlewoods	449	127
Strawberry souffle	St Michael	191	54
Strawberry Sparkles	Wall's		per portion 30
Strawberry split	Wall's		per portion 80
Strawberry supershake	Eden Vale	75	21
Strawberry Supreme Delight	Safeway	431	122
Strawberry Swiss roll	Tesco	367	104

Product	Brand	Calories per 100g/ 100ml	Calories per oz/ pack/ portion
Strawberry tartlets biscuits	St Michael	386	109
Strawberry Topsy Turvy	Ambrosia	103	29
Strawberry trifle	Eden Vale	160	45
	Littlewoods	138	39
	St Ivel	143	41
Real	Young's	150	43
Strawberry yogurt	Gold Ski	116	per 150g pack 174
	Mr Men	90	26
	Munch Bunch	100	per 125g pack 125
	Raines	80	23
	Safeway	95	27
	Ski	81	per 150g pack 122
	St Ivel Rainbow	70	20
	St Ivel Real	80	23
	St Ivel Shape	40	11
	St Michael	95	27
	St Michael Lite	39	11
creamy	Waitrose	140	per 125g pack 175
French style	Littlewoods	102	per 150g pack 153
	St Michael	103	29
Funtime	Safeway	90	per 150g pack 135
low fat	Diet Ski	55	per 150g pack 83
	Littlewoods	84	per 150g pack 126
	Tesco	88	25
	Waitrose	95	per 150g pack 143
whole milk	Safeway	59	per 146g pack 86
	Waitrose	115	per 150g pack 173
Strawberry yogurt dessert	Cow and Gate Heinz Baby	62	per 110g jar 68
	Foods	70	per 128g jar 90
Strawberryade	Corona	25	7

Product	Brand	Calories per 100g/ 100ml	Calories per oz/ pack/ portion
Strike cola	Barr	30	per 250ml can 75
Strong ale		72	20
Strongbow cider	Bulmer	36	per half pint 102
1080	Bulmer	49	per half pint 140
Stuffed olives	Tesco	160	45
Stuffed plaice	St Michael	109	31
Stuffed pork roll	Tyne Brand	153	43
Stuffed turkey roll	Tyne Brand	144	41
Stuffing mixes: *see flavours*			
Suet			
block		895	254
shredded		826	234
	Safeway	826	234
	Tesco	797	226
shredded beef	Tesco	797	226
shredded beef	Waitrose	850	241
Suet dumpling and pudding mix (as sold)	Granny Smiths	341	per 314g pack made up 1070
Suet pudding, steamed		333	94
Sugar			
Demerara		394	112
white		394	112
Demerara		394	112
white		394	112
brown, dark, soft	Safeway	394	112
	Tate and Lyle	380	108
	Tesco	383	109
	Waitrose	380	108
brown, light, soft	Safeway	394	112
	Tate and Lyle	384	109
	Tesco	371	105
	Waitrose	380	108

Product	Brand	Calories per 100g/ 100ml	Calories per oz/ pack/ portion
Sugar			
candy	Tesco	371	105
coffee crystals	Safeway	394	112
Demerara	Holland and Barrett	380	108
	Safeway	394	112
	Tate and Lyle	394	112
	Tesco	371	105
Demerara, dark	Waitrose	389	110
Demerara, light	Waitrose	389	110
for coffee	Tesco	371	105
fruit	Dietade	394	112
golden granulated	Tesco	371	105
icing	Tate and Lyle	392	111
Molasses	Waitrose	351	100
Muscovado	Safeway	394	112
	Tesco	383	109
Muscovado, dark	Waitrose	360	102
Muscovado, light	Waitrose	378	107
white, caster	Tate and Lyle	394	112
white, cubes	Tate and Lyle	394	112
white, granulated	Tate and Lyle	394	112
white, preserving	Tate and Lyle	394	112
Sugar flakes	Tesco	367	104
Sugar free muesli	Holland and Barrett	380	108
	Prewetts	340	96
Sugar letters	Littlewoods	375	per 92g pack 345
Sugar Puffs		348	99
Sugar strands			
assorted	Tesco	370	105
chocolate	Tesco	423	120
Sugared almonds	Littlewoods	417	118
	St Michael	460	130

Product	Brand	Calories per 100g/ 100ml	Calories per oz/ pack/ portion
Sultana and bran biscuits, handbaked	Boots	485	137
Sultana and cherry cake	St Michael	273	77
Sultana and spice creams	Waitrose	499	141
Sultana and syrup pancakes	St Michael	280	79
	Tesco	293	83
Sultana bar	Cadbury's	450	128
Sultana Bran	Kellogg's	298	84
Sultana cake			
cut	Safeway	360	102
large	Safeway	360	102
whole	Waitrose	347	98
Sultana cookies	Tesco	475	135
Sultana scones	Tesco	310	88
Sultanas			
dried		250	71
	Holland and Barrett	240	68
	Safeway	250	71
	Tesco	256	73
	Whitworths	250	71
Australian	Waitrose	250	71
Greek	Waitrose	250	71
Summer County dairy spread	Van den Berghs	650	184
Summer fruit lattice pie	Waitrose	340	96
Summer fruit trifle	St Michael	145	41

Product	Brand	Calories per 100g/ 100ml	Calories per oz/ pack/ portion
Summer fruits pure juice	Cow and Gate	40	per 125g jar 50
Summer harvest mix vegetables	Findus	72	20
Summer mixed vegetables (canned)	Tesco	50	14
Summer Orchard	Kellogg's	320	91
Sundae Cups chocolate	Lyons Maid		each 156
raspberry	Lyons Maid		each 89
Sundaes apricot	Lyons	396	112
blackcurrant and apple	Lyons	389	110
Sunflower fruit and nut bar	Shepherd Boy Bars		per bar 204
Sunflower margarine	Safeway	735	208
salt-free	Safeway	735	208
Sunflower oil	Boots	899	255
	Flora	900	255
	Holland and Barrett	720	213
	Safeway	900	266
	St Michael	900	255
	Sunwheel	900	255
	Tesco	875	248
	Waitrose	900	266
Sunflower seed bar, natural	Boots	464	132
Sunflower seeds	Holland and Barrett	560	159
Sunflower spread	Sunwheel	576	163

Product	Brand	Calories per 100g/ 100ml	Calories per oz/ pack/ portion
Sunfruit drink	St Michael	47	13
Sunny sauce	O.K.	85	24
Sunsnack, peanut	Sunwheel	622	176
Supa 5 chews	Trebor	364	per sweet 16
Super Fries			
salt and pepper	Hunters	441	per 24g pack 106
tomato ketchup	Hunters	441	per 24g pack 106
Super juice bar	Lyons Maid		each 50
Super Noodles, all flavours	Batchelors	465	per pack as sold 460
Super triple choc	Lyons Maid		each 277
Superfine biscuits	Rakusen	347	per biscuit 74
Supermousse tub dessert (Birds Eye): *see flavours*			
Supershake (Eden Vale): *see flavours*			
Superwhip tub dessert	Birds Eye		per tub 855; per level 10ml tsp 12
Supreme (Eden Vale): *see flavours*			
Supreme Delight (Safeway): *see flavours*			
Supreme style pot meal	Boots Shapers	328	93
Surprise vegetables (Batchelor): *see Peas, etc*			
Swede diced	Bejam	21	per 57g portion boiled 12
Swedes			
boiled		18	5
raw		21	6
Sweet and savoury biscuits	Holly Mill		per biscuit 25

Product	Brand	Calories per 100g/ 100ml	Calories per oz/ pack/ portion
Sweet and sour chicken	St Michael	99	28
	Vesta	362	per 281g pack for two as served 1018
Sweet and sour Chinese stir fry vegetable dish	St Michael	25	7
Sweet 'n' sour Chinese-style meal			
chicken	Bejam		per serving baked 145
pork	Bejam		per serving baked 338
Sweet and sour fried special savoury rice	Batchelors	465	per 143g sachet 665
Sweet and sour pickle	Pan Yan	139	39
Sweet and sour pork with rice	Waitrose	88	per 340g pack 300
	Birds Eye MenuMaster		per pack 670
Sweet and sour pork balls	St Michael	131	37
Sweet and sour pork vegetable mix	Ross	70	20
Sweet and sour prawns and rice	St Michael	100	28
Sweet and sour sauce	St Michael	38	11
Cook in	Homepride	53	per 376g pack 199
Cooking-in	Baxters	94	per 425g can 400
Pour Over	Crosse & Blackwell	112	32
Sweet and sour sauce mix			
Cook In	Colman's	320	91
Pour Over	Colman's	320	91
Sweet and sour savoury rice	Safeway	342	per 125g pack 428

Product	Brand	Calories per 100g/ 100ml	Calories per oz/ pack/ portion
Sweet corn			
canned kernels		76	22
on the cob, kernels only, raw		127	36
immature baby corn, canned, drained		21	6
on the cob, boiled		123	35
on the cob, raw		127	36
	Bejam	109	per 85g portion boiled 93
	Birds Eye	106	30
	Findus	127	36
	Ross	95	27
	Safeway	127	per 227g pack 288
	St Michael	83	24
	Tesco	101	29
	Waitrose	90	26
canned	Tesco	100	28
canned, golden, no salt added	Del Monte	101	29
on the cob, fresh, boiled	Tesco	124	boiled
with peppers	Waitrose	81	23
Sweet corn and peppers (canned)	Tesco	90	26
Sweet corn, peas and carrots	Birds Eye	53	15
Sweetcorn relish	Branston	132	37
	Crosse & Blackwell	133	38
	Tesco	109	31
Sweetcorn soup, low calorie	Knorr Quick Soup	364	103

Product	Brand	Calories per 100g/ 100ml	Calories per oz/ pack/ portion
Sweetcorn with red peppers salad	Littlewoods	159	45
Sweet military pickle	Haywards	130	37
Sweet peanuts	Trebor	406	per sweet 26
Sweet piccalilli	Waitrose	48	14
chunky	Safeway	98	28
Sweet pickle	Branston	131	37
	Littlewoods	160	45
	Safeway	91	26
	Waitrose	215	61
low calorie	Boots Shapers	66	19
Sweet pickled onions	Safeway	36	10
Sweet potatoes			
boiled		85	24
raw		91	26
Sweet Trolley Italiano ice cream: *see flavours*			
Sweetbread, lamb			
fried		230	65
raw		131	37
Sweetener, diabetic	Boots	360	102
Sweetex			
granulated	Crookes		per teaspoon
liquid	Crookes		per 4 drops
Sweetmeal biscuits, wheaten	St Michael	453	128
Swiss black cherry conserve	Safeway	248	70
	St Michael	240	68
Swiss black cherry jam reduced sugar	Waitrose	124	35
Swiss cheese with ham crepes	Findus	182	52

Product	Brand	Calories per 100g/ 100ml	Calories per oz/ pack/ portion
Swiss cup, instant	Granose	6	per cup 2
Swiss Gruyere cheese	St Michael	400	113
	Waitrose	272	77
Swiss gruyere spread	Tesco	306	87
Swiss mountain chocolate bar	St Michael	550	156
white	St Michael	562	159
Swiss muesli cereal	Waitrose	382	108
Swiss pies	St Michael	296	84
Swiss roll: *see flavours*			
Swiss style breakfast	Tesco	374	106
Swiss-style cereal	Safeway	473	134
Swiss style chocolate cake mix (as sold)	Green's	401	made up per portion 300
Swiss style muesli bar	Boots	350	99
Swiss style potato cake	Findus	80	23
Swiss style potato fry	Waitrose	135	38
Swiss white chocolate	St Michael	172	49
Syrup			
golden		298	84
golden	Tate and Lyle	298	84
pouring	Tate and Lyle	284	81
Syrup biscuits, Kennett	Huntley & Palmer	500	per biscuit 63
Syrup pancakes	Tesco	304	86
Syrup sponge pudding	Safeway	372	105
	St Michael	375	106
	Tesco	358	101

Product	Brand	Calories per 100g/ 100ml	Calories per oz/ pack/ portion
Szechuan spicy Classic			
Chinese sauce	Homepride	108	per 383g pack 413
Table salt			
Table crackers	Jacobs	431	per biscuit 33
	Safeway	431	per biscuit 8
Table jellies			
all flavours	Chivers	290	per portion 100
all flavours	Littlewoods	260	per 128g pack 333
Table jellies: see also flavours			
Tabouleh Salad	Waitrose	141	40
Taco filling, beef	Old El Paso	176	per 205g can 361
Taco sauce			
hot	Old El Paso	39	11
mild	Old El Paso	39	11
Taco shells	Old El Paso	490	per 125g pack 613
Tagliatelle	Buitoni	350	99
	St Michael	369	105
	Waitrose	378	107
new style	St Michael	142	40
wholewheat	Signor Rossi	275	78
Tagliatelle bianche	Signor Rossi	272	77
	Waitrose	222	63
Tagliatelle nicoise	Waitrose	170	48
Tagliatelle verde	Buitoni	340	96
	Signor Rossi	309	88
egg, cooked	Tesco	118	33
egg, uncooked	Tesco	336	95
Tagliolini			
bianchi	Signor Rossi	272	77
verdi	Signor Rossi	309	88
Tahini sesame cream	Harmony	560	159

Product	Brand	Calories per 100g/ 100ml	Calories per oz/ pack/ portion
Take-off bar	Hellas		per bar 170
Tamari sauce	Sunwheel	86	24
Tamarind leaves, raw		73	21
Tamatar Madras curry sauce	Sharwood	126	36
Tandoori chicken masala	Waitrose	376	107
Tandoori chicken masala soup, dried	Waitrose	376	per 44g pack 165
Tandoori Coat and cook sauce	Homepride	180	per 43g pack 77
Tandoori cutlet mix, vegetarian	Tomorrow Foods	318	90
Tandoori flavour chicken	St Michael	240	68
Tandoori marinade	Knorr	211	60
Tandori Dish of the Day	Crosse & Blackwell	461	131
Tangerine flavour jelly	Waitrose	272	per 142g pack 386
Tangerine jelly	Safeway	268	per 142g pack 381
	Tesco	57	16
Tangerine luxury cheesecake mix	Tesco	347	98
made up	Tesco	273	77
Tangerines			
raw		34	10
raw (with peel and pips)		23	7
fresh, without skin	Littlewoods	34	10

Product	Brand	Calories per 100g/ 100ml	Calories per oz/ pack/ portion
Tangy lemon cheesecake mix (as sold)	Green's	429	made up per portion 240
Tangy orange and apple bubble gum	Wrigley Hubba Bubba		per chunk 15-24
Tangy pickle spread	Heinz Ploughman's	118	33
Tapioca			
raw		359	102
cooked	Tesco	121	34
raw	Tesco	330	94
seed pearl	Safeway	359	102
seed pearl and medium pearl	Whitworths	359	102
Tapioca, creamed	Ambrosia	83	24
Tapioca pudding	Whitworths	131	37
Taramasalata		446	126
	Tesco	435	123
Taro tuber, raw		94	27
Tartare sauce	O.K.	255	72
	Safeway	255	72
	Tesco	279	79
	Waistline	138	39
	Waitrose	283	80
Tartare sauce dressing	Safeway	222	63
Tartaric acid	Boots		
Tartex			
herb	Vessen	233	per 180g pack 420
plain	Vessen	244	per 180g pack 440
Tartlet cases biscuits	St Michael	488	138
Tastex	Granose	208	59

Product	Brand	Calories per 100g/ 100ml	Calories per oz/ pack/ portion
Tea			
Indian		108	31
Indian, infusion		-1	
black, leaves, dried		293	83
green, leaves, dried		300	85
Indian, leaves, dried		108	31
Pakistani, infusion only		46	13
all flavours, dry	Waitrose	108	per 125g pack 135
all flavours, infused	Safeway	1	
infused	Littlewoods	2	1
Tea cakes	St Michael	270	77
	Tesco	270	77
chocolate coated	Tesco	432	122
toasted	Bassett's	441	125
Tea cakes mix	Tesco	372	105
lemon (as sold)	Tesco	422	120
lemon (made up)	Tesco	355	101
made up	Tesco	378	107
Tea crackers	Rakusen	347	per biscuit 17
Teabreak biscuits	Nabisco	420	per biscuit 38
wholewheat	Nabisco	388	per biscuit 38
Teddy bear gums, real fruit	St Michael	340	96
Ten fruits juice cocktail	Waitrose	38	11
Tendale cheese			
blue	Dairy Crest	252	71
Cheddar-like	Dairy Crest	253	72
Tendale Cheese			
Cheshire-like	Dairy Crest	246	70
Tender bits	Granose	79	22

Product	Brand	Calories per 100g/ 100ml	Calories per oz/ pack/ portion
Tequila sunrise cocktail	Lyons Maid		each 38
Terror Curses chews	Trebor	364	per sweet 16
Terror Rats and Bats	Trebor	600	per sweet 66
Thick chicken soup, dried	Safeway	350	99
made up	Chef Box	30	9
Thick country vegetable soup, dried (made up)	Chef Box	32	9
Thick garden vegetable soup, dried (made up)	Chef Box	25	7
Thick green bean soup, dried	Boots Second Nature	313	89
Thick onion soup, dried (made up)	Chef Box	29	8
Thick pea soup, dried (made up)	Chef Box	26	7
Thick potato soup, dried	Boots Second Nature	313	89
Thick vegetable soup dried	Tesco	50	14
	Littlewoods	356	per 37g pint packet 132
Things	Trebor	714	per sweet 45
Thistle shortbread biscuits	Tesco	513	145
Thousand island dressing	Duchesse	33	10
	Heinz All Seasons	282	80
	Kraft	393	116
	Safeway	224	66

Product	Brand	Calories per 100g/ 100ml	Calories per oz/ pack/ portion
Thousand island dressing			
	Tesco	384	109
Thousand island dressing cream	Waitrose	194	55
Thousand island dressing			
fresh	St Michael	281	80
low calorie	Boots Shapers	196	56
Thousand islands Prawnaise	Lyons Seafoods	150	43
Three bean salad	St Michael	148	42
Three fruit cocktail drink, long life	Waitrose	41	12
Three fruits marmalade	Baxters	248	70
thick-cut	Waitrose	248	70
Tigertots	Rowntree Mackintosh	380	per 43g bag 165
Tilsiter cheese	Waitrose	390	111
Tin roof dairy ice cream	Safeway	242	72
Tinda (round gourd)			
canned, drained		12	3
fresh, raw		21	6
Tiny tots	Littlewoods	315	89
Tip Top dessert topping	Nestle	110	31
Tizer	Barr	37	per 330ml can 122
	Littlewoods	39	per 330ml pack 129
Toad in the hole	Findus	207	59
Toast Toppers (Heinz): *see flavours*			
Toasted bran	Meadow Farm	360	102

Product	Brand	Calories per 100g/ 100ml	Calories per oz/ pack/ portion
Toasted bran farmhouse	Weetabix	300	85
Toasted tea cakes	Bassett's	441	125
Toffee almond ice cream, American style	St Michael	225	64
Toffee and almond ice cream	Tesco	202	57
Toffee and banana mousse	Waitrose	151	43
Toffee and chocolate Megabite	Wall's		per megabite 120
Toffee and mallow	Rowntree Mackintosh		per sweet 45
Toffee apple roll	Trebor	346	per sweet 14
Toffee biscuits	Littlewoods	485	per biscuit 76
Toffee bon bons	Tesco	417	118
	Trebor	403	per sweet 27
Toffee brazils	Tesco	442	125
Toffee caramello Supermousse tub dessert	Birds Eye		per tub 120
Toffee creams	Tesco	454	129
Toffee crisp	Rowntree Mackintosh	510	per 44g bar 225
Toffee crumble	Lyons Maid	303	each 171
Toffee crunch	Trebor	429	per sweet 27
Toffee cup	Rowntree Mackintosh		per sweet 40
Toffee de luxe	Rowntree Mackintosh		per sweet 45

Product	Brand	Calories per 100g/100ml	Calories per oz/pack/portion
Toffee dessert	Waitrose	444	126
Toffee finger	Rowntree Mackintosh		per sweet 30
Toffee fudge ice cream			
scooping	Wall's Italiano	110	per 1/40 4-litre pack 110
Sweet Trolley	Wall's Italiano	110	per 1/10 litre pack 110
Toffee pat	Rowntree Mackintosh		per sweet 30
Toffee ripple ice cream, soft scoop	Lyons Maid	180	51
Toffee rolls, chocolate coated	Tesco	458	130
Toffee yogurt	St Michael	112	32
low fat	Tesco	106	30
Toffees, assorted	Rowntree Mackintosh	470	per toffee
Toffees, mixed		430	122
Toffo, plain and mint	Rowntree Mackintosh	455	per sweet 25
Tofu (soya bean curd)			
steamed		70	20
canned, fried		302	86
	Morinaga	54	per 297g pack 160
Chinese	Granose	60	17
in savoury bean sauce	Granose	120	34
in tomato sauce	Granose	90	26
Tofu dressing	Duchesse	33	10

Product	Brand	Calories per 100g/ 100ml	Calories per oz/ pack/ portion
Tofu spread			
with garlic	La Source de Vie	285	81
with paprika	La Source de Vie	285	81
Tofu with Chinese vegetables	Granose	60	per 435g pack 260
Tom and Jerry	Wall's		per portion 55
Tomato and beef soup, low calorie	Waitrose	20	per 295g can 59
Tomato and cheese pizza	Birds Eye MenuMaster	290	per 93g pizza 270
	Birds Eye MenuMaster	276	per 227g pizza 630
	Ross	220	62
	St Michael	221	63
French bread	Findus	228	65
	Waitrose	220	per 130g pizza 286
wholemeal	Ross	230	65
Tomato and chilli chutney	Sharwood	92	26
Tomato and chilli relish	Safeway	118	33
	Tesco	109	31
Tomato and herb Dish of the Day	Crosse & Blackwell	377	107
Tomato and mushroom spaghetti sauce	Campbell's	68	19
Tomato and onion Cook in Sauce	Homepride	57	per 376g pack 214

Product	Brand	Calories per 100g/ 100ml	Calories per oz/ pack/ portion
Tomato and onion spread	Heinz	218	62
Tomato and pepper relish	Crosse & Blackwell	126	36
Tomato and vegetable soup, dried	Knorr	300	85
	Tesco	329	93
instant	Tesco	355	101
instant special (made up)	Safeway	45	13
made up	Chef Chunky	37	10
with croutons	Batchelors Cup-a-Soup Special	394	per 33.5g pack as sold 132
Tomato 'n' vegetable soup			
with croutons	Batchelors Snack-a-Soup	327	per 42.5g sachet as
Tomato, cheese and onion pizza	St Michael	203	58
Tomato chutney		154	44
	Waitrose	154	44
Tomato cream soup	Knorr "No Simmer"	459	130
Tomato dressing for seafoods and salads	Waistline	144	41
Tomato fruit juice	Heinz	22	7
Tomato juice canned		16	5
Tomato juice	Boots	16	5
	Britvic	25	per 170ml can 42
	Libby	20	6
	Volonte	16	5
	Waitrose	16	5
long life	Safeway	16	5

Product	Brand	Calories per 100g/ 100ml	Calories per oz/ pack/ portion
Tomato juice			
long life	Tesco	21	6
	Waitrose	17	5
Tomato juice cocktail	Britvic	25	per 113ml pack 28
	Hunts	16	5
	Stchweppes	17	5
Tomato ketchup		98	28
	Crosse & Blackwell	118	33
	Heinz	97	27
	Libby	106	30
	Safeway	95	27
	Tesco	100	28
	Waistline	57	16
	Waitrose	112	32
Tomato ketchup Super Fries	Hunters	441	per 24g pack 106
Tomato Pasta Choice	Crosse & Blackwell	353	100
Tomato paste		67	19
	Tesco	68	19
Tomato pickle	Baxters	140	40
	Heinz Ploughman's	95	27
Tomato puree		67	19
	Buitoni	72	20
	Tesco	71	20
	Waitrose	86	24
with basil	Waitrose	56	16
Tomato relish	Branston	129	37
	Crosse & Blackwell	131	37
	Safeway	118	33

Product	Brand	Calories per 100g/ 100ml	Calories per oz/ pack/ portion
Tomato relish	Tesco	93	26
Tomato rice soup, condensed	Campbell's	96	27
Tomato sauce		86	24
	Signor Rossi	35	10
Tomato sauce crisps	Christies	520	per 26g bag 130
	Hunters	520	per 26g bag 130
Tomato sausage	Littlewoods	275	78
Tomato savoury rice	Safeway	330	per 140g pack 462
Tomato soup			
dried, as served		31	9
dried		321	91
Tomato soup	Campbell's Bumper Harvest	59	17
	Granny's	40	as served 27
	Littlewoods	55	per 425g can 234
	Littlewoods	335	per 37g/1@oz pint
canned, low calorie	Heinz Weight Watchers	25	per 300g can 75
	Waistline	22	6
	Waitrose	18	per 29g can 53
condensed	Campbell's	65	18
dried	Batchelors Cup-a-Soup	350	per 24g sachet as sold 84
	Hera	364	103
	Knorr Quick Soup	395	112
	Prewetts Soup in Seconds	313	89
	Safeway	339	96
	Tesco	348	99
	Waitrose	334	per 56g pack 187
dried (made up)	Chef Box	36	10

Product	Brand	Calories per 100g/ 100ml	Calories per oz/ pack/ portion
Tomato soup			
dried, instant (as sold)	Safeway	338	96
dried, low calorie	Batchelors Slim-a-Soup	271	per 14g sachet 38
	Knorr Quick Soup	353	100
Tomato Super Noodles	Batchelors	465	per packet as sold 460
Tomato, vegetable and beef soup with croutons	Knorr Quick Soup	332	94
Tomatoes			
canned, drained		12	3
fresh, raw		14	4
fried		69	20
canned	Tesco	21	6
crushed	Waitrose	21	6
fresh	Littlewoods	14	4
whole peeled plum	Waitrose	21	per 227g can 48
Tomme de neige cheese	Waitrose	390	111
Tomor margarine	Van den Berghs	740	210
Tongue			
canned		213	60
lamb, raw		193	55
ox, boiled		293	83
ox, pickled, raw		220	62
sheep, stewed		289	82
ox	Waitrose	143	41
ox, sliced	St Michael	170	48
	Tesco	280	79
pork	Waitrose	176	50

Product	Brand	Calories per 100g/ 100ml	Calories per oz/ pack/ portion
Tongue			
pork, pressed, sliced	St Michael	152	43
Tongue and ham paste	Littlewoods	230	per 35g pack 81
Tongue and turkey paste	Littlewoods	210	per 35g pack 74
Tongue Twister	Wall's		per portion
Tonic-flavoured concentrate	Safeway	166	49
Tonic water	Safeway	28	8
	Schweppes	20	6
	Waitrose	27	8
low calorie	Safeway Diet Schweppes	1	
	Slimline	1	0.61
	Waitrose	4	1
Tonic Wine	Phosferine	137	41
Toor dahl cooked dish		109	31
Tooty Frooties	Rowntree Mackintosh	415	per sweet 8
Tooty Minties	Rowntree Mackintosh	425	per sweet 9
Top cream toffees	Trebor	439	per sweet 36
Topic	Mars	496	141
Tops cake mix (as sold)			
butterfly	Granny Smiths	432	per 363g pack made up 1568
chocolate	Granny Smiths	354	per 307g pack made up 1088
lemon	Granny Smiths	355	per 311g pack made up 1104
Topsy Turvy (Ambrosia): *see flavours*			

456

Product	Brand	Calories per 100g/ 100ml	Calories per oz/ pack/ portion
Tortelloni			
spinach, with ricotta			
filling	Signor Rossi	286	81
with meat filling	Signor Rossi	300	85
Tortilla chips	Old El Paso	272	per 150g pack 408
	St Michael	498	141
	Tesco	502	142
chilli	Trappers	492	per 50g pack 246
Tortillas	Old El Paso	497	141
Toss 'n' serve dressing,	Crosse &		
classic	Blackwell	219	62
herb	Crosse &		
	Blackwell	11	3
Tostada shells	Old El Paso	459	130
Tots			
Bunnytots	Rowntree Mackintosh	420	per 43g bag 180
Candytots	Rowntree Mackintosh	400	per 44g bag 175
Jellytots	Rowntree Mackintosh	345	per 46g bag 160
Tigertots	Rowntree Mackintosh	380	per 43g bag 165
Traditional mixes (Colman's): _see flavours_			
Trail bar snack bar,	Sunwheel		
carob coated	Kalibu	417	per 30g bar 125
Treacle			
black		257	73
	Tate and Lyle	257	73
Treacle baked roll	Waitrose	379	107
Treacle cookies	Waitrose	511	145

Product	Brand	Calories per 100g/ 100ml	Calories per oz/ pack/ portion
Treacle crunch biscuits	Peek Frean	436	per biscuit 29
Treacle crunch creams	Tesco	485	137
	Waitrose	495	140
Treacle Granymels	Itona	400	113
Treacle roly poly	Ross	390	111
Treacle scones	Tesco	293	83
Treacle sponge pudding	Heinz	288	82
Treacle sponge pudding mix (as sold)	Green's	394	made up per portion 334
Treacle tart		371	105
	Waitrose	371	105
Treacle toffee	Littlewoods	451	128
Trebor mints	Trebor	371	per sweet 6
Treets	Mars	515	146
Trellis bramley apple tart	St Michael	223	63
Trifle		160	45
mixed fruit	Young's	150	43
Trifle: see also flavours			
Trifle sponge	Waitrose	309	88
Trifle sponge pack of 8	Safeway	325	per sponge 24
Trifle tub dessert	Birds Eye		per tub 120
Trio biscuits	Jacobs	530	per biscuit 127
Tripe			
dressed		60	17
stewed		100	28
Triple choc	Lyons Maid		each 220

Product	Brand	Calories per 100g/ 100ml	Calories per oz/ pack/ portion
Tropical coconut cookies	Barbaras		per biscuit 220
Tropical double decker	St Michael	124	35
Tropical drink long life	Tesco	44	13
	Waitrose	43	13
Tropical 8 drink	Tesco	52	15
Tropical fruit and nuts	Waitrose	480	136
Tropical fruit cocktail	Del Monte	82	23
Tropical fruit drink	Safeway	46	14
	Waitrose	44	13
low calorie, carbonated	Boots Shapers	1	
low calorie, dilutable	Boots Shapers	8	2
Tropical fruit flavour cordial	Quosh	115	34
Tropical fruit flavour drink	Corona	26	8
	Quosh	34	10
Tropical fruit juice	Britvic	49	per 113ml pack 55
Tropical fruit lattice pie	Waitrose	340	96
Tropical fruit Pavlova	Bejam		per 1/8 Pavlova 183
Tropical fruit squash	Boots	167	49
Tropical fruit treat	Boots Baby Foods	380	108
Tropical fruit yoghurt whole milk	Safeway	101	per 150g pack 152
	Waitrose	115	per 150g pack 173
Tropical fruit yogurt	St Ivel Shape	41	12

Product	Brand	Calories per 100g/ 100ml	Calories per oz/ pack/ portion
Tropical Frutie	Wall's		per portion 55
Tropical muesli	Prewetts	340	96
Tropical Spring	Schweppes	30	9
Tropical supreme	Eden Vale	116	per 125g pack 145
Tropic-Ora drink, concentrated	Kia-Ora	131	39
Trout almande	Young's	160	45
Trout, brown			
steamed		135	38
steamed (with bones)		89	25
Trout fillets	Waitrose	135	38
fresh	Young's	134	38
Trout pate	Tesco	260	74
Trout, rainbow	Bejam		per trout grilled 196
large	Bejam		per trout grilled 249
whole	Waitrose	130	37
with mushrooms and onion stuffing	Waitrose	244	69
Trout, smoked	Bejam		per trout as sold 157
Trout veronique	Young's	130	37
Trout with savoury stuffing	Waitrose	189	54
Truffle and nougat	Rowntree Mackintosh		per sweet 50
Tub desserts (Birds Eye): see flavours			
Tuna			
canned in oil		289	82

Product	Brand	Calories per 100g/ 100ml	Calories per oz/ pack/ portion
skipjack chunks in vegetable oil	St Michael	288	82
skipjack in brine	Waitrose	117	per 99g can 116
skipjack in oil	Waitrose	278	per 99g can 275
skipjack steak in brine	Armour	97	per 200g can 194
skipjack steak in oil	Armour	237	per 200g can 474
skipjack steak in oil (Ivory Coast)	Armour	289	per 83g can 240
skipjack/Bonita chunks in brine	Armour	95	per 185g can 176
skipjack/Bonito chunks in oil	Armour	233	per 185g can 431
Tuna and prawn luxury pizza (frozen)	Safeway	198	56
Tuna and tomato quiche	St Michael	247	70
Tuna mayonnaise and tomato sandwich	Waitrose	226	64
Tuna pate	Tesco	387	110
Tuna sandwich	St Michael	240	68
Tunes	Mars	363	103
Turia: see Gourd, ridge			
Turkey			
raw, dark meat		114	32
raw, light meat		103	29
raw, meat and skin		145	41
raw, meat only		107	30
roast, dark meat		148	42
roast, light meat		132	37
roast, meat and skin		171	48
roast, meat only		140	40

Product	Brand	Calories per 100g/ 100ml	Calories per oz/ pack/ portion
Turkey	Waitrose	145	41
breast	Tesco	95	27
breast	Waitrose	130	37
breast with chestnuts	St Michael	232	66
breast with stuffing, cooked	Littlewoods	129	37
breast, cooked	Littlewoods	100	28
breast, roast, with stuffing	Waitrose	155	44
breast, sliced	Tesco	94	27
cured, smoked, cooked	Littlewoods	123	35
diced, boneless, casseroled	Bejam	141	40
livers (frozen)	Waitrose	145	41
oven ready	St Michael	157	45
prime slices	Tesco	94	27
roast, sliced	St Michael	121	34
steaks, breaded	St Michael	212	60
steaks, Goldenbake	Bejam		per piece baked 164
Turkey and ham pie	Waitrose	221	63
buffet	Bejam		per pie as sold 308
plate	St Michael	220	62
Turkey and ham sandwich	St Michael	190	54
Turkey and ham Toast Topper	Heinz	85	24
Turkey and vegetable broth, condensed	Campbell's	76	22
Turkey, bacon and salad club sandwich	Waitrose	226	64

Product	Brand	Calories per 100g/ 100ml	Calories per oz/ pack/ portion
Turkey bites	Bejam		per bite baked 42
Turkey breast roll	Waitrose	136	39
Turkey, cheese and tuna brioche	Waitrose	311	88
Turkey crunchies pie	Tesco	293	83
Turkey dinner	Heinz Baby Foods	54	per 128g can 69
Turkey ham, cooked	Waitrose	130	37
Turkey paupiettes	St Michael	74	21
Turkey pie, rich pastry	St Michael	318	90
Turkey ragout	Findus	138	39
Turkey recipe sausages	Wall's Light and Lean	199	per sausage 99
Turkey roll, stuffed	Tyne Brand	144	41
Turkey with asparagus en-croute	Bejam		per serving baked 409
Turkish delight without nuts		295	84
	Cadbury's	360	per 51g bar 185
Turmeric powder		354	100
Turnip tops, boiled		11	3
Turnips boiled		14	4
raw		20	6
fresh, boiled	Tesco	14	4
Tuscany Prego sauce	Campbell's	106	30
Tutti frutti chews	Trebor	379	per sweet 36

Product	Brand	Calories per 100g/ 100ml	Calories per oz/ pack/ portion
Tutti frutti Cornetto	Wall's		per super cone 240
Tutti Frutti ice cream			
dairy	Lyons Maid Napoli	199	56
Tutti frutti ice cream			
scooping	Wall's Italiano	110	per 1/40 4-litre pack 110
Sweet Trolley	Wall's Italiano		per 1/10 litre pack
TVP			
beef	Itona	250	per 113g pack 282
chunks	Itona	250	71
minced	Itona	250	per 113g pack 282
strips (vegetarian)	Boots	329	93
TVP mince			
vegetarian	Boots	329	93
Twango	Lyons Maid		each 120
Twiglets			
large	Peek Frean	400	per biscuit 6
small	Peek Frean	400	per biscuit 2
Twix	Mars	499	141
Ugli, fresh	Tesco	50	14
Umbongo fruit drink	Libby	41	12
Urad dahl, duhli (cooked dish)		88	25
Urad gram, whole (cooked dish)		85	24
V8 Juice	Campbell's	20	6
Valor beans: *see Balor beans*			
Vanilla and caramel choc ices	Safeway	259	77
Vanilla and chocolate ice cream	Tesco	180	51

Product	Brand	Calories per 100g/ 100ml	Calories per oz/ pack/ portion
Vanilla and mint choc ices	Safeway	259	77
Vanilla arctic circles	Birds Eye		per piece 155
Vanilla bar	Lyons Maid		each 72
Vanilla blancmange (dry)	Brown and Polson	328	93
Vanilla choc crunch ice cream	Lyons Maid Napoli	219	62
Vanilla choc flake ice cream	Lyons Maid Gold Seal	219	62
Vanilla choc ices	Safeway	259	77
Vanilla cup	Lyons Maid		each 84
Vanilla dessert	Waitrose	444	126
Vanilla ice cream	Lyons Maid	182	52
	Safeway	182	per family brick 883
	Tesco	182	52
	Waitrose	171	51
	Wall's		per slice 65
	Wall's Alpine		per 1/10 pack 125
	Wall's Blue Ribbon		per tub 105; 1/5 pack 85
Cornish cream of Cornish dairy	Tesco	181	51
	Wall's		per 1/5 pack 95
	Bertorelli	202	57
	Lyons Maid Napoli	183	52
	Safeway	230	68
economy	Bejam	123	35
mini milk	Wall's		per portion 35
non-dairy	Tesco	179	51
soft	Waitrose	155	46

Product	Brand	Calories per 100g/ 100ml	Calories per oz/ pack/ portion
Vanilla ice cream			
soft scoop	Lyons Maid	181	51
	Safeway	169	50
	St Michael	183	52
	Wall's Blue Ribbon		per 1/40 4-litre pack 90
		90	
white	Bejam	159	45
Vanilla King Cone	Lyons Maid		per cone 203
Vanilla real milk ice	Lyons Maid		each 50
Vanilla sandwich mix (as sold)	Tesco	417	118
Vanilla super cup	Lyons Maid		each 116
Vanilla yogurt, French style	Littlewoods	102	per 150g pack 153
Veal			
cutlet, fried		215	61
fillet, raw		109	31
fillet, roast		230	65
jellied, canned		125	35
Veal, ham and egg slicing pie	Waitrose	221	63
Veg 'n' rice mix	Bejam	48	per 113g portion boiled 54
Vegebanger			
herb	Real Eats	828	235
spicy	Real Eats	828	235
Vegeburger			
chilli	Real Eats	200	per 70g burger 140
herb and vegetable	Real Eats	200	per 70g burger 140
no salt	Real Eats	200	per 70g burger 140

Product	Brand	Calories per 100g/ 100ml	Calories per oz/ pack/ portion
Vegetable and bacon risotto	Heinz Baby Foods	69	per 128g can 88
Vegetable and beef soup			
dried	Batchelors	273	per 52g pint pack as sold 142
	Batchelors Cup-a-Soup	379	per 24g sachet as sold 91
dried (made up)	Chef Chunky	41	12
dried, low calorie	Batchelors Slim-a-Soup	300	per 13g sachet 39
dried, with croutons	Batchelors Cup-a-Soup Special	373	per 26g pack as sold 97
low calorie	Heinz Weight Watchers	23	per 304g can 70
Vegetable and chicken stock cubes	Bovril	190	54
Vegetable and leek soup	Knorr	313	89
Vegetable and meat stock cubes	Bovril	200	57
Vegetable and rice casserole	Cow and Gate	64	per 110g jar 70
Vegetable and spicy sausage pizza	Tesco	225	64
Vegetable and steak pie	Fray Bentos	185	52
Vegetable and steak pie filling	Fray Bentos	115	33
Vegetable and steak pudding	Fray Bentos	215	61
Vegetable bake	St Michael	126	36
Vegetable Bolognese	Hera	333	94

Product	Brand	Calories per 100g/ 100ml	Calories per oz/ pack/ portion
Vegetable broth with beef	Granny's	35	as served 23
Vegetable burger mix	Boots	281	80
Vegetable casserole with pasta	Cow and Gate	66	per 150g jar 99
Vegetable chilli	St Michael	95	27
Vegetable chilli mix	Hera	350	99
Vegetable cubes	Knorr	308	87
Vegetable curry	Boots Ready Meal	84	24
	Hera	338	96
	Prewetts Ready Meals	75	21
medium	Hofels	73	21
mild	Hofels	73	21
with pilau rice	Birds Eye MenuMaster		per pack 400
Vegetable curry mix	Prewetts	297	84
Vegetable dip, fresh	St Michael	718	204
Vegetable drink	Knorr	248	70
Vegetable flan, fresh	St Michael	228	65
Vegetable goulash mix	Hera	352	100
	Prewetts Ready Meals	57	16
Vegetable juice	Prewetts	25	7
Vegetable lasagne	Bejam		per serving baked 374
	Birds Eye MenuMaster		per pack 280
	Prewetts Ready Meals	91	26
	St Michael	113	32

Product	Brand	Calories per 100g/ 100ml	Calories per oz/ pack/ portion
Vegetable lasagne	Waitrose	106	30
Vegetable oil		899	255
	Safeway	900	255
	Spry Crisp 'n' Dry	900	255
	Waitrose	900	266
pure solid	Waitrose	900	255
Vegetable pasta	Birds Eye	141	40
Vegetable pate	Granose	296	84
Vegetable pear: see Cho cho			
Vegetable Provencal mix	Prewetts	301	85
Vegetable pulao	Waitrose	135	per 320g pack 432
Vegetable salad	Eden Vale	141	40
	Heinz	152	43
	Littlewoods	146	41
	Safeway	208	59
	Tesco	122	35
in reduced calorie dressing	Tesco	76	22
mild	Eden Vale	208	59
other recipes	Tesco	98	28
Vegetable samosa	St Michael	186	53
	Waitrose	226	64
Vegetable sausage mix	Boots	468	133
Vegetable soup *canned, ready to serve*		37	10
	Campbell's Bumper Harvest	40	11
	Crosse & Blackwell	48	14
	Granny's	30	as served 26

Product	Brand	Calories per 100g/ 100ml	Calories per oz/ pack/ portion
Vegetable soup	Heinz Big Soups	39	11
	Heinz Ready to Serve	37	10
	Heinz Weight Watchers	22	per 295g can 65
	Littlewoods	37	per 425g can 157
	Safeway	39	per 425g can 166
	Tesco	36	10
	Waitrose	44	per 425g can 187
condensed	Campbell's	67	19
dried, made up	Chef Chunky	41	12
low calorie	Waistline	22	6
	Waitrose	22	per 295g can 65
Vegetable stock cubes	Safeway	295	per 11.5g cube 34
Vegetable with beef soup, dried (made up)	Chef Box	26	7
Vegetable, yogurt, cheese and onion dip	Waitrose	311	88
Vegetables au gratin	Bejam		per serving baked 285
Vegetarian Burgamix	Ranch House Meals	538	153
Vegetarian canelloni	Prewetts Ready Meals	103	29
Vegetarian casserole mix	Hera	351	100
Vegetarian cheese	Tesco	405	115
Vegetarian jumbo grills	Protoveg Menu	251	71
Vegetarian mince beef flavour	Direct Foods	273	77

Product	Brand	Calories per 100g/ 100ml	Calories per oz/ pack/ portion
Vegetarian mince natural flavour	Direct Foods	250	71
Vegetarian sizzles	Protoveg Menu	587	166
Vegetarian Tandoori cutlet mix	Tomorrow Foods	318	90
Velvet black cherry yoghurt	Safeway	98	per 150g pack 147
Velvet strawberry yoghurt	Safeway	99	per 150g pack 149
Velvet tropical yoghurt	Safeway	104	per 150g pack 156
Venison, roast		198	56
Vermicelli raw		355	101
	Buitoni	350	99
	Tesco	348	99
cooked	Tesco	104	29
Vermouth dry		118	33
sweet		151	43
Vesta meals (Batchelors): *see flavours*			
Vichyssoise	Baxters	53	per 425g can 230
	Waitrose	54	15
specialty soup	Crosse & Blackwell	47	13
Victoria plum yoghurt low fat	Waitrose	85	per 150g pack 128
Victoria plums	Waitrose	80	23
Victoria sponge mix, classic (as sold)	Green's	430	made up per portion 179
Viennese chocolate sandwich biscuit	St Michael	510	145

Product	Brand	Calories per 100g/ 100ml	Calories per oz/ pack/ portion
Viennese whirls	Lyons	516	146
Viennetta dessert log	Wall's		per 1/6 log 135
Vimto	Barr	26	per 330ml can 85
	Littlewoods	24	per 330ml can 79
Vinaigrette, reduced calorie	Kraft	88	26
Vinaigrette salad, diet	Eden Vale	33	9
Vindaloo Classic curry sauce	Homepride	118	per 383g pack 452
Vine leaves		15	4
Vinegar		4	1
all varieties	Boots	4	1
cider	Safeway	3	1
distilled	Safeway	4	1
malt	Safeway	4	1
	Waitrose	4	
red wine	Safeway	7	2
white wine	Safeway	6	2
	St Michael	6	2
Vinegar and oil dressing, low calorie	Safeway	155	44
	Waistline	150	43
Vino bianco Prego sauce	Campbell's	43	12
Vintage orange marmalade	Baxters	248	70
Virginia sweetcorn soup	Knorr	368	104
Vitafood	Boots	445	126
Vol au vent pastry cocktail	Jus-Rol	393	111
	Bejam		per vol au vent baked 43

Product	Brand	Calories per 100g/ 100ml	Calories per oz/ pack/ portion
Vol au vent pastry			
medium	Bejam		per vol au vent baked 69
Vol au vent pastry cases	Birds Eye		per case 70
Wafer Club biscuits	Jacobs	517	per biscuit 100
Wafers			
filled		535	152
	Safeway	505	143
milk chocolate	Littlewoods	530	per wafer 104
Waffles	Safeway	216	61
potato	Ross	190	54
Waldorf salad	Tesco	180	51
other recipes	Tesco	126	36
Walnut and apple salad	Safeway	114	32
Walnut cheese spread, processed	St Michael	310	88
Walnut flavour cake mix (as sold)	Green's	399	made up per portion 259
Walnut halves	Whitworths	525	149
Walnut layer cake	Littlewoods	424	120
	Waitrose	372	105
Walnut supreme ice cream	St Michael	239	68
Walnut thins	St Michael	504	143
Walnut Whip, milk chocolate			
coffee flavour	Rowntree Mackintosh	480	per whip 170
vanilla flavour	Rowntree Mackintosh	480	per whip 170

Product	Brand	Calories per 100g/ 100ml	Calories per oz/ pack/ portion
Walnut Whip, plain chocolate			
vanilla flavour	Rowntree Mackintosh	465	per whip 165
Walnut whips	St Michael	474	134
Walnuts		525	149
(with shells)		336	95
	Haywards	80	23
	Holland and Barrett	520	147
	Tesco	542	154
kernels	Littlewoods	525	149
shelled	Whitworths	525	149
Water biscuits		440	125
	Jacobs	394	per biscuit 31
	Safeway	394	per biscuit 8
	St Michael	395	112
	Tesco	412	117
high bake	Jacobs	394	per biscuit 31
	Safeway	390	111
high baked	Tesco	402	114
rich table	Jacobs	411	per biscuit 30
small	Safeway	394	per biscuit 5
thinner	Jacobs	387	per biscuit 27
Water chestnuts, canned, drained		49	14
Watercress			
raw		14	4
	Tesco	14	4
Water ice			
lemon	Bertorelli	109	31
orange	Bertorelli	110	31
raspberry	Bertorelli	101	29
Watermelon			
raw		21	6

Product	Brand	Calories per 100g/ 100ml	Calories per oz/ pack/ portion
Watermelon raw (with skin)		11	3
	Tesco	21	6
Weetabix		340	96
	Weetabix	335	95
Weetaflakes	Weetabix	335	95
Weetaflakes 'n' raisin	Weetabix	345	98
Weight Watchers ice cream	Lyons Maid	97	27
Welsh rarebit		365	103
Wensleydale cheese	Dairy Crest	375	106
	Safeway	375	106
	St Ivel	375	106
	Tesco	400	113
	Waitrose	390	111
West Countryman cheese	Dairy Crest	286	81
West Indian bread		284	81
Wheat bulgur	Holland and Barrett	370	105
cracked	Holland and Barrett	311	88
Wheat bran	Holland and Barrett	210	60
	Waitrose	248	70
Wheat crackers	Safeway	490	139
	Tesco	466	132
	Waitrose	454	129
with bran	Tesco	418	119
Wheat crispbread	Tesco	390	111
Wheat crunchies	Sooner	483	per 30g pack 145

Product	Brand	Calories per 100g/ 100ml	Calories per oz/ pack/ portion
Wheat crunchies	Waitrose	482	137
Wheat flakes	Holland and Barrett	343	97
	Waitrose	335	95
whole	Safeway	312	88
Wheatears	St Michael	432	122
Wheateats	Allinson	429	per 21g pack 90
Wheaten matzo crackers	Rakusen	340	per biscuit 17
Wheaten sweetmeal biscuits	St Michael	453	128
Wheatgerm	Holland and Barrett	230	65
natural	Jordans	325	92
stabilized	Boots Second Nature	379	107
Wheatgerm bread, sliced	Vitbe	230	per slice
Whelks			
boiled		91	26
boiled (*with shells*)		14	4
Whipped dairy cream tub dessert	Birds Eye	203	60
Whisky and American ginger ale	Britvic Drivers	31	per 180ml pack 57
White bread mix (as sold)	Granny Smiths	248	per 480g pack made up 1190
White Cap cooking fat	Van den Berghs	900	255
White chocolate	St Michael	172	49
White chocolate and croquant sticks	St Michael	565	160

Product	Brand	Calories per 100g/ 100ml	Calories per oz/ pack/ portion
White currants			
raw		26	7
stewed without sugar		22	6
stewed with sugar		57	16
White fish, dried, assorted, raw		148	42
White grape juice	Schloer	48	14
	Waitrose	59	17
sparkling	Schloer	49	15
White Lymeswold cheese	Dairy Crest	425	120
White marzipan	Waitrose	408	116
White pepper	Tesco	275	78
ground	Safeway	380	108
White pudding		450	128
White rum and cola	Britvic Driver's	37	per 180ml pack
White sauce			
savoury		151	43
sweet		172	49
White sauce, dessert	Ambrosia	97	27
White sauce mix	Safeway	366	104
Pour Over	Colman's	380	108
savoury	Knorr	360	102
White Stilton cheese	Dairy Crest	360	102
	St Ivel	360	102
White vanilla ice cream	Bejam	159	45
White wine			
dry		66	19
medium		75	21
sparkling		76	22
sweet		94	27

Product	Brand	Calories per 100g/ 100ml	Calories per oz/ pack/ portion
White wine Cook in Sauce	Homepride	83	per 376g pack 312
White wine Cooking-in Sauce	Baxters	91	per 425g can 387
White wine sauce mix	Knorr	426	121
White wine vinegar	St Michael	6	2
Whitebait, fried		525	149
Whiting			
fried		191	54
fried (with bones)		173	49
steamed		92	26
steamed (with bones)		63	18
	Tesco	105	30
cutlets, poached	Bejam	92	26
fillets	Ross	80	23
fillets	Young's	73	21
fillets, breaded	St Michael	118	33
ovencrisp	St Michael	238	67
smoked fillets	Ross	80	23
Whiting fillets, breaded, **deep-fried**	Bejam	215	61
Whole drinks: *see flavours*			
Whole grain mustard	Colman's	145	41
powder	Colman's	505	143
Whole grain rice: *see Rice, whole grain*			
Whole green chillies in brine	Old El Paso	25	per 113g can 28
Whole milk yogurt natural, French	St Michael	68	19
set with mango	St Michael	103	29
Whole nut chocolates	Nestle	557	158

Product	Brand	Calories per 100g/100ml	Calories per oz/pack/portion
Wholegrain fruit muesli	Granose	408	116
Wholemeal/wholewheat bread: see Bread			
Wholemeal bran biscuits	Littlewoods	431	per biscuit 62
	Safeway	432	122
	St Michael	433	123
	Tesco	471	134
Wholemeal crackers	St Michael	459	130
Wholemeal flour: see Flour, wholemeal			
Wholemeal food	Boots Second Nature	306	87
Wholemeal fruit and nut loaf mix (as sold)	Green's	370	made up per portion 150
Wholemeal mince pies	Waitrose	401	114
Wholemeal muffins	Sunblest Muffin Man	214	per muffin 154
Wholemeal scone mix, classic (as sold)	Green's	434	made up per portion 134
Wholemeal shortbread fingers	Tesco	505	143
	Waitrose	500	142
Wholemeal slab cake	Tesco	294	83
Wholemeal spaghetti	Holland and Barrett	350	99
Wholemeal toasties	Granose	407	115
Wholenut bar	Cadbury's	555	per 55g bar 305
Wholewheat breakfast biscuit cereal	Safeway	344	98
Wholewheat breakfast cereal	St Michael	333	94

Product	Brand	Calories per 100g/100ml	Calories per oz/pack/portion
Wholewheat cereal	Tesco	360	102
Wholewheat cereal biscuits	Waitrose	335	per biscuit 60
Wholewheat cheese crisps	Nature's Snack	550	per 20g pack 110
Wholewheat crispbread	Allinson		per biscuit 90
Wholewheat crisps	Nature's Snack	550	per 20g pack 110
Wholewheat flakes	Tesco	360	102
Wholewheat fruit munch biscuits	Moorlands		per biscuit 60
Wholewheat macaroni: *see Macaroni*			
Wholewheat muesli	Tesco	346	98
Wholewheat pasta shells in spicy tomato sauce	Heinz	65	18
Wholewheat pasta spirals	Signor Rossi	275	78
Wholewheat ravioli: *see Ravioli*			
Wholewheat spaghetti: *see Spaghetti*			
Wholewheat teabreak biscuits	Nabisco	388	per biscuit 30
Wholewheat with raisins	Kellogg's Nutrigrain	326	92
Wieners	Soyapro	210	60
Wild berry crumble ice cream	Safeway	233	69
Wild bramble jelly preserve	Baxters	255	72
Wine gums	Bassett's	324	92
	Littlewoods	311	88

Product	Brand	Calories per 100g/ 100ml	Calories per oz/ pack/ portion
Wine gums	St Michael	342	97
	Tesco	372	105
	Waitrose	342	97
mini	Tesco	381	108
Wine, red		68	19
Wine, white			
dry		66	19
sparkling		76	22
sweet		94	27
medium		75	21
Winkles			
boiled		74	21
boiled (with shell)		14	4
Wisebuy children's mix	Wilkinson	345	98
Wispa	Cadbury's	565	per 35g bar 200
Wizard mousse			
raspberry	St Ivel	183	52
strawberry	St Ivel	183	52
Wood ear: see Jew's ear			
Woodpecker cider	Bulmer	29	per half pint 82
dry	Bulmer	30	per half pint 84
Woppas, orange/ strawberry	Wall's		per woppa 40
Worcester apples	Tesco	46	13
Worcester sauce crisps	Christies	520	per 26g bag 130
	Hunters	520	per 26g bag 130
Yam			
boiled		119	34
raw		131	37
Yeast			
bakers', compressed		53	15

Product	Brand	Calories per 100g/ 100ml	Calories per oz/ pack/ portion
Yeast			
dried		169	48
Yeast extract	Waitrose	224	64
Yellow pepper, fresh	Tesco	35	10
Yellow Quick-Set Jel	Tesco	365	103
Yoga biscuits	St Michael	518	147
Yoghurt, natural	Safeway	47	per 150g pack 71
Yogurt: see also flavours			
Yogurt, flavoured			
low fat		81	23
Yogurt, French style			
all varieties	Eden Vale	87	25
Yogurt, fruit			
low fat		95	27
cow's milk	Holland and Barrett	95	27
Yogurt, hazelnut			
low fat		106	30
Yogurt, low fat			
natural set	Waitrose	59	per 150g pack 89
Yogurt, natural		52	15
low fat		52	15
	Eden Vale	70	per 150g pack 105
	St Ivel	60	17
	St Michael	69	20
cow's milk	Holland and Barrett	50	14
low fat	Tesco	64	18
	Waitrose	47	per 150g pack 71
unsweetened	Raines	55	16
whole milk, French	St Michael	68	19

Product	Brand	Calories per 100g/ 100ml	Calories per oz/ pack/ portion
Yogurt, natural set whole milk	Waitrose	75	per 150g pack 113
Yogurt, whole milk set with mango	St Michael	103	29
Yogurt and chive dressing	Heinz All Seasons	291	82
Yogurt and cucumber crisps, natural	Hedgehog	407	per 27g pack 110
Yogurt and gram flour raita		94	27
Yogurt coated nuts and fruit	Waitrose	570	162
Yogurt coated peanuts and raisins, no added sugar	Sunwheel	477	135
Yogurt coated peanuts, no added sugar	Sunwheel	559	158
Yogurt coated raisins	Tesco	451	128
no added sugar	Sunwheel	396	112
Yogurt coated snack bar banana	Sunwheel Kalibu	323	per 30g bar 97
raisin	Sunwheel Kalibu	340	per 30g bar 102
Yorkie almond	Rowntree Mackintosh	530	per 66g bar 350
milk chocolate	Rowntree Mackintosh	525	per 61g standard bar 320
raisin and biscuit	Rowntree Mackintosh	470	per 55g bar 260
Yorkshire pudding		215	61

Product	Brand	Calories per 100g/ 100ml	Calories per oz/ pack/ portion
Yorkshire pudding and pancake mix (as sold)	Granny Smiths	267	per 243g pack made up 648
	Whitworths	348	99
Yule log cake	Tesco	448	127
giant	Safeway	428	121
Zoom	Lyons Maid		each 38
Zucchini: *see Courgettes*			
Zucchini lasagne	Findus Lean Cuisine	82	23
Zywiecka	Waitrose	358	101